Textbook of Social Administration
The Consumer-Centered Approach

Textbook of Social Administration
The Consumer-Centered Approach

John Poertner
Charles A. Rapp

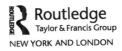

Routledge
Taylor & Francis Group

NEW YORK AND LONDON

First Published by

The Haworth Press, Inc. 10 Alice Street, Binghamton, NY 13904-1580.

Transferred to Digital Printing 2009 by Routledge
270 Madison Ave, New York NY 10016
2 Park Square, Milton Park, Abingdon, Oxon, OX14 4RN

For more information on this book or to order, visit
http://www.haworthpress.com/store/product.asp?sku=5802

or call 1-800-HAWORTH (800-429-6784) in the United States and Canada
or (607) 722-5857 outside the United States and Canada

or contact orders@HaworthPress.com

PUBLISHER'S NOTE
The development, preparation, and publication of this work has been undertaken with great care. However, the Publisher, employees, editors, and agents of The Haworth Press are not responsible for any errors contained herein or for consequences that may ensue from use of materials or information contained in this work. The Haworth Press is committed to the dissemination of ideas and information according to the highest standards of intellectual freedom and the free exchange of ideas. Statements made and opinions expressed in this publication do not necessarily reflect the views of the Publisher, Directors, management, or staff of The Haworth Press, Inc., or an endorsement by them.

A version of this book was previously published by Pearson Education, Inc.

Cover design by Jennifer M. Gaska.

Library of Congress Cataloging-in-Publication Data

Poertner, John.
    Textbook of social administration : the consumer-centered approach / John Poertner, Charles A. Rapp.
       p. cm.
    Includes bibliographical references and index.
    ISBN: 978-0-7890-3177-8 (case 13 : alk. paper)
    ISBN: 978-0-7890-3178-5 (soft 13 : alk. paper)
    1. Social work administration—United States. I. Rapp, Charles A. II. Title.

HV95.P645 2007
361.3068'4—dc22

2006035937

To my parents, Charles and Carmella Rapp,
to whom I owe everything.

Charles Rapp

To all of those social administrators
who taught me about consumer-centered management.

John Poertner

ABOUT THE AUTHORS

John Poertner, DSW, is Professor Emeritus in the School of Social Work at the University of Illinois at Urbana-Champaign, where he was Associate Dean and Director of the Children and Family Research Center. He has more than 25 years of experience in teaching, research, writing, and social administration. Dr. Poertner has also conducted research and written on public child welfare.

Charles A. Rapp, PhD, is Professor and Director of the Office of Mental Health Research and Training at the University of Kansas in Lawrence. He has been teaching social work administration courses for 25 years, as well as providing training and consultation to human service agencies. He has conducted extensive research and written on mental health, including policy and administration.

CONTENTS

Foreword

About fifteen years ago Charles Rapp and John Poertner authored a book that helped facilitate a significant shift in the understanding of the role of the human service agency manager. This shift included the recognition that the purpose of management in the human services was the attainment of client, or consumer, outcomes. Rapp and Poertner drew a fundamental distinction between management technology borrowed from other contexts and the skills required to be effective in the human services. Their text articulated a unique technology for leaders of human service agencies.

The hallmark of that text, and of this subsequent offering, are twofold: that human service agencies exist for the attainment of client outcomes and that management performance is identical to agency performance. The changes they advocated in their first text were slow to emerge. It remained difficult to engage agency administrators and students in a discussion of client outcomes. Both audiences struggled to grasp their contribution to those elusive constructs, and their responsibility for obtaining and monitoring client outcomes. In their paradigm, management was accountable for efficient processes, balanced budgets, and consistent adherence to well-articulated procedures. Outcomes were assumed and anecdotal at best, or perceived as out of the control of the program manager. It was a rare agency that made efforts to monitor the effect of their interventions upon clients, except perhaps in the domain of client satisfaction.

However, the outcomes landscape changed as agencies were increasingly held accountable for client outcomes. Many funders now tie continued fiscal support to the achievement of some minimal benefit for the agency's clients. That shift in funding has gone a long way to move the agenda toward a client outcomes approach. Yet the increasingly espoused emphasis on a client outcome framework falls far short of the consumer-centered approach advocated here by Poertner and Rapp. Although the increased monitoring and emphasis on client outcomes is a good start, in many cases that emerging emphasis is, in practice, more a product of a resource acquisition activity than of a focus on achieving client outcomes.

Textbook of Social Administration: The Consumer-Centered Approach
© 2007 by The Haworth Press, Inc. All rights reserved.
doi:10.1300/5802_a

Many human service agencies engage in this new behavior as an organizational maintenance function rather than as a result of having embraced the important principles articulated in this text.

In this book, Poertner and Rapp advocate a framework for consumer-centered practice that transcends an emphasis on measuring and reporting upon consumer outcomes to obtain funding. Defining their consumer-first perspective, Poertner and Rapp note that "consumer-centeredness is the degree to which consumers and their well-being intrude on or flavor all aspects of the agency." This represents a value-based approach that substantially surpasses a mere pay-for-performance approach to client outcomes. This book's emphasis on the core values of human service management is a unique and inspiring approach and one that evokes passion and purpose in a discipline at risk of falling victim to policies, procedures, and organizational maintenance.

Their value-based approach alone would make for a refreshing approach to human service management. However, the great strength of this text is that Poertner and Rapp only begin with the notion of a value-based approach to human service management. Having established the value context, Poertner and Rapp proceed to place a strong emphasis on the notion that management is action, and is best understood as a definable set of behaviors. Perhaps my favorite quote in this book was the author's lament that "discussing issues or problems at a theoretical level often passes for doing work." These authors support their advocacy for management as performance with a clear prescription for day-to-day management behavior that extends well beyond conducting a lively meeting.

The most important asset a manager possesses is his or her ability to influence others. No idea, regardless of its potential impact, will see the light of day in an organization lest the manager has the ability to understand the work culture and possesses the skills to influence its members. Certainly the value-based approach advocated in this book will go a long way toward helping a manager create an environment where workers strive to engage in consumer focused behavior. However, in their useful approach to articulating both values and knowledge for practice, Poertner and Rapp take the wizardry out of organizational change, and articulate the skills to make all managers effective change agents. In the chapters on organizational change and personnel management, Poertner and Rapp provide clear instructions for a theoretically based approach to organizational influence and change.

Human services occur in the context of a program. No level of commitment or passion for the consumer can withstand an inadequately designed program. Poertner and Rapp provide a straightforward approach to grounding consumer needs and subsequent interventions in the context of a social problem. This connection increases the likelihood of designing an effective intervention. Their approach to program design retains from their first text an emphasis on evidence-based practice, a component of program design they articulated long before that term became commonplace.

In a time where agencies are drowning with information, Poertner and Rapp provide a framework for using information as a management tool. Although the task at one time was locating useable program information, today's challenge is more often deciding what information to ignore. Again their approach is simple, and powerful. An effective information system is driven by a well-articulated program design. Poertner and Rapp also recognize that information is not benign; they provide a useful framework for using information to create a learning organization.

This text is bereft of jargon, which makes it both a pleasure to read and substantially increases the likelihood that it will impact practice. Poertner and Rapp have demystified human service management without oversimplifying or trivializing the practice. Occasionally when teaching their approach to human service management I have encountered a student, or community practitioner, who has criticized this consumer-centered framework as naive, and out of touch with the "real world." These critics argue that the exigencies of the "real world" render many of Poertner and Rapp's prescriptions unrealistic. I have always assumed that Poertner and Rapp would take the label of naive and unrealistic as a compliment, rather than as the intended criticism. Conceding the limitations of the "real world" is anathema to the consumer-centered social administration. To the extent that naive means aspiring to lofty goals for clients, being naive is the minimum requirement to work as a human service manager under the Poertner and Rapp schema. To be labeled naive is to embrace Poertner and Rapp's healthy disrespect for the impossible, a central principle of their consumer-centered management.

In this text, Poertner and Rapp have created a framework for human service management that is at once both passionate and informed. Their approach venerates the consumer, and celebrates those who would help the client move toward their desired outcomes. Their provision of both a value context for practice and well-informed knowledge base for doing the work of management makes this text a significant achievement and a gift to those who would practice social administration on behalf of their consumers.

Tom Gregoire

Acknowledgments

As in any effort of this scope, numerous people have influenced the conception and content of this book. Our students deserve credit for their audacity in demanding clarity and coherence in our lectures. Our students operate in a wide variety of agencies in virtually all fields of practice, and they have demanded that our teaching be applicable for all of them. Their demands were our encouragement. They urged us to write this book, and their successful application of the ideas in it to the exigencies of real-life human service organizations gave us confidence. Their encouragement became our inspiration. As they graduated and assumed management positions themselves, we have been able to see their difficulty in moving their agencies to increased levels of client-centeredness, but despite numerous obstacles, many of them have prevailed—and they have demonstrated that consumer-centered management will produce more humane and effective service to clients. Many of our students became our heroes.

We also owe a debt of gratitude to those social administrators who may never have heard of consumer-centered management. So many ideas gleaned from their practice have found their way into this text. These managers have made a profound difference in the lives of their clients, often in the face of limited resources and indifferent or unsupportive environments. Our contact with them often has been based on their requests for our help through consultation, training, systems development, and so on; we only hope that we have given them half of what we received in return.

We would like to acknowledge the generous contribution of our colleagues Terry Moore, Tom McDonald, Linda Carlson, Rick Goscha, Doug Marty, and Eric Van Allen. They have devoted a portion of their careers to the application of consumer-centered management in child welfare and mental health. We borrowed their ideas, lessons learned, and adapted materials that they have developed.

A special recognition goes to Rino Patti and Tom Gregoire. Rino, Professor Emeritus of the School of Social Work at the University of Southern

Textbook of Social Administration: The Consumer-Centered Approach
© 2007 by The Haworth Press, Inc. All rights reserved.
doi:10.1300/5802_b

California, is among the most respected scholars in human service management. When we were not sure we had anything to say, he told us we did. He encouraged, stimulated, and helped us to become clearer about our recommendations for this complex field. Tom Gregoire, Associated Dean at the Ohio State School of Social Work, was first our student and then taught alongside us as we continually struggled to further develop the ideas and methods of the approach. Not only did his ideas inform our work but he graciously agreed to write the foreword to this book.

To each of these people we extend our sincerest thanks, and it is our hope that this book does justice to all of them.

Introduction

Consumer-Centered Social Administration: What This Book Is About and How to Use It

Since the publication of our first management book, there have been several significant developments in the field. First, a client outcome orientation to service delivery has been commonplace but far from ubiquitous. Fourteen years ago, there were precious few arguing for such a stance. Second, many social policies now explicitly identify the desired results for clients and some include mechanisms for holding service providers accountable for these outcomes. Third, fourteen years ago, there was virtually no social administration research that linked management and organizational behavior to client well-being. There is now a beginning base on which to build. Finally fourteen years ago, evidence-based practice was not a term in common usage and the amount of practice research available was small. In fact, in some areas today, there are multiple replications demonstrating improved client outcomes upon which to erect our services. All these developments support the concept that social administration is defined by producing results for consumers.

Suggestion

You may be tempted to skip this introductory chapter—DO NOT! A quick read will give you a good overview of what is ahead.

Textbook of Social Administration: The Consumer-Centered Approach
© 2007 by The Haworth Press, Inc. All rights reserved.
doi:10.1300/5802_01

ASSUMPTIONS, PRINCIPLES, AND PERFORMANCE EXPECTATIONS OF CONSUMER-CENTERED SOCIAL ADMINISTRATION

Results for those people who are served through social programs whether they are called clients or consumers remain at the center of our approach to social administration. Social policies that demand results, evidence-based practices, outcome-based contracting systems, and the NASW Code of Ethics also place consumers at the center of management attention. Through the years social administration scholars have struggled to identify the roles and responsibilities of managers with little or no empirical evidence linking administrators to results for consumers. There is now an emerging body of research that links management behavior to results for consumers that as it grows will further inform the field on what it is that social administrators do to make a difference to consumers. Results of this research to date are integrated into this text.

Consumer-centeredness is the degree to which consumers and their well-being intrude on or flavor all aspects of agency behavior.

The consumer's first perspective is the assumption that forms the basis of this text. A consequence of this is that consumers are the linchpin of all management activities. Conversations with staff, board members, and key actors in the community are all dominated by concerns for producing results for consumers. The third assumption is that the social service organization is judged according to results it produces for consumers. The social service organization is not judged by the number of staff or clients served or dollars acquired. If consumer benefit is the criteria by which organizations are to be judged, it only follows that this is the same criteria by which social administrators are judged.

Assumptions of Consumer-Centered Management

Assumption #1: Consumers are the "reason for being" of social agencies and the social administration of those agencies.

Assumption #2: Therefore, consumers should be the linchpin of all activities including direct service, management, and relations with the organization's external environment.

Assumption #3: The ultimate criterion of organizational performance is producing consumer benefits—consumer outcome.

Assumption #4: Managerial performance is identical to organizational performance; there is not a separate set of criteria.

These assumptions are laudable but insufficient. Social administrators need to know how to practice in ways that are consistent with these assumptions. Given the complex world that social administrators operate within, throughout this book we provide managers a large number of conceptual and practice skills. To assist managers in learning and organizing this information we follow our assumptions with four principles of consumer-centered practice. In Chapter 1 we begin the process of identifying the behaviors that follow from the assumptions. Each principle is explained in terms of implications for management practice.

Principles of Consumer-Centered Social Administration Practice

Principle #1: Venerating the people we call consumers or clients
Principle #2: Creating and maintaining the focus
Principle #3: A healthy disrespect for the impossible
Principle #4: Learning for a living

A third element of our model is recognition that managers' success in demonstrating outcomes for consumers is primarily accomplished through the work of front-line staff. Social administrators need to recruit, train, and maintain staff and provide them with the tools to do their job. Managers need to understand, help structure, and support the service events where workers engage consumers to achieve mutually desired goals. This leads to reminding managers that there are five areas of performance.

Management Performance Area

- *Consumer or client outcomes*
- *Service events*
- *Resources*
- *Staff morale*
- *Efficiency*

FRAMEWORKS FOR ORGANIZING SOCIAL ADMINISTRATION SKILLS

The consumer-centered model of social administration follows assumptions, principles, and performance expectations with the behaviors that implement these important ideas. One element of the principle of a healthy disrespect for the impossible is the idea that managers must see themselves as powerful and responsible. This power is derived less from the traditional hierarchy of the bureaucracy and more from the recognition that it is the manager's knowledge and skills practiced on a daily basis that produce results. Social administrators achieve results through their interactions with people over time. Managers use their considerable set of skills in consistent interactions with staff, others within the agency, and key actors in the broader community including colleagues in other agencies, those responsible for funding social programs, and those who form and monitor social policy.

Social administrators achieve results through their interactions with people over time.

One result from the beginning body of research linking management behavior to results is that of Corrigan, Lickey, Campion, and Rashid (2000) who found that consumers of services from teams whose leaders rated them more highly on the dimension of laissez-faire reported lower quality of life. In other words, not only can management behavior make a positive difference in people's lives, but staying out of the way of workers and allowing them to "do their own thing" can produce harm.

Identification of social administration behavior that helps consumers is organized in this text under three frameworks that are integrated through the concept of the inverted hierarchy. The first framework is strategies for exercising influence. Social administrators' power comes primarily from their knowledge and skills that are practiced through daily interactions with people. A manager's ability to use interpersonal abilities to exercise influence requires grounding in these important change skills. The second framework is a structure for understanding the various elements of social programs and how to use them to aid consumers. Evidence-based practices identify what interventions are most effective in helping consumers achieve desired outcomes. Social administrators understand the complexity of these interventions. The program framework helps managers recall critical dimensions of social programs and how to manage them for consumer benefit. The third framework helps managers keep the social program on course. That is, guiding the program to results for consumers and improving performance. Finally all of these concepts and skills are integrated into daily practice through the idea of the inverted hierarchy.

Frameworks for Identification of Social Administration Behavior That Helps Consumers

- *Strategies for exercising influence*
- *A structure for understanding the elements of social programs and how to use these to aid consumers*
- *Keeping the social program on course*

Strategies for Exercising Influence

Social administrative power, in part, derives from a manager's ability to exercise influence. In Chapter 2, we use a model of influence, the theory of behavioral intention that is drawn from social psychology that has a substantial base of empirical support. For each element of the framework there are multiple skills or strategies for influencing change. We demonstrate the use of these skills in a variety of administrative contexts. Administrators operate at multiple levels and need skills to influence funding sources, policymakers, and others exerting influence on the social program as well as workers and colleagues. It is our belief that the skill set applies across the contexts in which social administrators work.

Theory of Behavioral Intention

Behavior or action is influenced by a person's intention to act, which is influenced by their

- *perceived behavioral control;*
- *attitudes; and*
- *cultural, personal, and organizational norms.*

Framework for Program Analysis and Management

Consumers of social services achieve desired outcomes by engaging and working with social workers. This interaction occurs within and is influenced by a variety of environments that are subject to management influence. In this text, one way to manage these environments is to specify the elements of the social program. A social program is a set of people, resources, and behaviors that are directed at producing an outcome or result with a consumer. The program includes the behaviors of workers, administrators, and others who are essential to producing desired results. It is the social program that is established and shaped by social policy as well as by our understanding of consumers and their desires. For social administrators to successfully achieve desired outcomes with consumers, they must understand the transaction between the consumer and the worker as well as other components of the social program. It is through careful consideration of various program elements that managers use their skills to shape responses that produce results.

This text presents an analytic framework for the social program as a tool for social administrators in Chapter 3 through 5. To function as a tool we include in each chapter a section giving examples of how managers use the relevant program specifications to enhance outcomes for consumers. This involves application of the influence skills provided in Chapter 2 and also anticipates the skills identified in Chapters 6 through 8.

Framework for Program Specifications

- *Problem analysis*
- *Identifying the beneficiary of the program*
- *Determining the social work theory of helping*
- *Specifying the stages of helping*
- *Identifying key people required to produce the consumer benefit*
- *Specifying the helping environment*
- *Identifying the actual helping behaviors*
- *Specifying the most likely emotional reactions and the most effective responses*

Framework for Keeping the Program on Course

By now it is clear that social administrators need a large number of conceptual and practice skills. One way to help managers organize these skills is through a framework for piloting the program toward its goal of achieving results for consumers. The all important service transaction occurs between a social worker and a consumer. Consequently, the skills of acquiring and directing staff are critical. Skills in acquiring and using information act as the gauges in the cockpit of an airplane helping the manager/pilot keep the program on course. Managers need skills in acquiring and using resources in addition to people and information. Finally, all of this activity occurs within an organizational context that the administrator structures to produce maximum consumer benefits. In addition, to providing examples of these skills linked to each program framework element, we include chapters on each of these critical skills.

Administrative Skills for Keeping a Social Program on Course

- *Acquiring staff and directing people*
- *Acquiring and using information*
- *Acquiring and using other resources*

Acquiring Staff and Directing People

Consumers achieve the benefits of social services through their interaction with social workers. The questions addressed here are as follows:

- How do social administrators assure that the best people are working with consumers?
- How does the social administrator insure that staff are doing what they need to do to produce the benefit of the service transaction?

Consumers need social workers with the knowledge, skills, and values to engage with them in helpful ways. Social administrators need to make certain that they are hiring people with the requisite knowledge, skills, and values. Administrators need to work with staff so that they receive rewards for their good work, are empowered to solve problems, and motivated to acquire new skills as needed.

Acquiring and Using Information

Information is the tool through which managers know if they are successful. It is impossible for the manager to observe every worker and consumer to determine whether they are achieving the desired benefits. Just as the gauges in the cockpit of an airplane provides the pilot information on where he/she is headed, program information is an essential tool for keeping the program operating as intended. The questions addressed in this section are as follows:

- What information does a manager need about a program to be assured that it is performing as intended?
- What does a manager do with this information to maintain or increase positive outcomes for consumers?

Managers need information of several types. By now it is evident that, in our approach, managers need information on results for consumers. Recognizing that outcomes for consumers occur through the interactions of workers and consumers, managers need information on these interactions or what are called service events. These interactions and the results do not occur unless there are resources or program inputs of the right types. Managers also need information about a broad range of resources.

Specification of the information needed to keep the program on track is just part of the story. It is the use of this information that can have an important impact on program operations. One of the unique perspectives of this volume is its focus on manager use of information. Social administrators use information to reinforce practices that are in line with expectations and redirect activities when performance indicates its need. The presentation of information in a manner that speaks for itself, either in rewarding staff for their efforts or pointing out a need for redirection, is a powerful administrative tool that requires skill and thoughtfulness.

Acquiring and Using Other Resources

What resources do managers need to acquire and how can they use them to maximize benefits to consumers? Social programs cannot produce benefits for consumers without resources of many different types. In addition to funds and staff, necessary resources include community goodwill, technology of a variety of types, space, and so on. The number and types of resources is so large that social administrators may even view resource acquisition as their major responsibility, leaving little time for other functions.

The efficient use of these resources is yet another skill. There are always more people with needs than available resources. The more efficiently that managers can use precious resources, the more consumers who may be helped. In addition, some recent funding mechanisms put programs at financial risks, leading to inefficient use of resources that can result in financial loss and eventual closing of the program.

STRUCTURING THE ORGANIZATION FOR MAXIMUM CONSUMER BENEFIT: THE INVERTED HIERARCHY

How does a social administrator structure the organization so that consumers achieve desired benefits and the work gets done in an efficient manner? Bureaucracies dominate social services despite recent emphasis on organizations with few levels. Assuring that decisions are made in a consistent manner seems to conflict with the need to allow workers to be creative in working with consumers. Social administrators need ways to think through these apparent dilemmas, place consumers at the pinnacle of the organization, and organize the work of the program.

The inverted hierarchy (Chapter 10) provides social administrators a variety of tools for structuring the organization and integrating the vast number of skills identified in this text. This management behavior uses opportunity finding as a way to guide action. These opportunities are ubiquitous in the social service organization, and are used to enhance performance by providing direction and tools to do the job as well as removing obstacles and influencing the organizational culture in positive ways. Finally three practice mechanisms for pulling all of this together are detailed. These are field mentoring, group supervision, and performance-enhancement teams.

The Inverted Hierarchy

Opportunity finding
Using opportunities to enhance performance by

providing direction;
providing the needed tools;
removing obstacles; and
shaping the organizational culture.

Integrating social administration skills through

field mentoring;
group supervision; and
performance-enhancement teams.

A NOTE TO READERS ON HOW TO USE THIS BOOK

This book contains more information than can be absorbed in one reading, one course, or one year. Just as we encourage social administrators to put the helping transaction under a microscope to identify ways to improve results for consumers, we have put social administrative practice under the microscope. The result is recognition of the complex world of social administration and the myriad of skills that it requires. This text focuses on skills that are best mastered through practice.

One way to use this book is to link chapters to semester-long courses. For example, at the University of Kansas where we implemented the entire curriculum, Chapter 2 was one course. The chapters on program specification (3, 4, 5) were covered in one course. A semester course in information management used the content of Chapters 6 and 7. Each of the last three chapters was a separate course: Personnel Management, Resource Management, and The Inverted Hierarchy. The field practicum component was designed so that students could practice the skills acquired in the classroom in the "real" world.

In an ideal world the reader would

- learn and practice interpersonal influence skills;
- have an opportunity to specify all of the elements of a program and shape it to match the ideal through practicing influence skills;
- design an information system for a program and practice using it;
- practice the six tasks identified for personnel management;
- analyze the fiscal environment in which the program operates including recognition of financing incentives;
- practice finding opportunities and implementing the strategies for turning opportunities into improved performance;
- practice field mentoring, group supervision, and performance enhancement teams; and
- practice creating and maintaining an organizational culture that is consumer-centered, reward-based, and learning.

What is outlined here is a career in social administration. As someone once said, an MSW degree is like a learner's permit for driving. It is the beginning of a career of learning new concepts and practices. These skills can only be learned and mastered through repeated practice. The authors do not pretend to have mastered all of the skills included in this text and continue to refine them through practice.

For most readers it is likely that you will only have time initially to read part of this text. In that case we suggest that you read the first two chapters and then dive into the section of your choice. Our aforementioned outline of courses indicates which chapters go together. When approaching a section, take time to command the content by applying the ideas of the section to your agency or program. For example, when reading the section on program specifications (Chapters 3 through 5) it is useful to write a description of each program element as it applies to a program that you use or have worked with. Finally, connect the content of the section to performance outcomes and practice the influence skills of Chapter 2.

For the benefit of all of our consumers we wish you well in learning and practicing consumer-centered social administration. We seek feedback on your experiences with this text and its application. We seek your administrative successes and failures so that we can all learn together.

Chapter 1

Consumer-Centered Social Administration

We have devoted a considerable portion of our careers to the premise that social administrators make a difference in the lives of the people we call clients or consumers of social work services. We believe this because we have known administrators who had a positive effect on consumers through their efforts in directing resources toward this end. We can now say that there is a beginning body of research that supports this position.

Argyris (1999) says that managing is creating intended consequences. In social work, the intended consequences are results for consumers. Managing is the behavior that creates these results. Many people who have studied social administration have attempted to identify management behavior. They catalog daily management activities and group them into different types of social work management tasks. Patti (1977) was one of the first to take this approach. Recently Menefee (2000) has pursued this line of research in social work and determined that managers must be

- effective communicators within the organization;
- boundary spanners;
- innovators;
- organizers;
- resource administrators;
- evaluators;
- policy practitioners;
- advocates;
- supervisors;
- facilitators; and
- team builders.

Textbook of Social Administration: The Consumer-Centered Approach
doi:10.1300/5802_02

Another line of scholarly activity is determining the fit between organizational theories and social welfare management. Hasenfeld (2000) has written extensively and draws connections between organizational theories and administrative activities. One way that he makes these connections is by taking administrative tasks and identifying the corresponding organizational theory. This includes:

Task	Organizational Theory
Goal attainment	Rational-legal, scientific management
Management of people	Human relations, feminist perspective
Proficiency and efficiency	Contingency
Adaptation and mobilization of resources	Political economy
Founding and survival	Population ecology
Institutionalization	New-Institutionalism
Integration and social cohesion	Culture, sense-making
Knowledge, power, and control	Neo-Marxist, postmodern, structuration
Social change	Critical theory, radical feminism (p. 91).

Determining what social administrators do and the organizational theories that link to these behaviors is useful. However, the consumer is missing from both of these approaches. The work on identifying management tasks has not focused on those behaviors that produce the benefit to consumers. Organizational theories have more to do with understanding the organization than its results.

For us, it is imperative that social administration begins with outcomes for consumers, determines management behavior that results in these intended consequences, and uses research and theory to create the conditions for consumer success. By beginning with consumer results, we propose an approach that puts beneficiaries of our services first. This is consistent with social work history and values.

Consumer-centeredness is the degree to which consumers and their well-being intrude on or flavor all aspects of agency.

This consumer-first approach allows a more directed inquiry into the tasks of social work managers. We argue that the most important administrative tasks are those that produce results for consumers while keeping the organization functioning. We also believe that theory can usefully guide management practice and we shall rely on theory either explicitly or implicitly throughout this text. We agree with Patti when he says:

> In the long term, however, as I have argued elsewhere (Patti, 1985; Patti et al., 1988), all of these goals should be considered instrumental or intermediate purposes, essential but not sufficient to achieving the basic mission of the organization, which is to change people's lives and social circumstances. (Patti, 2000, p. 23)

Consumer-Centered Social Administration Learning Objectives

1. *Based upon the existing research, identify the ways that supervisors affect consumer outcomes.*
2. *Based upon the existing research, identify other organizational arrangements that affect consumer outcomes.*
3. *State the four assumptions underlying consumer-centered social administration.*
4. *State the principles of consumer-centered administrative practice and give examples of each.*
5. *State the five management performance areas.*

SOCIAL ADMINISTRATION AND OUTCOMES FOR CONSUMERS: WHAT WE KNOW*

There is a beginning body of research that links organizational characteristics and management behavior to results for consumers. In part, the scarcity of this type of management research is due to the difficulty in conducting it. There are many methodological problems. With the unit of interest being a work group or an organization rather than a person, statistical power requires many agencies to participate to generate significant findings. In addition, organizations are complex entities with many elements and relationships between them. Relevant research must account for a number of these elements or variables. As a general rule, the more variables that

---

*Much of this section is based on Poertner, J. (in press). Social Administration and outcomes for consumers: What do we know? *Administration in Social Work*. Reprinted with permission.

a researcher brings into a study the more research subjects are needed to help explain the impact of these variables. Not only must the study include a large number of organizations or units, it must also use reliable and valid measures. Seldom are there well-established measures for these variables.

However, studies now exist that link organizational variables to client outcomes. Some are published in administrative journals but more often they appear in other fields such as child welfare or mental health. Consequently, they are difficult to find. This may be, in part, because there has been more public policy emphasis on client outcomes in some fields than others. For example, the Adoption and Safe Families Act of 1997 and the Foster Care and Independence Act of 1999 established safety, permanency, and child well-being as the desired outcomes for children vulnerable to abuse and neglect. This emphasis encourages research that helps explain how programs can obtain desired results. Although this research is not typically intended as management research, it includes organizational variables in a larger context to help explain results for consumers. This scattering of the research makes it difficult to stay current on research linking management to outcomes.

We reviewed the research that we knew of linking management behavior to outcomes for consumers of social work services. This review is both imperfect and incomplete. We encourage readers to identify this type of research in their field of practice and send the reference to one or both of the authors. Although standard bibliographic databases were searched, few of these studies were found in this traditional manner. Social administration scholars and researchers in the fields of child welfare and mental health who were known to have an interest in the link between organizational variables and client outcomes were asked to identify such studies. For each article, identified references within it were also checked for additional studies. This process resulted in the identification of ten studies.*

Later in this text we discuss evidence-based practices. When the reader comes to that part of the text, you will see that the social administration research summarized here does not meet the standard for the highest level of evidence. This is another reflection of the beginning nature of this research. We hope and expect that research more strongly linking management behavior to consumer outcomes will emerge. In the mean time, this body of research provides useful insights.

---

*This section only includes results of nine of the ten studies. For purposes of brevity we have eliminated nonsignificant findings. Grasso (1994) found no significant relationships between study variables and consumer outcomes.

Supervisors Make a Difference to Consumers

Supervisory behavior has been shown to be positively associated with consumer outcomes (Table 1.1). Although this may be reassuring to those who have been or intend to be supervisors, it should be noted that supervisory behavior has also been shown to be negatively related to consumer outcomes. In other words, making a difference to consumers can be positive or negative.

A recent study that demonstrated this was by Corrigan, Lickey, Campion, and Rashid (2000), who used the transformational leadership model developed by Bass to link team leader behavior to consumer satisfaction and quality of life. This study had 143 leaders and 473 subordinates rate the leadership style of the team leader on the 3 dimensions of the Bass model. Transformational leadership was defined as situations where the leaders' goal was to improve programs. Transactional leaders used feedback and reinforcement to maintain effective programs. Laissez-faire leadership was a hands-off leadership style.

In this study, subordinates, the researchers' term for those working directly with consumers, identified leadership behaviors that were associated with consumer satisfaction with their quality of life. Subordinates who viewed their leaders as charismatic, inspiring, and considerate of the interests of individual staff members were more likely to work in programs that had consumers with higher quality of life. Subordinates who ranked their leaders high on management-by-exception worked in programs where consumers reported low satisfaction.

Leaders who rated themselves high in inspiration, those who were more frequent users of contingent rewards with their staff, and those who ranked themselves low in passive management by exception and laissez-faire leadership worked in programs with consumers who reported high satisfaction. Other study findings included an association between subordinates' age (inverse relationship) and education level (positive relationship) with consumers' satisfaction.

Ahearn (1999) had 100 supervisors and a sample of their child welfare workers rate their client-centeredness and interpersonal skills. The outcome of interest was children achieving permanency (i.e., reunification, adoption, or guardianship). Higher workers' ratings of supervisor client-centeredness and higher supervisory assessment of their interpersonal skills were associated with higher permanency rates. Her findings included that larger caseloads were associated with lower rates of permanency.

Harkness (1997) and Harkness and Hensley (1991) compared normal supervision in a mental health center, which was a mixed focus on adminis-

TABLE 1.1. Supervisory Behavior that Makes a Difference to Consumers

Study	Supervisory Behavior	Link to Consumer Outcomes
Corrigan, Lickey, Campion, and Rashid (2000)	Team leaders' ratings of passive management by exception, contingent rewards, and subordinates' ratings of leaders' active management; subordinates' ratings of consideration of the interests of individual staff members	• Subordinates who ranked their leaders as high on active management-by-exception worked in programs where consumers reported low satisfaction • Subordinates who viewed their leaders as charismatic, inspiring, and considerate of the interests of staff members were more likely to work in programs that had consumers with higher quality of life • Leaders who rated themselves high in inspiration, those who were more frequent users of contingent rewards with their staff, those who ranked themselves low in passive management by exception and laissez-faire leadership worked in programs with consumers who reported high satisfaction • Subordinates' age was inversely related to client satisfaction • Subordinates' education level was positively associated with consumers satisfaction
Ahearn (1999)	Supervisors being client centered (as rated by workers) and supervisors self-rated on interpersonal skills	• Workers' ratings of supervisor client centeredness and supervisory assessment of interpersonal skills were positively related to higher permanency rates. • Larger caseloads were related to lower rates of permanency (i.e., reunification, adoption, or guardianship)

Harkness (1997) Harkness and Hensley (1991)	Supervisors asked mental health counselors questions about client outcomes and interventions related to outcomes	• Increased client satisfaction • Increased goal attainment
Harkness (1995)	Relationship between worker and supervisor and the supervisor's problem-solving skills as rated by workers	• Supervisory relationship positively associated with client goal attainment and generalized contentment • Supervisory empathy positively associated with client report of generalized contentment and goal attainment • Supervisory trust not associated with either client outcomes • Supervisory problem solving positively associated with goal attainment but not generalized contentment • Supervisory helpfulness positively associated with client-generalized contentment and goal attainment.
Sosin (1986)	Supervisors reminded workers that child welfare case reviews were needed	• Fewer children were in care for long periods of time

Note: For purposes of brevity Tables 1.1 and 1.2 only include statistically significant findings. Nonsignificant findings are also important and readers are encouraged to read the original research reports.

trative issues, training, and clinical supervision with client-focused supervision. Clinicians were asked questions about client problems and staff's attempts to address them. Client outcomes were assessed using measures of generalized contentment, client satisfaction, and goal attainment. They found that when a supervisor used client-focused supervision, adult outpatients reported increased goal attainment and greater satisfaction with counseling. In a replication of the original study, Harkness (1995) found positive associations between workers' report on their relationship with their supervisor and supervisory problem-solving skills with client goal attainment. Workers' ratings of supervisory empathy and helpfulness were also positively associated with clients' generalized contentment and goal attainment.

In an early study, Sosin (1986) studied variation between Wisconsin counties in permanency outcomes. He found that where supervisors reminded workers that child welfare case reviews were needed, fewer children were in care for long periods. He also found that caseload size, another organizational characteristic, did not reduce length of stay.

Other Organizational Characteristics that Make a Difference to Consumers

Management literature frequently mentions the importance of teams to organizational outcomes. However, evidence of a link between teams and consumer outcomes is meager (Table 1.2). Yeaman, Craine, Gorsek, and Corrigan (2000) conducted a study of the implementation of performance-enhancement teams using the concepts of empowerment and delegating responsibility for change. Consumer satisfaction, changes in their knowledge of key illness-management skills, and aggressive incidents were the dependent variables. After three months of operation, the performance-enhancement teams demonstrated a pre/post increase of 42 percent in consumer satisfaction, 25 percent increase in their knowledge of key skills, and a 50 percent decrease in aggressive incidents.

A study by Glisson and Hemmelgarn (1998) is in many ways a model of useful management research. Although it is widely recognized that the environment influences what occurs within the organization, it is rare to find research that includes this as a variable. Glisson and Hemmelgarn (1998) examined the environmental variable of interorganizational service coordination on child behavioral outcomes. They found that increased service coordination was related to reduced service quality and that this had no effect on service outcomes. However, this study also found that office climate was positively associated with improvement in child behaviors. Office climate

TABLE 1.2. Organizational Variables that Make a Difference to Consumers

Study	Organizational Variables	Consumer Outcomes
Yeaman, Craine, Gorsek, and Corrigan (2000)	Performance-enhancement teams using team empowerment and delegating responsibility for change	• 42 percent pre/post increase in consumer satisfaction • Consumers showed a 25 percent increase in knowledge in key skill areas including medication skills, symptom management, and leisure skills • Nearly 50 percent reduction in aggressive incidents
Glisson and Hemmelgarn (1998)	Organizational climate included fairness, role clarity, role overload, role conflict, co-operation, growth and advancement, job satisfaction, emotional exhaustion, personal accomplishment and depersonalization. Service coordination included the number of authorizations needed to obtain a service, the number of people responsible for services that were delivered, the proportion of those monitoring services for a child who also provided service	• Service coordination had the largest effect on service quality, increased service coordination was related to reduced service quality—defined as service comprehensiveness, continuity, and responsiveness • Positive organizational climates was associated with both better service quality and better service outcomes
Martin and Segal (1977)	Organizational structure defined to include complexity (number of titles and levels of supervision), decentralization, impersonality of interpersonal relations, technical qualifications of staff, number of members and staff/client ratio	• Under certain conditions organizational complexity, decentralization, and impersonality were positively associated with staff ratings of client independence • Greater organizational size was negatively associated with client independence • Higher staff to client ratio was positively associated with client independence

in this study included the dimensions of fairness, role clarity, role overload, role conflict, cooperation, growth and advancement, job satisfaction, emotional exhaustion, personal accomplishment, and depersonalization.

It was surprising to find a study as early as Martin and Segal (1977). This study examined the relationship between clients' independence and organizational structure and size. Client independence was measured through workers' ratings. Although the hypothesized relationships were not strong, key findings included that staff expectations of clients were positively associated with greater organizational complexity, as measured by the number of occupational titles and supervisory levels, decentralization when staff size was controlled, and higher staff/client ratios.

The research literature that is beginning to link management behavior to results for consumers suggests that managers and characteristics of social service programs make a difference. Although this research in not sufficient to classify any behavior at a high level of evidence-based practice, it points managers in useful directions. The reader does not need to commit these findings to memory at this point. This research will be repeated in several places throughout this text as warranted by the topic at hand.

ASSUMPTIONS OF CONSUMER-CENTERED MANAGEMENT

The consumer-centered approach to social administration is based on the following four assumptions:

1. Consumers are the "reason for being" of social agencies and the social administration of those agencies.
2. Therefore, consumers should be the linchpin of all activities including direct service, management, and relations with the organization's external environment.
3. The ultimate criterion of organizational performance is producing consumer benefits and outcomes.
4. Managerial performance is identical to organizational performance; there is not a separate set of criteria.

Consumers Are the "Reason for Being" of Social Agencies and the Social Administration of Those Agencies

Social agencies are created and sustained by a society's citizenry to care for people who need protection (e.g., child protective service) or who need some additional or specialized help to attain a minimal standard of health and decency, or to participate fully in our society. Although societies vary on the generosity with which they support human services, all societies have made some level of commitment.

The social work profession grew out of such a commitment and reflects it. The primacy of consumers is found in the very first ethical principle of the Code of Ethics: "Social workers primary goal is to help people in need and to address social problems." If the central purpose of the professional and of the social agency is consumers' well-being, then the central purpose of social administration is, likewise, consumers.

Consumers Should Be the Linchpin of All Activities Including Direct Service, Management, and Relations with the Organization's External Environment

If assumption #1 can be accepted, then consumers should be the linchpin of all activities. This is what we refer to as consumer/client-centeredness. Consumer-centeredness is the degree to which they and their well-being intrude on or flavor all aspects of agency behavior. This is easily understood in considering the agency's direct services where staff use their skills and resources to help consumers succeed. Consumers should also be the linchpin of management and organizational behavior. For example, information systems should be designed to capture and report on consumer outcomes and key service events that lead to those outcomes. Employee-performance appraisal systems should emphasize worker skills and behavior that directly affects consumer success. Policies and procedures are developed to facilitate the work with consumers and consumer achievement, rather than act as impediments. Meetings focus on topics that relate to the quality of consumer services or, even better, the results of meetings contribute to consumer's being "better off."

The interactions and work between social administrators and the agency's multiple constituencies (e.g., judges, funders, employers, other agencies) should also be focused on behavior that contributes to consumers' well-being. Social administrators operate in multiple environments and each of these is an opportunity to put consumers first. The relationships, partnerships, and agreements with these environments should create more synergistic efforts to help consumers.

The Ultimate Criterion of Organizational Performance Is Producing Consumer Benefits and Outcomes

The ultimate criterion of organizational performance is producing consumer benefits or what we call outcomes. Agencies also need to acquire resources, serve adequate numbers of consumers, maintain records, document activities, recruit and sustain talented staff, and maintain congenial relationships with the agency's multiple constituencies. These dimensions of performance are important but secondary or supportive of the ultimate purpose: producing consumer outcomes.

Consumer outcomes are as much the "bottom-line" for human services as profit is in business. No successful business manager would assume that the business was profitable merely because the enterprise was producing enough widgets (e.g., cars, clothes), employees were working hard, or the business occasionally received favorable articles in the media. In human services, an agency could be serving a lot of consumers with contented employees and a nice story occasionally printed in the local newspaper, but the number of consumers achieving the desired outcomes could be woefully small.

Managerial Performance Is Identical to Organizational Performance; There Is Not a Separate Set of Criteria

If the first three assumptions are accepted, then managerial performance should be viewed as identical to organizational performance. If the ultimate performance criterion is consumer outcomes, why would an organization hire someone to be a manager if the hiring was not the best use of funds to produce consumer outcomes? With few exceptions, we believe that you cannot be a "good" or "effective" manager of a team that is producing inadequate levels of consumer outcomes. Similarly, you cannot be a "bad" manager if the team's results for consumers are exceptional.

Assumptions of Client-Centered Management

1. *Clients are the "reason for being" of social agencies and the social administration of those agencies.*
2. *Therefore, clients should be the linchpin of all activities including direct service, management, and relations with the organization's external environment.*
3. *The ultimate criterion of organizational performance is producing client benefits–client outcome.*
4. *Managerial performances are identical to organizational performances; there is not a separate set of criteria.*

PRINCIPLES OF CONSUMER/ CLIENT-CENTERED PRACTICE

The first definition of principle at Dictionary.com is "a basic truth, law, or assumption." We think that our principles fit this broad definition rather well. The principles included in our previous text were derived, in part, from a study conducted by Elizabeth A. Gowdy and Charles A Rapp entitled, "The Common Denominators of Effective Community-Based Programs." Unfortunately, both our other work and a lack of resources have prevented us from continuing this line of research to strengthen the evidence for these principles or to revise them. Over the years these principles have received wide acceptance from students and practicing managers alike. We have also observed managers who exemplified consumer-centered practice that embodied these principles. Their acceptance and these examples are another type of evidence. In addition, as we will point out, these principles are supported by other research or social work values.

Principles of Consumer-Centered Management

1. Venerating the people we call consumers or clients
2. Creating and maintaining the focus
3. A healthy disrespect for the impossible
4. Learning for a living

Principle #1: Venerating the People We Call Consumers or Clients

We have already argued for the development of social administration from a consumer results perspective. This is not a difficult argument to make for any social worker. The very first sentence of the Code of Ethics of the National Association of Social Workers states: "The primary mission of the social work profession is to enhance human well-being and help meet the basic human needs of all people, with particular attention to the needs and empowerment of people who are vulnerable, oppressed, and living in poverty" (www.socialworkers.org). The very first ethical principle of the Code states: "Social workers' primary goal is to help people in need and to address social problems." The first standard is "commitment to clients." Clearly social administrators fulfill their professional ethical obligations when they venerate consumers.

Venerating consumers is similar to staying close to the customer in private enterprise. Businesses that sell products or services quickly learn about the importance of staying close to the customer because they generate the revenue that maintains the business. Social services are different in that public funds are allocated to address a social problem. Although newer forms of contracting are attempting to align consumer outcomes with revenue, consumers are still often the least powerful part of the agency. Although business managers have a natural fiscal interest in consumers, social administrators must make a conscious decision to value consumers.

Two tools that managers have for venerating consumers are language and operating from a consumers' strengths' perspective. (More tools will be presented throughout the rest of this text.) What an administrator says makes a difference. The words chosen to talk about consumers communicate organizational values and norms. If consumers are described as dysfunctional, codependent, crazy, or messed up, that is how most people in the organization will describe them. If this is the language used by a social administrator when interacting with people in the community, this is likely to be the image that important groups in the community will have of consumers. For years, advocates for people with many types of disabilities have pointed out that a person may be visually impaired, have schizophrenia, or a developmental disability, but that is just one of his or her characteristics.

In this text, we use both the terms clients and consumers. It is likely that Mary who is struggling with a major mental illness would say that she is neither a client nor a consumer but a person by the name of Mary. She is correct. For the purposes of this text we need a term that designates the people who are beneficiaries of social services. Many people believe that consumer is a better term than client. We use both because they are widely used in the field.

Recognizing that consumers have many various characteristics is the beginning of operating from the strength's perspective. In addition to a condition that may have led someone to seek social work services, consumers have strengths that Rapp (1998) defines as their aspirations, competencies, and confidence. It is these characteristics that consumers and workers employ to achieve desired outcomes. In the daily stressful work of school social work, such as trying to keep a child in her or his classroom while the family is without housing, a parent is recently out of jail, or the mother is afflicted with an alcohol addiction, it is easy to be overwhelmed by these conditions and lose sight of the child's abilities in music, the parents' aspirations to keep a job and pay rent, or the mother's history of contacting her sister when she needs someone to take care of her children. The social administrator who is venerating consumers uses the language of consumers, aspirations, and competencies. She or he asks workers what the consumer would like to achieve and what they have achieved. Social administrators venerate consumers when they

1. know consumers;
2. promote the idea that consumers are heroes; and
3. act as consumer advocates.

Social administrators get to know consumers by name. They spend time with Mary and Joe to find out about their lives and what they would like to achieve. They seek Nancy's and Henry's perspectives on how agency staff are working with them to achieve their goals. They demand this same respect, friendliness, and consideration from everyone in the agency.

Managers who know consumers as individual people are continually acquiring knowledge of consumers' cultural heritage that are important to achieving results. The hospital social worker who gets to know Henry finds out that the Native American Nation he is a member of regards burning sage as a healing ceremony. This leads to dedicating a room in the hospital to this ceremony.

Venerating the People We Call Consumers or Client (Some Beginning Tools)

1. *Careful use of language*
2. *Strengths perspective*
    a. *Know consumers*
    b. *Promote the idea that consumers are heroes*
    c. *Act as consumer advocates*

Managers who venerate consumers talk about them as heroes. They know what consumers have achieved and the obstacles that they have overcome. They conduct award ceremonies for consumers who have achieved significant milestones. For example, a judge holds a ceremony when a child abuse and neglect case is closed with the parent(s) and others who have had a significant role in the success. In this celebration of what the parent(s) have achieved, they are given a rose and asked to identify the contributions of others who contributed to the success.

Recognizing consumers as heroes is an important dimension of a consumer-centered organizational culture. Within a culture, heroes help define desired results and paths to success. Heroes describe what is achievable. In the midst of a challenging situation that looks like it is doomed to failure, heroes remind everyone that success is not only possible but occurs on a regular basis.

Social administrators venerate consumers when they advocate for them on a daily basis both within the agency and community. Several examples of advocating for consumers have already been mentioned. Advocacy or speaking with and for consumers is a natural outgrowth of getting to know consumers and operating from the perspective of consumer strengths. Advocacy occurs in the reminder to workers of what Nancy (a consumer) has achieved. Advocacy occurs when administrators select evidence-based interventions that have documented success in achieving consumer goals. Advocacy occurs when the administrator shares an agency information system report on consumer outcomes. Advocacy occurs when the shelter administrator accompanies consumers to the city council meeting to speak on proposed ordinances aimed at "problems caused by the homeless."

Exercise

Using a social service organization that you are familiar with, perform the following:

1. *Identify five to ten examples that you saw which demonstrated the principle of venerating the consumer.*
2. *Brainstorm five to ten ways that you think would be ways to venerate consumers.*

Principle #2: Creating and Maintaining the Focus

The successful organization is one that has a clear focus defined through its mission statement with its resources (e.g. knowledge, staff, information, funds) directed at achieving that end. The world is a complex and demanding place with many interests seeking to influence the use of resources. Without attention to maintaining the organizational focus on consumer well-being, resources will be scattered in many different directions. Diffusion of resources results in insufficient effort to achieve any end. For example, a manager may see the organization as so dependent on the environment for survival that he or she may strive to maintain legitimacy by satisfying a select group of people in the community, chasing every new service delivery idea in hopes of attracting new dollars, and doing everything possible to keep staff happy. With this busy agenda, consumers often get lost.

For the social welfare organization the focus is results for consumers. This is a clear reference back to venerating consumers. An organization without results for consumers as the central theme of its mission is not venerating consumers. Increasingly, public policy supports this same notion. The Adoption and Safe Families Act specifies that the outcomes of public child welfare are to be the safety, permanency, and well-being of abused and neglected children. The No Child Left Behind Act, although controversial, seeks to hold public school accountable for children learning and school social workers play a critical role in making this work for "at-risk" children. In mental health, the evidence-based practice movement in many states is, at its core, an effort to improve outcomes such as reduction in psychiatric hospitalization, increase in employment, and recovery from substance abuse and psychiatric disability.

Creating and Maintaining the Focus on Consumer Outcomes

1. *Make certain that the organizational mission has the consumer outcome as a central theme.*
2. *Avoid implementing organizational activities that do not contribute to consumer outcomes.*
3. *Eliminate organizational activities that do not contribute to consumer outcomes.*
4. *Make the consumer outcome focus a commitment by directing meetings, memos, information, and rewards (more to follow) toward the consumer outcome.*

It is the job of the social administrator to create and maintain the consumer outcome focus of the organization. Fortunately, many managers are already working within an organization that has a consumer outcome focus. This may be related to public policy or the legacy of another social administrator. In some cases, a manager may assume the leadership of an organization and be able to create or recreate a consumer results oriented focus. In still other cases, a manager may find herself or himself responsible for a team or a program within a larger organization that does not have a consumer focus. In these cases, it is the manager's challenge to define the focus for his or her unit and advocate for a change in the organization mission or insulate the unit from distracting elements in the organization.

Maintaining the consumer results focus requires elimination of other goals and activities. Maintaining the focus is bringing all available resources to bear on the desired outcome. Other ends and activities may be worthwhile and even important but if they do not contribute to the consumer outcome they sap available organizational strength. An organization dedicated to the safety, permanency, and well-being of abused children may be presented with an opportunity to operate a nutrition program for poor children. These are important programs and there is a high correlation between poverty and children who are identified as abused or neglected. Nutrition is certainly an important aspect of child well-being. However, operating this program will direct organizational attention away from safety, permanency, and well-being. The social administrator presented with this opportunity may seek other organizations in the community to assume responsibility for this program while maintaining her or his focus.

Maintaining the focus also means eliminating organizational activities that do not contribute to the outcome. This increases the resources that are available to produce desired results. This is easier said than done. Certainly a level of organizational maintenance (e.g., office of personnel management, accounting, purchasing) is necessary or there would be no resources for consumer results. There are also activities in every organization that if refocused could make a significant contribution to consumer outcomes. For example, as some public child welfare agencies contract for services to families, they may maintain a caseworker for each child. With legal responsibility for the child resting with the public agency, they feel obligated to maintain this level of staffing. Consequently, each family or child has two caseworkers. This redundancy is not only an added personnel expense, it also increases both agencies' time for communication between the caseworkers, and confusion on the part of judges and other service providers as to who is in charge and has the latest correct information.

A commitment to the consumer outcome focus is the beginning of identifying worthwhile activities as well as distractions. Meetings within the organization and the community discuss consumers' goals, successes, and challenges. Memos discuss consumer goal achievement and related barriers. Information system reports center on outcomes for consumers. Rewards, both formal and informal, are linked to consumer achievements. These are just a few examples of management behaviors that demonstrate a commitment to a consumer outcome focus.

Exercise

Use the example of a social service organization that you know and perform the following:

1. *Identify the desired outcome and organizational mission. Does the mission include the outcome?*
2. *Identify three to five activities that you think could be eliminated because they do not seem to contribute to the consumer outcome. Explain your reasoning for your choice of activities.*
3. *Identify ten to twelve behaviors that a social administrator (you) could use to demonstrate a commitment to the consumer outcome focus. Explain your reasoning for each.*

Principle # 3: A Healthy Disrespect for the Impossible

Protecting children who are vulnerable to abuse or neglect, enhancing the living condition of a person with psychiatric disabilities, keeping a child exhibiting difficult behaviors in a normal classroom, arranging supports enabling an elderly person with multiple needs to remain at home are just a few of the very difficult situations confronted by social workers on a day-to-day basis. Too often our social programs are asked to produce wonderful results for consumers with inadequately tested and funded interventions. Frustrated workers then come to their supervisor, who has limited time due to ill-focused organizational and community meetings, and the demands of fund-raising. A quick look at the policy manual suggests little flexibility, few possibilities, more requirements, and hints at what cannot be done.

When confronted with seemingly impossible consumer situations, it is no wonder that so many managers yield supervision to the policy manual, trying to minimally satisfy the most influential key actors or management by exception. The policy manual becomes the document that specifies what we cannot do, under the assumption that if the manual does not say that something could be done then it should not be done. The consumer is never an influential key actor and is never accommodated. Management by exception has been shown to result in negative outcomes for consumers (Corrigan, Lickey, Campion, & Rashid, 2000).

Although agreeing that something is impossible may be a rational response to a demanding and difficult situation, it does not benefit consumers. In fact, not knowing what can or ought to be done in a difficult consumer situation may engender feelings of impotence or hopelessness, but recognizing that something can be done is the first step in creating possibilities.

Snyder (1994) has done extensive research on the concept of hope and concludes that hope includes the idea that we have goals and the confidence to pursue them. The hopeful social administrator starts by disrespecting the impossible.

Characteristics of Managers Who Disrespect the Impossible

1. *A perception of self as powerful and responsible in the situation*
2. *Highly developed problem-solving skills with a premium on partializing*
3. *The ability to blend agendas of seemingly disparate interests*
4. *Persistence*

Perception of Self as Powerful and Responsible

The child welfare supervisor, is confronted by an increasing number of intakes that do not include abused and neglected children, identifies the source as local police responding to situations late at night and on the weekend, and believes that something can be done to change this situation. The case management supervisor attempting to get employment for consumers in times of high unemployment believes that work opportunities can be found. The school social worker who is working with the youth dismissed from his classroom for the fifth and "final" time believes that he can be reintegrated and his troublesome behavior can be altered. In all these instances, the belief that the current situation can be changed is the beginning of disrespecting the impossible.

Belief in the possibility of change is one aspect of the perception of self. The second is the sense of personal responsibility. This is a natural consequence of venerating consumers and focusing on outcomes. When we believe that our job is to achieve results for consumers, then whatever gets in the way of this occurring becomes an obstacle that needs to be overcome. Corrigan, Lickey, Campion, and Rashid (2000) found that subordinates who viewed their leaders as charismatic and inspiring worked in programs where consumers attained a higher quality of life. Although these characteristics were unlikely to be sufficient to produce these results, we contend that they are necessary. How can anyone expect workers to continually confront challenging consumer situations if their supervisors do not believe that something can and should be done?

Highly Developed Problem-Solving Skills
with a Premium on Partializing

The Harkness (1995) finding that workers' ratings of supervisors' problem-solving skills were positively related to consumers' goal attainment supports this aspect of disrespecting the impossible. Overwhelming consumer problems almost always appear as large tangled webs of barriers. Confronting seemingly insurmountable consumer problems by breaking them down into manageable pieces and thinking about them creatively can make many positive outcomes possible.

Finding a starting point by partializing or breaking down the problem into smaller parts is an essential first step.

A child welfare supervisor finds that there are a large number of children being placed into custody by police. Upon investigation by protective service workers, many of these children are deemed to be safe or in situations where an in-home safety plan is feasible and desirable. However, by this time the legal process is well down the road that most often results in the child being placed in foster care and leaves the parents angry and alienated. This is supported by a public perception that more children in this community should be removed from their homes. Police are important people in this community, with wide public support, and enjoy a better relationship with the county attorney than do current protective service workers. There are many dimensions to this problem that could lead this supervisor to throw up her hands and feel helpless.

However, consistent with disrespecting the impossible, this supervisor feels responsible for this situation and he or she feels that there is a starting point somewhere. Upon further investigation, the supervisor finds that there is a particular group of children who are placed into custody when police respond to calls regarding domestic violence. Police officers say that they frequently find children from these households wandering the streets, and therefore the children are placed into protective custody due to neglectful behavior on the part of the parents. The officers also feel that being in a household where there is domestic violence is harmful to children.

The supervisor is not sure how to respond but now she can focus on part of the problem. The situation is put on the agenda for the next team meeting and the supervisor gets quick agreement that some of the children are being abused and should be taken into custody. The team also agrees that what appears to the police as neglectful behavior on the part of the mother is, in some cases, protective behavior—the mother sends the child to play outside when she senses a violent episode is about to occur. They also agree that educating police officers about which situations present a safety risk to the child and which do not will be difficult. They agree that officers are more likely to learn these distinctions from real-life cases than from training. Brainstorming by the team results in generating three possible next steps: First, ask police to call protective services when they receive a domestic violence call in a household with children, and a worker will respond immediately. One of the workers who has a good relationship with a police officer agrees to talk with him about how to best proceed on this idea. Second, approach the local domestic violence agency to develop community guidelines on protecting children in households experiencing domestic violence. The supervisor agrees to take the first step on this one. Historically, protective service workers and domestic violence advocates have been at odds in this community. Third, hire a former battered woman who lost her children to protective services but now is successfully parenting them to be a parent advocate when a child is placed into custody due to domestic violence. She has been talking about trying to find a way to help others who were in her situation. The supervisor will find the funds for this and the mother's caseworker, who has a great relationship with her, will talk with her about this idea.

Exercise

Describe a very difficult consumer situation that you experienced in an agency that you are familiar with.

1. *Identify three ways to partialize or break the problem down into manageable pieces.*
2. *Identify two or three interest groups concerned with this problem and identify their goals and interests in resolving this problem.*

This example demonstrates the supervisor's hopefulness or belief that she can and should do something about this situation. She learns enough about the problem to break it down to identify a seemingly feasible starting point. She keeps the focus on the safety and permanency of the children. She draws upon the experience of her workers to brainstorm feasible next steps.

This example also demonstrates the supervisor's ability to be flexible and inventive. Hiring a consumer is going to be difficult given the bureaucratic personnel system. She will need to use her best influence skills to get the police chief to agree to his officers calling a protective service worker in domestic violence situations. She also recognizes that all of these efforts may fail, in which case she will restart the problem-solving process.

The Ability to Blend Agendas of Seemingly Disparate Interests

Difficult consumer situations are frequently described in terms of particular interests that appear to conflict. Disrespecting the impossible includes the skills to see beyond these single interests to find common ground and meet the needs of a variety of key actors within the community. The community and its police force in the aforementioned example want children in domestic violence households to be placed into foster care. Child protective service workers want to keep as many children within their own home as possible. Mothers who are victims of domestic violence want their children with them. Domestic violence advocates want victims to be able to be safe.

By focusing on the safety of the child and mother, the supervisor finds a highly regarded value that all of these groups can agree upon. This allows all of the groups to begin to identify ways that this can be accomplished. Although there are situations where interest groups have goals that may not be able to be blended, more often than not common ground can be found.

Blending agendas begins with many basic social work skills, such as listening, respect, and reframing. Careful listening to the police officers revealed that their primary concern was for the safety of the children. Listening to the domestic violence advocates revealed that their primary concern was the safety of the mother. Listening to mothers revealed that their concern was keeping their children safe and with them. Given these concerns it was not difficult to approach the situation from the perspective of child safety and permanency.

Persistence, Persistence, Persistence

Disrespect for the impossible includes not giving up when someone says: "It can't be done." Given the intractable nature of many challenges faced by consumers, a supervisor's feelings of powerfulness and responsibility can easily be followed by fatigue and frustration. Removal of one barrier can reveal several new ones. The creative paths to success generated by a team may all fail. Demands to address other problems, such as funding or personnel, can draw energy and focus away from the difficult consumer problem.

The consumer-centered social administrator does not give up in the face of continued road blocks and other demands. This is frustrating and difficult work. One way to manage the frustration is to understand how people and systems change and develop. As social workers we use concepts such as socio-ecological models to understand human development within complex environments.

One of the socioecological models adopted by many social workers is that of Urie Bronfenbrenner (1995a) He proposed a rather simple way to understand developmental processes. His model is called the person-process-context-time (PPCT) model of human development, which includes the interactions between characteristics of the person, the social context within which that person is operating, and the developmental process that the person is undergoing, along with the realization that social roles, relationships, and resources change over time (Moen, Edler, & Lüscher, 1995). Bronfenbrenner (1995a) explains his paradigm as follows:

> Human development takes place through processes of progressively more complex reciprocal interaction between an active, evolving biopsychological human organism and the persons, objects, and symbols in its immediate environment. To be effective, the interaction must occur on a fairly regular basis over extended periods of time. Such enduring forms of interaction in the immediate environment are referred to as proximal processes. (p. 60)

This somewhat theoretical language simply states that development or change happens through a person's continuous interactions (proximal processes) with other people over time. The context of these interactions also influences these interactions and includes the environments of the organization, community, and policy. This means that social administrators produce change through persistent and focused interactions with key actors. There are many implications of this idea for social administrators but these are beyond the scope of this section. These will be revisited in Chapter 2. Recognizing that change and development is a slow process that takes place through repeated interactions with others can help a consumer-centered social administrator to respond to the natural frustration that occurs as a result of roadblocks to progress.

Principle # 4: Learning for a Living

If we knew exactly how to help every person with a psychiatric disability to maintain a good quality of life in the community, social workers would not be needed. If we knew exactly how to maintain abused and neglected children safely within their family, we would not be needed. If no child were left behind by our schools, we would not be needed. Clearly, we do not know enough and, given the dynamic nature of society, we will never know enough.

Someone once said that a social work degree was equivalent to a learner's permit issued to beginning drivers who have enough information about driving to continue to learn by doing. Social workers confront new situations nearly daily. Being inquisitive about consumers' situations, new helping technologies, and new policies is a prerequisite to working with people in a dynamic society.

Social administrators take this passion for learning to the organizational level. They demand continued learning from themselves and from everyone else in the organization. They create or foster a climate of seemingly contradictory ideas of supreme confidence in what is being done and doubt as to its effectiveness.

A number of years ago Argyris and Schon (1978) developed the idea of double loop learning that continues to be useful (Argyris, 1999). Their idea was to help explain how organizations detect and correct errors in values, objectives, and standards of performance. This is now more popularly labeled as organizational learning.

It is interesting to note that learning starts by detecting errors. This is consistent with social administrators' passion for understanding the reasons why more of our consumers are not achieving desired results. There are a variety of errors, including wrong standards or incorrect objectives. These and other important organizational components are discussed in further detail later in this book.

Argyris and Schon (1978) and Argyris (1999) identify characteristics of organizations and managers required for this "double loop" learning. The organization must have information systems that provide valid data to detect these errors. It must allow free choice of options but these choices must be informed and based upon the best possible information. There must be commitment to a chosen path, and monitoring and evaluation of its implementation.

Managers in these organizations produce action strategies such as combining advocacy with inquiry. In other words, they are comfortable with seemingly contradictory ideas. While advocating for an option they recognize that they do not have all the needed information and simultaneously support acquiring additional information. They make statements that can be tested and confirmed or disconfirmed. They identify and test their own inferences. They inquire into the reasoning of others.

This learning for a living creates or fosters an organizational climate where everyone has a sense of safety so that experimentation is encouraged and errors are tolerated. There is an atmosphere of openness and accountability. New ideas are tried, monitored for results, and if they are not found to be successful they are abandoned. These conditions are created in part by everyone in the organization, making judgments based upon reason and substance rather then personality. There is a sense that everyone is equal in their quest for knowledge and commitment to learning.

MANAGEMENT AS PERFORMANCE

Given the consumer-centered emphasis of this text up to this point, it is not surprising that we say that the manager's job is to use her or his skills to produce results for consumers. However, social administrators cannot manage by principles alone! Social work values and ethics are important. Specification of consumer-centered principles that places values and ethics in the context of social administration is useful and necessary but not sufficient. Social administrators also need an array of tools to use on a day-to-day basis that yield results. Much of this text presents the tools that we have found necessary to be a consumer-centered manager. We have also found that it is useful for managers to see their responsibility as producing results in five areas: consumer or client outcomes, service events, resources, staff morale, and efficiency.

Consumer or Client Outcomes

We have presented our case for consumer results being the driving force behind social programs. Social work values and ethics dictate that we work to "help people in need and address social problems." Society is increasingly focused on results by including this in social policy. For example, society is now demanding child safety and permanency in public child welfare. We have also found it useful to classify the various types of outcomes that social policy and consumers are seeking. We have identified five types of consumer outcomes. These are changes in affect, knowledge, behavior, status, and environment. Although this list may not be exhaustive, we have found that it covers nearly all types of consumer outcomes.

Consumer-Centered Social Administration Performance Results

1. Outcomes for consumers
2. Service events
3. Resources
4. Staff morale
5. Efficiency

Service Events

Many evidence-based practices are a mixture of structural elements and direct service (clinical) elements. Structural elements include such dimensions as caseload size, composition of teams, nature of supervision, and location of work (e.g., outreach). Clinical elements reflect the intervention done with and on behalf of consumers. Service events are the occurrence of these elements of the intervention. Examples could include a home visit, completion of a strengths assessment, acquiring resources, a class session, a home-delivered meal, a job development contact with a potential employer, and so on. These service events are the key program activities that directly lead to the consumer outcomes.

Social administrators that consider this helping transaction, the service event, as one of the results of their efforts are also putting the principles of consumer-centered management into practice. Seeking to produce the most effective service events *venerates consumers,* obsessing about the quality of service events *maintains the program's focus* on the results of these interactions, recognizing that existing service events are not always effective for a particular consumer and worker pushes managers to *learn* more about these situations and *to attempt what seems to be impossible.*

The social administrator's attention to the most powerful service events also means that she or he is constantly searching for practices with the highest level of evidence to indicate the production of the intended results. It is likely that the reader has encountered the term *evidence-based practice.* However, this has come to mean many different things to different people. We discuss our understanding of this important concept later in this text. For now we simply say that social administrators continually seek out interventions that have demonstrated the ability to produce the desired consumer outcomes.

Resources

Broadly speaking, resources include everything needed for the social program to produce the consumer benefit. Of course, money is first on any administrator's list of resources. It is likely that a majority of many administrators' time is devoted to acquiring the funds to keep the program operating. Resources also include staff, consumers, effective interventions and methods, and goodwill of the community.

Money is the lifeblood of the organization because it makes the acquisition of other resources more possible. If consumers achieve results primarily through their work with staff, then it is the frontline worker who vies with money as an important resource. The largest component of the budget for social services is for personal costs frequently amounting to 85 percent of the budget. Although a program supervisor in a large public bureaucracy may have little to do with budgeting or acquiring funds, they are responsible for the transaction between frontline staff and consumers and, therefore, have a major interest in and hopefully a role in the acquisition of staff. Matching the person to the consumer, program, and agency involves careful consideration of the skills, values, and interests of those who are called direct service workers. It is common to not only seek to match the skills and values of workers with the agency but also to assure that staff reflect the cultural and ethnic composition of the population of consumers. Having the program operated by the best staff is an important and complex resource acquisition responsibility.

However, a program without consumers will have staff drawing salaries with no meaningful result. Although it may seem ludicrous in a time of many social problems and few resources to think of a social program with too few consumers, it happens. To produce consumer benefits, social programs need to match an intervention to consumers of sufficient number with specific characteristics. A poorly designed program can result in a service designed for a consumer population so rare that there are not sufficient numbers in the community to justify hiring staff. Similarly a poorly designed program's intervention may require abilities of consumers that they are not likely to have. For example, many life skills programs for teens growing up in foster care are designed for learning complex behavioral skills by listening rather than by doing. This represents a mismatch between consumer skills and program requirements. A program may also lack consumers because the agency has lost or never acquired credibility in the community. Consumers are unlikely to flock to an agency with values that do not match those of the community, whose staff do not appear to be like most members of the community, or whose reputation has been damaged by some scandal.

As the independent living skills example demonstrates, workers' behavior when they engage consumers is yet another resource. Frontline supervisors are particularly attuned to their role in assuring that workers are engaging with consumers in the intended manner. This can be thought of as a helping technology and is every bit as important, if not more so, than any other technological resource. In social work, helping technologies are evidence-based practices that have been tested and produce evidence for their efficacy. In their resource acquisition role, social administrators continually scan the intervention research in their field of practice and seek to transfer those practices with the highest level of evidence from current research to the interaction between workers and consumers.

The acquisition of funds, staff, and consumers are all related to public support or community standing. Some people call this community "goodwill" and it is another critical resource. The social administrator that has excellent interpersonal influence skills is more likely to be successful in acquiring funds. The agency with a positive reputation in the community is likely to have consumers. The agency with a positive reputation among professionals is likely to have more applicants for jobs.

However, there is another dimension to this public support resource. Managers with excellent interpersonal influence skills (Chapter 2) are also more likely to be able to obtain support from key individuals in the community. The child protection supervisor with good influence skills is more likely to achieve desired changes in child abuse referrals from police officers. The mental health case management supervisor with influence skills is likely to receive a positive response from the local chamber of commerce about implementing a supported employment program for people with serious mental illness.

However, this discussion of resource acquisition as a management performance area is necessarily incomplete. There are many types of resources needed by social programs. The social administrator's job in this area is to acquire the resources needed to make the interaction between the worker and the consumer as effective as possible in achieving desired results.

Staff Morale

Social administrators are responsible for the job satisfaction of their staff. We see this as a valued result in and of itself regardless of any research connecting job satisfaction to outcomes for consumers. Social programs should contribute to the personal fulfillment of staff as they work with consumers.

Although there is not a body of research that meets the standard of a high level of evidence that connects worker satisfaction with consumer outcomes, the emerging research linking organizational variables to outcomes is beginning to show a connection between workers' feelings about the job and results. Glisson and Hemmelgran (1998) included job satisfaction as part of organizational climate that showed a positive relationship to service outcomes. The performance-enhancement teams of Yeaman, Craine, Gorsek, and Corrigan (2000) included team empowerment and after three months of operation found a positive pre/post relationship to consumer satisfaction and outcomes. The work of Harkness (1995), Ahearn (1999), and Corrigan,

Lickey, Campion, and Rashid (2000) all included some aspects of the supervisor–worker relationship that was positively associated with results for consumers.

The Gallup Organization has conducted organizational research over many years that led to the publication of *First, Break All the Rules: What the World's Greatest Managers Do Differently* (1999) by Marcus Buckingham and Curt Coffman. A major conclusion of this body of research is that great managers attract, focus, and keep the most talented employees. When the researchers then sought to determine what made a difference to these employees they came up with the following measuring stick.

1. Do I know what is expected of me at work?
2. Do I have the materials and equipment I need to do my work right?
3. At work, do I have the opportunity to do what I do best every day?
4. In the last seven days, have I received recognition or praise for doing good work?
5. Does my supervisor, or someone at work, seem to care about me as a person?
6. Is there someone at work who encourages my development?
7. At work, do my opinions seem to count?
8. Does the mission/purpose of my company make me feel my job is important?
9. Are my co-workers committed to doing quality work?
10. Do I have a best friend at work?
11. In the last six months, has someone at work talked to me about my progress?
12. This last year, have I had opportunities at work to learn and grow? (p. 28)

This is an impressive list of what many people would agree constitutes job satisfaction or leads one to be satisfied with their work. We will not discuss this list here but return to staff morale throughout this text. For now, we simply want to emphasize the importance of the social administrators' role in producing a high level of staff morale.

Efficiency

Finally, we propose efficiency as a social administration performance area. Efficiency is simply a ratio of resources acquired (inputs) and activity (outputs). The cost of a unit of service is an example.

The rationale for efficiency is straightforward. There are never enough resources to achieve all of the desirable consumer outcomes. The social administrator can use a focus on efficiency to redirect resources to produce better results or to work with more consumers.

Without a focus on efficiency, organizations can trap resources and use them for maintenance with little or no benefit for the intended beneficiaries. Think about how time can get wasted in organizations in which you have worked. People, for example, suggest that there should be a meeting about this question or that with little thought to the time this takes away from consumers. Social work achieves outcomes when direct service personnel spend time with consumers. When these social workers are engaged in staff meetings, this time is no longer available to consumers. A powerful efficiency measure is the percentage of time that workers spend with consumers and this is a measure that every social administrator should manage to achieve maximum benefit to consumers.

Chapter 2

Initiating Change Through Persuasion: The Microskills Approach

Change is a central concept in social work whether it is individual, organizational, or societal. The preamble to the NASW Code of Ethics states:

> Social workers promote social justice and social change with and on behalf of consumers. "Consumers" is used inclusively to refer to individuals, families, groups, organizations, and communities. Social workers are sensitive to cultural and ethnic diversity and strive to end discrimination, oppression, poverty, and other forms of social injustice. These activities may be in the form of direct practice, community organizing, supervision, consultation, administration, advocacy, social and political action, policy development and implementation, education, and research and evaluation.

The social administrator promotes social justice and change on behalf of consumers in a variety of contexts. Administrators work with program and agency staff and key individuals in the community who play an essential role in results for consumers. These individuals may be policy makers, people responsible for funding social programs, key decision makers such as judges, or the larger community.

Within the social administration literature change is normally discussed at the organizational level. There are many models proposed to aid a manager to guide change efforts. Felice Perlmutter (2000) summarizes the literature on initiating and implementing change and identifies the work of Patti and Resnick (1985) and Kotter (1996) as two models that focus primarily on the administrative role in managing change.

Textbook of Social Administration: The Consumer-Centered Approach
doi:10.1300/5802_03

Patti and Resnick (1985) discuss the types of leadership that are needed to direct change. Using a traditional problem-solving approach they identify the steps in each of three phases of change. The planning phase includes identification of the problem, analysis of the problem, determining whether the problem is internally or externally induced, clarifying the objective, and selecting a course of action. The implementation phase consists of consideration of communication, allocation of roles, and provision of resources. The evaluation phase allows for feedback to maintain, modify, or abandon the change effort.

Kotter (1996) presents an eight-step model of organizational change. These steps are as follows: establishing a sense of urgency, creating the guiding coalition, developing a vision and strategy, communicating the change vision, empowering broad-based action, generating short-term wins, consolidating gains and producing more change, and anchoring new approaches in the culture.

These models, like the broader management literature, are helpful in providing ways of thinking about organizational change. At the same time these models tend to be linear and abstract, and place less emphasis on the context of change beyond the organization. The world of the social administrator is more complex and requires daily attention to change through the normal interactions with a variety of people. Social administrators interact with people on a daily basis to reward a behavior or to influence them to do something differently. In this text, we focus on administrative behavior or the microskills that managers need in these daily contexts to foster change on behalf of consumers.

Change and Social Administration: Learning Objectives

1. *Recognize that change begins by identifying the person to be influenced and their desired behavior.*
2. *Identify and apply the components of the theory of behavioral intention to a social administration context.*
3. *Describe the importance of gender and cultural differences to influencing behavior.*
4. *Describe and demonstrate the strategies to enhance perceived behavioral control.*
5. *Describe and demonstrate the strategies to change an attitude toward a behavior.*
6. *Describe and demonstrate the strategies to change the normative component.*
7. *Describe and demonstrate the strategies to move from intention to behavior.*

It is also our view that change is the responsibility of every administrator and not the exclusive domain of top management. In Gummer's (2001) review of recent management literature, he finds that innovators in organizations tend to be career public servants, frontline staff, and middle managers. This suggests that although top management has a role in the efforts to bring about change, they may not be the most important people in identifying and implementing change on behalf of consumers.

The model used in this book is firmly rooted in the bioecological model of growth and development (Bronfenbrenner, 1995a,b). Our experience is that change occurs through the behavior of administrators exhibited in interchanges with other people over time. This is consistent with the bioecological model of growth and development that understands growth and change as resulting from proximal processes. These proximal processes are interchanges between people that occur consistently over time. The young person, for example, learns to manage money through interchanges with someone (conversations) who also structures practice through something like an allowance. The social administrator likewise promotes change by structured interchanges with people, which occur on a consistent basis over time.

An important finding from developmental psychology is that these proximal processes are more effective if the person directing the process believes that they are effective. Change occurs when social administrators believe that the interchanges in which they are engaged with a person over time will result in the person adopting a different behavior or attitude. These interchanges are directed at attempting to influence another person to do something differently that is linked to improved outcomes for consumers. With interpersonal influence being the primary mechanism for producing change, the research on persuasion is the basis for identifying the mechanisms and behaviors to help people change their attitudes, intentions, and behavior.

The bottom line for the social administrator is behavior. Social administrators start change by identifying the behavior that will produce the increase in performance. Every change effort begins with the identification of the person and their behavior as the focus of attention. Lack of clarity on who is needed to perform what action will doom many change efforts.

Change Begins with Answering Two Questions:

What is the behavior that is needed to improve results for consumers?
Who needs to exhibit this behavior?

The model of change presented in this chapter is complex, befitting the nature of change. The model relies on microskills or discrete strategies and behaviors that managers use to bring about change. Each of the fourteen to eighteen (if you count subcategories) skills presented is explained in detail with an example. The model of change and the associated skills are presented as one of the first chapters so that the use of these skills can be illustrated as management topics are presented. These features may present some challenges for using this chapter. In addition, for social workers with extensive clinical skills, some of the skills will appear to be nearly second nature and the detailed presentation may be seen as tedious.

The authors suggest considering different ways that this chapter can be used before proceeding. One approach is to first learn the model of persuasion and then practice each skill in a setting where performance feedback can be provided and adequate time can be devoted to discussion of the skill, its fit with the model, and potential use in a social administration context. This could be the basis of an entire semester's practice course in social administration.

Another approach is to learn the change model, skim the fourteen to eighteen skills, and identify those that the reader would like to practice. The identified skills can then be practiced as in the first approach. Still another approach is to learn the model and skim the skills and proceed with the rest of the text. As the change model and accompanying skills are presented in subsequent chapters, the model can be reviewed and selected skills practiced. Regardless of the readers' approaches to this material we encourage review of the model and skills as they are integrated into the material throughout this text. The model and its components should become second nature to the social administrator.

PERSUASION: SOME BASICS

Much of what social workers do is to try to persuade someone to exhibit a behavior. Workers try to persuade consumers to think differently and do something differently. These same workers advocate for consumers with others in the community such as landlords, other service providers, or judges. Similarly, social administrators try to influence people who control resources to provide increased or stable funding for a program.

There are many theories and definitions of persuasion (Seiter & Gass, 2004). One definition that is succinct and incorporates the most important ideas is the one put forth by O'Keefe (2002), "Persuasion is a successful intentional effort at influencing another's mental state through communication

in circumstances in which the persuadee has some measure of freedom." (p. 5). Gass and Sieter (2004) review nine theories of persuasion leading O'Keefe (2004) to observe that no single theory of persuasion is likely to provide a complete and detailed account of every persuasion circumstance.

Although no single existing theory explains all types of persuasion in all circumstances, the Theory of Behavioral Intention is probably the most widely accepted theory and is supported by an extensive research base (Gass & Sieter, 2004; Hale, Householder, & Greene, 2002). This theory suggests targeting another's mental state because it is through change of attitudes that behavior is most likely to change. The relationship between attitudes and behaviors is complex but, in general, behaviors are consistent with attitudes (O'Keefe, 2002; Sieter & Gass, 2004). However, there are important factors that can moderate the connection between attitudes and behaviors, including

- the amount of effort required to exhibit the behavior;
- having a vested interest in a position;
- the manner in which the attitude was formed; and
- perceived relevance of attitude to action.

Social administrators engage in influence when they communicate with a person to influence that person to think differently about something and exhibit behavior that is consistent with this attitude. This communication takes place in recognition of factors that influence behavior such as the person's current attitudes or position, the manner in which these were formed, the effort required to follow through, and the importance to the person of being consistent in their beliefs and actions (O'Keefe, 2002).

For example, a social administrator may be talking with a state legislator in an effort to influence him or her to vote for a piece of legislation that the administrator believes will contribute to improved outcomes for consumers. The administrator's communication is aimed at having the legislator think more positively about a bill and consequently vote for passage. The administrator takes into consideration the possible moderating factors. In this example, the behavior (voting) by itself is not difficult. However, the legislator's experience with the type of consumer that is to be benefited may be important. If the legislator has a family member who is this type of consumer, the vote may be more likely to follow. If, however, the legislator has had negative experiences with people in this condition, the vote will be more difficult to obtain. If the legislator voted for a bill that was substantially different from the one proposed, he may have a vested interest in the current situation and will be less likely to vote for the bill. Finally, if the legislator does not think that voters will be very interested in his or her vote on this one bill, it may not be important for the attitude and behavior to be consistent.

The link between attitude and action is a person's intention to perform a given behavior. This intention is considered the best predictor of actual behavior (O'Keefe, 2002; Sieter & Gass, 2004). This intention is a function of many variables including the person's attitude toward the behavior, their perception of the importance to others that the person performs the behavior, and the person's belief about the resources and obstacles to performance of the behavior (Figure 2.1).

For example, a program manager thinks that it is important for direct service staff to start talking with consumers about what is going well in their lives. The social worker's intention to start talking with consumers in this way is more likely to occur if they think that this is a good idea, if they think that the program manager is an important person, and if they think that there are no significant obstacles to this behavior. If this results in the worker having the intention to start this behavior, then it is more likely to occur.

The person's attitude toward the behavior is their belief concerning the outcome of the behavior (O'Keefe, 2002; Terry, Hogg, & White, 2000). The strength of this belief is also important. So in our example, if the social worker strongly believes that the result of this new practice will be beneficial, they are more likely to attempt it.

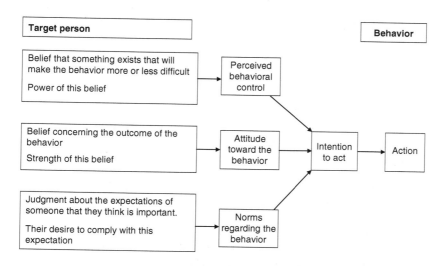

FIGURE 2.1. Theory of Behavioral Intention

The second component that explains the intention to behave is a little more complex and is called the person's subjective norms (Sieter & Gass, 2004; O'Keefe, 2002; Terry, Hogg, & White, 2000). Subjective norms are the person's perception of the importance of this behavior to significant others and their motivation to comply. So the following three things are important: (1) who is important to the individual; (2) the importance of this behavior to that person; and (3) how strong the motivation to comply is. In our example, the worker's subjective norms will be most favorable to trying the new behavior if he or she thinks that the program manager expects it, if the program manager is important to him or her, and if he or she wants to satisfy the program manager's expectations.

The third component of this model is perceived behavioral control (O'Keefe, 2002; Terry, Hogg, & White, 2000). This is (1) the person's belief that something exists that is either an obstacle to the behavior or a resource to facilitate the behavior and (2) the power of this "control factor" to inhibit or control the behavior. In our example, the behavior does not require new skills and is to be done in the normal interaction between consumer and worker, so it is likely that the worker would not perceive large obstacles to talking with consumers this way. However, if the behavior change was a new type of therapy that the worker had not been trained in, this would be an obstacle. If the behavior needed to be exhibited in a context that the worker could not control, such as a courtroom, this would also decrease the perceived behavioral control.

The relationship between attitudes, norms, and perceived control is complex. We probably have all experienced situations where people have done things that they thought were important regardless of what others expected and in the presence of significant obstacles. Similarly, you probably know of situations where someone has done something because it was important to someone else despite his or her own attitude toward the action. People weigh many variables to arrive at a decision to do something. On a day-to-day basis, it is unlikely that a manager can determine how a particular person will weigh various considerations and select a strategy specific to that person. Consequently, we suggest that people who are attempting to be persuasive target all three components: attitudes, norms, and obstacles.

GENDER AND CULTURAL DIFFERENCES IN PERSUASION

Linda Carli (2004) has reviewed the extensive research on gender differences in influence. Her unsettling conclusion will not be news to many of the women reading this text.

> The different distribution of men and women into social roles, accord-
> ing to which women are more often found in domestic and lower-
> status occupational roles and generally have lower overall status then
> men, has resulted in descriptive gender stereotypes that women are
> less competent and less legitimate than men as authorities and lead-
> ers. (p. 143)

Many of us had hoped that this was no longer a true statement. However, Carli has found this to be pervasive and current. She has found this effect repeatedly demonstrated among small children as well as adults. Unfortunately, these are findings that we all need to factor into our work. It may be that there is less of this stereotyping in social work settings because of our professional views of equality but this cannot be assumed. In addition, since so much of the work of a social administrator is in the community with nonsocial work audiences, these results cannot be taken lightly.

Research on influence shows that people who are perceived as competent and likable exert greater influence than those who do not (Carli, 2004). Perceptions of women in regard to the two key elements of competence and likablity make exercising influence more difficult for them. Research has shown that group members are more likely to attend to the ideas contributed by men and use them in problem solving than to acknowledge identical ideas contributed by women (Propp, 1995). Additional research has shown that even when the persuasive messages of men and women were identical, men remained more influential (DiBerardinis, Ramage, & Levitt, 1984).

So women must demonstrate exceptional competence to be seen as equal in ability as men. However, competent behavior of women may be resisted although competent behavior exhibited by men is widely accepted (Carli, 2004). Competent behavior can enhance women's influence by enhancing their perceived competence and at the same time lower their influence by decreasing their likeability. This is a classic double bind for women.

Carli (2004) finds that the characteristic of being likable is important to influence but with differential effects by gender. For women being likable is more highly correlated with influence than it is for men. So women must combine competence with behavior that communicates likeability whereas men can be mainly concerned about competence. This research suggests that likeability is enhanced by conveying concern for others and by showing a lack of interest in asserting personal status. This is particularly important when women are trying to influence men. Men typically resist messages from direct and competent women. The bottom line is that women are more influential when they combine communication in a warm style with out-standing competence.

Of course men can play roles in supporting women in their efforts to influence. First they need to examine their own responses to both women and men to see whether they are evaluating the argument or the person. Second, they can reinforce others' (particularly men) perceptions of the competence and likeability of the women with whom they work.

There is much less research on the effects of cultural characteristics on influence. This is not surprising given the vast number of cultural groups in this society and the cost and difficulty of conducting research on each of them. However, we believe that the research on gender differences is useful for consideration of cultural differences. It is likely that the larger society has negative stereotypes about any minority cultural group and that these will lessen their influence. They are likely to be viewed as less competent and less likeable. Until research identifies the relevant factors for each subculture, it is likely that attention to the dominant cultures' perceptions of others' competence and likeability should be of concern to all of us. In the meantime, the same aforementioned strategies in relation to women are likely to be useful in the context of different cultural groups.

STRATEGIES TO ENHANCE PERCEIVED BEHAVIORAL CONTROL

The theory of behavioral intention contends that action is preceded by intention to act. Intention to act is influenced by perceived behavioral control, the attitudes that a person has about the change, and the existing norms regarding the behavior. Although the theory targets change in attitudes in order to change behavior, research suggests that attitudes based on direct behavioral experience with the attitude object have been found to be more predictive of later behavior toward the object than are attitudes that are based on indirect experience (O'Keefe, 2002). In other words, it is more powerful to engage in behavioral strategies. Consequently we begin by focusing on behavioral strategies that enhance behavioral control.

Fortunately, there are at least five strategies available to the social administrator to enhance behavioral control. Each of these strategies is described in detail along with examples so that the social administrator will be able to implement it in efforts to influence peoples' perceptions about behavioral control. The strategies are as follows:

1. Obstacle removal
   a. Task groups
   b. Paperwork
   c. Education and training

2. Modeling
3. Behavioral rehearsal
4. Provide verbal encouragement
5. Provide information

Obstacle Removal

It comes as no surprise that removing obstacles is a major activity of social administrators. The research on persuasion indicates that this is an important element of influencing people's intention to act and their behavior. Not surprisingly, when people perceive obstacles to a new behavior, they are not likely to want to change. Similarly, when people perceive that there is nothing in the way of exhibiting the behavior, then they are more likely to have a positive attitude about the behavior. Directly removing obstacles is one strategy for enhancing perceived behavioral control (O'Keefe, 2002). In this section we present three primary tools for social administrators to use to remove obstacles. We have found all three of these to be powerful strategies and these will be revisited later in this book.

1. Leading a group in the task of identifying obstacles and developing plans for their removal
2. Paperwork
3. Education and training

Remove Obstacles Through a Group Task

One of the most powerful ways to engage in obstacle removal is to bring together key individuals to identify those factors that anyone in the group believes will make the behavior difficult (obstacles) and to work together to eliminate these conditions. All too often meetings in organizations are a waste of time. The agenda is unstructured or absent, and the desired outcomes are not specified. Few participants take responsibility for helping to structure or lead the meeting. When a meeting operates at an abstract level with vague verbal exchanges, few concrete results can be expected. Discussing issues or problems on a conceptual level often passes for doing work. However, when meetings are used to identify perceived obstacles to a change effort, accompanied by group plans for removing these conditions, they are productive, and change can occur. This requires involving the right people in this important group task.

Of course, group members must have the specific skills required to complete the task. The group may simply not have any history in doing work together, which may make it difficult to engage them in a task. The idea of identifying obstacles and ideas for their removal may be so new to the group members that they do not have the ability to complete the task. However, it is likely that the original tasks can be broken down into a small task or set of tasks that the group can successfully complete.

It may also be true that part of the task cannot be finished because someone needs to do work outside of the group meeting (e.g., checking case files or state policy). In this situation the work is delegated to group members. The more responsibility that each member takes for tasks, the more the benefits of this approach accrue. One advantage of delegating the tasks to be done outside of the group is the natural establishment of the agenda for the next meeting, as well as prior commitment to work at the next meeting. In short, managers who are skilled at leading groups in identifying obstacles to a change effort and developing plans for their removal are often quite successful in change efforts. And remember that change requires belief and persistence. The group will be more successful if the leader is persistent and believes that it will succeed. Change is the result of proximal processes taking place over an extended period of time. We will return to obstacle removal several times in this book, including in Chapter 10.

Paperwork

As people state their thoughts about being able to engage in a particular behavior they almost naturally identify obstacles. Paperwork or the perception that there will be a whole new set of forms to complete is often an identified obstacle, although this is not always openly stated. Reduction of paperwork or an improved integration of paperwork with practice is a valuable strategy and a continuing struggle for the social administrator.

Paperwork is the most onerous task for frontline practitioners; the burden can consume more than 35 percent of an agency's time and resources and the benefits accrued to the organization are slight even when identifiable. Paperwork is a major factor in reduced productivity, efficiency, job satisfaction, and even effectiveness. The reduction of paperwork, however, seems particularly difficult.

Paperwork is important and forms can serve legitimate purposes. First, forms provide the information needed for documentation, a record of what was done to whom. This information can help the agency meet professional standards set by accrediting bodies, protect the agency against complaints and lawsuits, and meet requirements for funding. The majority of forms in agencies are devoted to this purpose.

Second, forms can act as tools for staff to help prompt and guide their work. For example, a model of intervention depends on an assessment of consumer strengths. This requires an assessment device that helps guide the practitioner and consumer through this process. Consumer assessment and case planning forms are the most common manifestations of forms for this purpose.

Third, forms can act as a management tool used by a supervisor or through the collection of program performance information. Supervisors cannot possibly participate in every service transaction but they can, and in most cases should, read assessment or case planning documents. In addition, the data that is essential to knowing how the program is performing, particularly regarding outcomes for consumers, is primarily collected by workers through the service transaction.

Integration and elimination of forms is a strategy for enhancing behavioral control. Readers can probably identify paperwork whose purpose was unclear in agencies that they have known, and was therefore a candidate for elimination. Specific strategies for elimination of paperwork will be revisited in Chapter 10.

Education and Training

The second most dominant strategy for solving problems in social service organizations after developing a policy is to send people for training. In their usual forms, neither of these is effective and should be avoided. Just because there is a new policy for or against something does not mean that people will comply. Similarly, just because someone is sent off to training does not mean that they will change their behavior on the job. Yet a worker who is asked to use a new intervention must acquire the knowledge and skills to implement the new approach. Lack of skills is a real obstacle to change efforts and education and training does have an important role to play. The key is the proper selection, preparation, and use of training.

The concept of transfer of training or the conditions that are necessary before, during, and after the event for the skills to be acquired and then demonstrated on the job is seen as a possible answer to the inefficiency that normally accompanies training. The concern about the effectiveness of training is understandable in light of recent estimates of training expenditures and the extent to which transfer of training occurs. Baldwin and Ford (1988) estimated that organizations in the United States spend about 110 billion dollars annually, including 15 billion work hours on training. In 1994, Curry and his colleagues estimated that only 10 to 13 percent of skills learned in training are actually transferred back to the job. Although these findings are a little outdated, it is unlikely that these dismal results have changed much. To get the most out of any investment in training it is useful to focus on those conditions that are likely to maximize transfer of skills from the training event to the job.

One review of the transfer of training literature suggests that the following variables are related to people exhibiting behavior on the job following a training event (Gregoire, Propp, & Poertner, 1998).

Individual attributes of the training participant refers to the level of confidence that they feel in their ability to use skills, and their beliefs as to the relevance or applicability of the skills in the job situation. This is thought to include

- what participants expected to occur in training;
- participants' involvement in making decisions about training;
- participants' perceptions of acquiring sufficient skills to be able to use them; and
- participants' perceptions that they have sufficient control in the work environment to use the new skills (behavioral control).

Instructional design is the second major component that contributes to training transfer. An effective training curriculum is said to include

- clear behavioral objectives;
- content that is relevant to the work context;
- content that is presented in a variety of ways;
- trainers who have the skills or possess credibility from the trainee's point of view; and
- practice and performance feedback as part of the training event.

Organizational context is another factor in the transfer of training. This consists of the people, structure, cultural milieu, and the value that is placed on learning and development. This includes

- support from peers, supervisors, and managers;
- a reward system that encourages the changes that the new skills bring to the organization; and
- a supportive climate for learning.

Clearly the social administrator has a role to play to insure that the best possible conditions exist so that people who participate in training receive the maximum benefit and apply the behavior on the job. The social administrator makes certain that the training event is designed in line with the characteristics identified earlier. Before training occurs, the manager involves the participant in decision making about the training. The social administrator and the training participant have a conversation before the training event that includes the manager's reassurance that the skills to be acquired are important to success results for consumers, the development of an individualized learning plan that specifics the desired learning results, and other considerations that are important to the participant. Finally, the manager has the responsibility for creating the organizational context that promotes the use of new skills. There is nothing more destructive than co-workers who remind someone who has just returned from a training event that things are not done that way in this workplace. Rather, the manager has created a work environment where new learning is valued and co-workers ask the training participant what they learned, how it helps consumers, and how they will obtain the new skills. The manager also asks the training participant about the training event, including his or her perceptions of the trainers, activities, what he or she learned, how it is working with consumers, and what the participant needs to more effectively use the skills on the job. Training will be revisited several times in this text including in Chapter 8.

Modeling

As an influence strategy to enhance perceived behavior control, modeling is simply doing. If the behavior is acquired through training, modeling and practice should have been a part of the instructional design. However, modeling is also used in other situations, such as supervision. Modeling is a powerful strategy (O'Keefe, 2004; Anderson, 2000; Ng, Tam, Yew, & Lan 1999; Hagen, Gotkin, Wilson, & Oats, 1998). Seeing a peer perform the behavior makes it concrete and meaningful. For maximum effectiveness there are several considerations that need to be kept in mind.

Modeling recognizes that much of what we want people to do is a set of behaviors that are much too complex to explain or to attempt to talk people into doing. When a person does something (models), the individual components of the set of behaviors is demonstrated. This allows the audience to compare their behavior in similar situations to the demonstrated behavior. Not only are the behaviors demonstrated but so are the rewards possible or accruing from the behavior. This includes both extrinsic and intrinsic rewards. Modeling not only demonstrates the rewards available from others but also demonstrates the ways in which the behavior is intrinsically energizing or exciting.

The social administrator who uses modeling needs to consider several elements of this strategy to have maximum effect. The audience has to be able to see the behavioral components, the extrinsic rewards, and the intrinsic rewards. The audience has to believe that the rewards would be available to them. The audience has to believe that they could perform the behavior. These conditions mean that for modeling to be effective, the administrator who uses modeling must establish the conditions for modeling. The social administrator must make certain that the rewards are available to others who perform the same behavior and explicitly demonstrate the implicit rewards through demonstrating the excitement or joy felt by performing the behavior.

Modeling

- *Make certain that the audience sees the behavior.*
- *Make certain that the audience can identify the intrinsic rewards.*
- *Make certain that the audience sees the extrinsic rewards.*

Behavioral Rehearsal

People are not likely to feel that they have behavioral control if they have never exhibited the behavior. A secondary school language teacher frequently told her class to use the Spanish vocabulary that they knew because they could never use what they did not know. This simple truth is frequently overlooked. If the desired behavior is the subject of training, a well-designed curriculum will include behavioral rehearsal and feedback. However, leaving the acquisition of an important new skill to the limited practice that occurs in training is risky and there are many other situations where people would feel enhanced behavioral control through practice. Rehearsal has been found to be an effective persuasion strategy (O'Keefe, 2004; Yzer, Fisher, Bakker, Siero, & Misovich, 1998; Weise, Turbiasz, & Whitney, 1995; Mishra et al., 1998).

Behavioral rehearsal is simply performing the behavior in a situation where the person can feel free to risk failure and receive feedback on his or her performance. Consequently, the social administrator needs to construct these conditions. When the administrator consistently values learning to improve outcomes, people are more likely to take the risk of trying the new behavior. It is also important that feedback occur so that participants are likely to respond positively and continue to refine their behavior. For this to occur it is important for the source of the feedback to begin by telling the person what he or she did well. This can then be followed by suggestions for improvements in the behaviors in the future. The manager can also remind the person of the rewards linked to the new behavior to increase the likelihood of the behavior being repeated.

Behavioral Rehearsal

- *Have the person perform the behavior in a "safe" environment.*
- *Provide rewarding and correcting feedback on the behavior.*
- *Involve consumers whenever possible.*

This is also another good opportunity for consumer involvement. Inviting or hiring a consumer who can participate in the behavioral rehearsal can be very useful. The consumer can speak with more credibility about how they experience the behavior along with what seemed to be particularly helpful and suggest changes. Of course, this requires preparation of the consumer. If the behavior is a new intervention, it is unlikely that the consumer would have experience with it. Consequently, the consumer will need to understand what has led the program to attempt this change as well as its components.

Provide Verbal Encouragement

As the previous sections demonstrate, there is a great deal that a social administrator can do to enhance perceived behavioral control through obstacle removal, training, modeling, and behavioral rehearsal. These are powerful behavioral strategies. There are also strategies that are largely verbal that can also enhance perceived behavioral control. One of these strategies is verbal encouragement (Anderson, 1995). There are two sides to providing verbal encouragement. One is to provide encouragement or inducements to perform and then reward the behavior. The second is to recognize that inducements may backfire and result in resistance. Consequently, when using inducements it is important to avoid high-pressure tactics.

This strategy comes from the various behavioral psychology schools of thought. People exhibit behavior that they believe to be rewarding. There are two ways this happens. Conditions are established that assure the person of being rewarded or behavior is exhibited and rewards accrue. The rewards increase the frequency of the behavior. An important condition is that the link between the behavior and the inducement or reward must be explicit.

For inducements and rewards to work, they must be valued by the person and must be perceived as fair and not patronizing.

This strategy is yet another instance where the administrator must know what people value and what specific individuals find rewarding. Chapter 8 includes consideration of common job values and the reward-based environment. The administrator must also explicitly link the inducement or reward to the desired behavior. In many behavioral models, this is emphasized through temporal placement of rewards and behavior. That is, the reward occurs as soon as possible after the behavior.

In the use of this strategy in the day-to-day environment in which administrators operate, "being there" when the behavior occurs is unlikely. Consequently, the administrator needs to identify for the target person the link between the inducement, the reward, and the desired behavior. Linking rewards that come from the social administrator to rewards that normally occur within the environment also enhances their effect. Talking about the intrinsic rewards is one part of this strategy. Creating a reward-based environment is another. Administrators create a reward-based environment when they establish the conditions where co-workers reward each other for behavior that is the norm for that work unit. An important task of the social administrator is to make the rewarding of each other an expectation in the workplace and to clearly define the behavior that warrants these rewards.

Inducements and Rewards

- *Explicitly link rewards to desired behavior.*
- *Rewards must be valued by the person and perceived as fair and non-patronizing.*
- *Develop a reward-based environment in which everyone knows what the desired behavior is and rewards others when it occurs.*
- *Avoid what would be perceived by the person as being pressured to exhibit the behavior.*

Provide Information and Make It Comprehensible

Providing information to people involved in a change effort is yet another strategy for enhancing perceived behavioral control leading to action (O'Keefe, 2002). There are two primary considerations in providing information. First, the people involved must be able to understand the message. Our tendency to use jargon as verbal shorthand and the everyday pressures of work frequently result in miscommunication. People in agencies frequently think that they are communicating even though they are using different definitions for words. Some of our favorite undefined terms are "coordinate," "provide support," or "the system." It is worth the time and effort to arrive at common definitions of words and to use as specific a language as possible Second, remember to avoid high-pressure tactics. If people involved in a change effort feel threatened or pressured they are more likely to be resistant than cooperative.

The research finds that messages that are specific descriptions of the action to be taken are more persuasive (O'Keefe, 2002; O'Keefe, 1999; Frantz, 1994). That is, when the message is specific and behavioral, it is more likely to be understood. Specificity is a point of emphasis throughout this book. In addition to being behavioral, an important part of this specificity is presenting messages in a language that is readily understood by the target audience. Technical jargon should be avoided. People will not adopt a line of action that they do not fully comprehend. Simple, easily understood ideas are more likely to be accepted than complex and hard-to-follow arguments. Comprehension can sometimes be augmented with graphs, charts, or through site visits where the audience can view the innovation in action. Clarity and comprehension are important in enhancing a person's perceived behavioral control.

Provide Information

- *Consider the audience—make ideas comprehensible.*
- *Avoid high-pressure tactics.*

STRATEGIES TO CHANGE THE ATTITUDE TOWARD A BEHAVIOR

Recall that the model of behavioral intention contends that action is preceded by intention to act and that this is influenced by perceived behavioral control, the attitudes that the person has about the change, and the existing norms regarding the behavior. O'Keefe (2002) also emphasizes that messages targeted at specific attitudes rather than general ones tend to be more consistent with behavior. In other words, social administrators are likely to be more effective when focusing on an attitude about a specific behavior and not a general attitude about a social problem or group of consumers.

This chapter is necessarily written in a linear fashion; in reality the strategies that are suggested to enhance perceived behavioral control also impact attitudes and norms. Attitudes based on direct behavioral experience with the attitude object have been found to be more predictive of behavior than attitudes based on indirect experience (O'Keefe, 2002). In other words it is more powerful to engage in the behavioral strategies covered in the previous section than to rely on the verbal strategies identified here. However, ignoring components of the theory of behavioral intention would lessen and not strengthen a manager's change efforts.

This section focuses on presenting strategies for enhancing the person's positive attitude toward a specific behavior. There are three general strategies for influencing a person to change his or her attitude toward a behavior that are applicable to social administration.

1. Add a new reason to think positively about the behavior
2. Increase or decrease the importance of an existing belief about the behavior
3. Try it—"foot in the door technique"

Adding a Reason to Think Positively About the Behavior and Changing the Importance of an Existing Belief

We have chosen to group the first two general strategies together for practical reasons. In any given situation it may not be possible to determine whether a reason to think positively about the behavior is new or is simply being reinforced or increased. The specific strategies in this section may be the most common and comfortable for social administrators because they primarily rely on the verbal skills of social workers. These skills can be used for either adding a reason or changing the importance of a belief. The microskills are as follows:

- Emphasize advantages and rewards.
- Cite proven results/weight of the evidence.
- Specify the consequences of a stance.

Emphasize Advantages or Rewards

People are constantly processing the information available to them and making decisions. These analyses include how they might best satisfy their needs and achieve their goals. Research on persuasion finds that when messages match a person's function for an attitude, they are more effective for changing an attitude (O'Keefe, 2002; Maio & Olson, 1995). In other words, different attitudes meet different needs of people and when the persuasive message meets this need, it is more likely to be effective. Hence, the probability that individuals will change their behavior in response to a communication is increased when the message provides information indicating that the change will enable them to more effectively satisfy a need or desire. This is a verbal strategy that the social administrator implements by explicitly stating the advantages and rewards for adopting a new behavior. One good reason for doing so is because the new approach yields rewards at a level unavailable through existing practices or alternative action. Perhaps the most powerful of these rewards is improved outcomes for consumers.

Cite Proven Results or the Weight of the Evidence

The emphasis on evidence-based practice brings proven results to the forefront and is a natural element of the advantages and rewards. When the change is an evidence-based practice, one of the advantages is clearly that it has been demonstrated to produce the desired results. In addition, an improved outcome for consumers is a clear reward. Still, it is useful to be reminded of citing proven results as a separate strategy.

One way to implement this strategy is through documentation. That is, present all of the evidence for your position. This has the potential of helping people have a more positive attitude toward the change. Comparing the evidence for one position to the evidence for another position can also be used. Similar to a courtroom analogy, the position with more evidence tends to be sustained. Just like in court, you need to consider the nature of evidence. In court, there are specific rules of evidence. In the area of the social programs, evidence tends to come from empirical literature, theoretical literature, and the experiences of others.

Another way to implement this strategy is by conducting a trial of the innovation. An audience is more apt to accept an idea if they are reminded that its consequences have already been demonstrated or observed. When people can see the positive results of an action or procedure, they are more likely to adopt it. In addition to becoming part of the list of advantages and rewards, this suggests that a stepping stone approach is often an effective way of selling an idea. This is the strategy known as the "foot-in-the-door" technique, which will be presented shortly.

Specify the Consequences of a Stance

With this strategy, the audience is involved in exploring the consequences of a position through logical reasoning. When the consequences of the desired position are seen as more beneficial or more likely to satisfy a need, then the audience is likely to have a more positive attitude toward the behavior. This strategy involves thinking through positions and their consequences. It is very common to adopt a position without systematically thinking through the consequences. After all, we are all busy people with workloads that seldom allow time for reflection. In addition, all of the consequences can seldom be determined. Social policy analysts talk about unintended consequences of a policy. This is simply recognition that not all of the consequences of a position can be foreseen.

Specifying the consequences of a stance works best when the audience describes their position and its anticipated consequences. The leader's job is to help clarify the position and the consequences. Positive consequences for adopting the change result in a more positive attitude toward the change. However, the leader also has to assure that negative or possible undesired consequences are identified. Although this may result in a less positive attitude toward the change, these cannot be ignored. The leader can address these negative consequences as obstacles and begin the process of their removal.

For this strategy to be effective, the leader must have done his or her homework and be a skilled interviewer. The leader must be able to draw out people's thoughts and opinions and listen for negative and positive consequences. When the position and its consequences are clear, the leader points out how the positive consequences reinforce the change effort and then works to eliminate the negative consequences.

People may identify real negative consequences, or they may be saying things to try to prevent the change from occurring. In the event that something is said that is not a negative consequence, it is important for the leader to point this out. As O'Keefe (1999) states, it is best to meet the opposing arguments head on by refuting them.

Try it—*"Foot-in-the-Door Technique"*

Persuasion researchers have studied this technique for many years. Many of us have had some experience with this when a salesperson has asked us to comply with a small request (e.g., answering a couple of questions.), which leads to larger requests that we may be surprised to find ourselves agreeing to (e.g., buying something that we did not want). The term is derived from the days of door-to-door salespeople. The first request was to be allowed into the home so that the sales pitch could begin. Thus the name "foot-in-the-door."

Foot-in-the-door is used by asking for something small and when the person agrees to that request, one builds on that commitment to gain compliance with a larger and related request (Cialdini & Guadango, 2004; O'Keefe, 2002; Burger, 1999). In the context of the social administrator, she or he may ask staff to use a new intervention technique on just one or two consumers in the next week to see how it works. Or a funding body might be encouraged to fund a new program for just a few people or in just one or two areas of the community. In either case, the intent is to follow this up with expansion of the requested behavior or program.

Research has shown that there are several factors that explain the working of this technique (Cialdini & Guadango, 2004). The reason that this technique is in this section regarding influencing of attitudes is that one of these factors is self-perception. That is, when a person sees himself or herself as the type of person who engages in actions such as the initial request, he or she is then more likely to agree with the next request because of this self-perception. This self-perception was formed or changed when the person agreed to the initial request and found him or herself engaging in the behavior.

However, other factors also either enhance or reduce the effect of this strategy. When people comply with the initial request because the person making the request has done them a favor, then compliance with the second request is less likely to occur. For example, if a salesperson gives you a piece of candy and then asks you to answer a couple of questions, you may comply with this request but go no further because you have returned the favor.

Individual differences are important. If a person has a high need to be consistent in his or her behavior, he or she is more likely to comply with the second request. However, if this need does not exist, agreeing to the next request is less likely. Similarly, if the person sees compliance as attributing to an internal source, such as "this is the type of person that I am," he or she is more likely to agree to the follow-up request. However, if the person thinks that he or she complied for an external reason (e.g., the boss made me do it), then he or she is less likely to agree to the next request.

Finally, the more the person complying with the initial request was involved in it, the more likely he or she is to agree to the next request. In other words, if it is the worker who suggests trying the new intervention with a couple of consumers during the next week, he or she is more likely to view the effort positively (unless the effort goes terribly wrong) and agree to expansion of the effort. As can be seen, this strategy is complex. As a social administrator it is not possible to accurately predict when any strategy will work. This is precisely the reason why every administrator needs to be proficient in several different strategies and attempt to affect all of the elements of this change model.

STRATEGIES TO CHANGE
THE NORMATIVE COMPONENT

Desired behavior is preceded by the intention to act and this is influenced by perceived behavioral control, the person's attitude toward the behavior, and the norms that exist regarding the behavior. There is considerable controversy in the social psychology literature regarding the relative importance of attitudes or norms to influencing behavior (Terry & Hogg, 2000). However, most scholars agree that norms play a role in the influence process. Trafimow (2000) found that some people's behaviors are more controlled by attitudes and some are more controlled by norms. He found that individual differences and cultural background were important in distinguishing people whose behavior seemed to be more linked to attitude from those whose behavior seemed more linked to norms.

The study conducted by Glisson and Hemmelgarn (1998) in agencies working with troubled children demonstrated that the office climate was positively associated with the important consumer outcome of improvement in child behaviors. Norms in the workplace and community are a powerful influence on behavior in terms of encouraging or discouraging certain actions (Mackie & Queller, 2000; Terry, Hogg, & White, 2000). Norms are the informal rules in the workplace. For example, the understanding that consumers should be treated respectfully might be a norm. When this is highly valued in the workplace, staff will struggle to determine its behavioral meaning in a variety of circumstances and are more likely to act accordingly.

The social administrator consistently works to assure that the norms of the work group are consumer-centered. Consequently, the existing norms in the workplace are already likely to support whatever consumer-focused changes the manager is implementing. The research on influence suggests that persuasive messages are more effective when they engage in what people want rather than what they do not want, and people vary greatly in what they want (O'Keefe, 2002). Within the social work agency we are more likely to share values about consumers that may result in the normative component being more effective. However, when social administrators are engaged in the larger community, this is an important point to keep in mind. Community norms may not be as supportive of consumers and the social administrator may need to be more consciously aware of the normative component of influence. O'Keefe (2002) suggests the following as strategies to affect the normative component of influence.

1. Link message to a new important person.
2. Increase the importance of an existing key actor.
3. Change the belief attributed to a current key actor—either positive or negative.

Link Message to a New Important Person

Linking a message to an important person is in many ways a straightforward strategy. The reason for emphasizing a new person is that it is assumed that those who are already important are exerting their influence on the group norms. The strategy is for the social administrator to identify someone the audience sees as an important person who has not expressed support for the change and demonstrate that person's support to the audience to be influenced. Another part of this strategy that needs to be emphasized is "important." The new person must be important to the individual or group to be influenced. The person may be important to you but if he or she is not important to the individual to be influenced, the strategy will not work.

Although this strategy emphasized the role of a new person, it is also useful to remind people of compatible values of existing important people. Maybe there is a person who is important to those to be influenced who shares a value about a change, and who is not in the immediate environment exerting influence. In this case, the social administrator reminds people that this important person shares the norm that supports the change.

For example, Fred is advocating for his board of directors to approve the development of a new evidence-based program. The development of this program will result in the reduction in size or elimination of a very popular program that Fred has had concerns about since he came to the agency. The program has not produced the desired consumer outcomes and has consumed a large amount of resources, yet remains very popular in the community. Fred is using many of the strategies of the change model and is currently thinking about the normative component. Fred realizes that in terms of community norms he is not a very important person to most of his board members, so for each he makes a list of people he thinks are important to them. This list is derived from comments he has heard at board meetings, conversations he has had with board members, and what he has read in the local newspaper. This produces a list of existing important people who may be enlisted to support the new program. Fred also uses his knowledge of the board members and the community to list people who may fit the description of "new" important people. Among these individuals is a judge who has demonstrated a real concern for agency consumers because they frequently appear in his courtroom. Fred thinks that the judge's legal training makes her open to objectively evaluating the evidence for and against the existing and the proposed programs. Fred makes an appointment with the judge to make his case for trying the new program. If he is successful with the judge, he will then use the judge's support to shape the board's norms for the new program. Since he has been consistently working with the board to emphasize outcomes for consumer- and evidence-based practices, he thinks that he has a reasonable chance to be successful. This example illustrates the use of this strategy in an abbreviated form. It does not include all of what Fred would do to influence the board of directors but it does illustrate the basics of this strategy.

Increase the Importance of an Existing Key Actor

The three strategies identified in this section all involve the influence of a person important to those to be influenced. What is different in this strategy is changing the importance of someone who is already an important person.

If Fred is successful with the judge, it is unlikely that it would be necessary or possible to change the importance of the judge to the board. However, Fred's efforts to have the board make decisions based upon outcomes for consumers has resulted in garnering support from one board member who is fairly popular with the other board members. Since the time of year for election of officers is coming soon, Fred approaches the nominating committee as well as the selected board member about becoming board president. Although this does not really change this person's values or opinions or even power, it does change this person's importance to the rest of the board members. This example may seem contrived or trivial because Fred would want a person with compatible values as board president anyway. This is certainly true and illustrates how a social administrator works on a day-to-day basis to create the norms that support a consumer-focused agency. The research on influence simply supports these efforts and helps describe how they work.

Change the Belief (Positively or Negatively) Attributed to a Current Key Actor

This strategy may have been implied by the strategy of linking the support of the change effort to a new important person. In fact it is very similar. To enlist the influence of a new important person, the social administrator needs to determine this person's position and, if necessary, influence it for or against the change effort. In other words this key actor becomes a person to be influenced using all of the strategies available to the social administrator. This strategy uses the words attributed to the important person. This raises the possibility of not influencing the key actor but only what others attribute to this person. In our opinion this would be deceptive. In this text, we choose to use only positive growth-enhancing strategies and not deception. Enhancing organizational performance, consumer centeredness, and consumer outcomes comprises an attractive ideology and set of values that can be difficult, but far from impossible, to disagree with.

STRATEGIES TO HELP MOVE
FROM INTENTION TO BEHAVIOR

The link between intention to act and acting is not automatic. We all know people who say that they will do something and do not follow through. According to O'Keefe (2002) the link between intention and action can be enhanced by the following three strategies.

1. Enhance perceived relevance of behavior.
2. Encourage anticipation of feelings.
3. Induce feelings of hypocrisy.

Enhance Perceived Relevance of Behavior

In some ways, this is simply reminding the person of his or her intention to act and giving him or her a reason to follow through. With outcomes for consumers being the main reason why we are engaging in such efforts, it is easy to remind the person of the positive impact of the behavior on consumers. In the example of seeking to influence staff to practice a new evidenced-based practice, once all of the obstacles have been removed and attitudes and norms have been established valuing the new practice, staff may only need to be reminded that the relevance of this behavior is enhanced outcomes for consumers.

Encourage Anticipation of Feelings

Helping the person anticipate the good feelings associated with exhibiting the behavior is about the satisfaction arising from feeling of competence in being able to exhibit a new behavior, the satisfaction of "fitting in" with the unit by conforming to group norms, and the satisfaction of the consistency of one's attitudes and behaviors (McConnell et al., 2000; Hetts, Boninger, Armor, Gleichen, & Nathanson, 2000). In the social administration context, all this revolves around outcomes for consumers. Implementation of this strategy in the example of influencing workers to use an evidence-based practice may be as simple as asking them to think about how they will feel when they exhibit the behavior and achieve a positive result with a consumer.

Induce Feelings of Hypocrisy

This strategy comes from cognitive dissonance theory that says that when a person is aware of an inconsistency between attitudes and behavior, he or she is uncomfortable and seeks to resolve this feeling (dissonance) (Cooper & Stone, 2000). Resolution of dissonance feelings does not necessarily result in changes in behavior. Dissonance can be resolved in a variety of ways that cannot always be predicted. For example, dissonance can be resolved by changing attitudes. As with all aspects of influence theory, the effects are complex and many variables are important. However, O'Keefe (2002) suggests that there are two ways to work with cognitive dissonance to encourage movement from behavioral intention to behavior. One is to emphasize the importance of the attitude toward the behavior. The previous strategies for enhancing the attitude toward the behavior are useful here. This reinforcement of the importance of the attitude may be sufficient to move the person to resolve the dissonance through action.

Another way to induce feelings of hypocrisy or cognitive dissonance is to remind the person of previous support and remind the person of past failures to act (O'Keefe, 2002; Stone, Wiegand, Cooper, & Aronson, 1997). For example, a supervisor may accompany a worker to a session with a consumer to view the service transaction. During the session, the worker does not implement the new approach that has been the focus of research, discussion, and training. When the supervisor talks with the worker about the session, she or he gently reminds the worker of her or his previous statements in support of the new practice and points out that this did not occur in the session with the consumer. However, there is a danger of this being perceived by the worker as heavy-handed or a high-pressure tactic that may backfire by generating resistance. O'Keefe (2002) suggests that when using this strategy it is important to offer only enough incentive to induce compliance and let the dissonance reduction processes encourage subsequent attitude change. Once again this emphasizes the importance of knowing the person you are trying to influence so that the approach is tailored to the person.

SUMMARY

We have used the Theory of Behavioral Intention as a framework for assisting social administrators in producing change. This theory has strong empirical support and involves enhancing perceived behavioral control, attitudes toward the behavior, and norms that support the behavior. In this theory it is these factors that help explain a person's intention to act. This intention is then targeted to help move a person to action.

Change efforts begin by the social administrator identifying the behavior that will enhance program performance and the person who needs to perform this behavior. The social administrator then uses the components of the Theory of Behavioral Intention to help the person exhibit the desired behavior. One of the benefits of this approach to change is that fourteen to eighteen different strategies become available (Exhibit 2.1). The number of strategies may seem a bit overwhelming but many of them are already part of a social worker's training and experience.

EXHIBIT 2.1. Summary of Change Strategies

Strategies to enhance perceived behavioral control:

1. Obstacle removal
   a. Task groups
   b. Forms and paperwork
   c. Education and training
2. Modeling
3. Behavioral rehearsal
4. Provide verbal encouragement
5. Provide information

Strategies to change an attitude toward a behavior:

1. Add a new reason to think positively about the behavior
2. Increase or decrease the importance of an existing belief about the behavior.
   a. Emphasize advantages and rewards
   b. Cite proven results/weight of the evidence
   c. Specify the consequences of a stance
3. Try it—"foot in the door technique"

Strategies to affect the normative component:

1. Link message to a new important person
2. Increase the importance of an existing key actor
3. Change the belief attributed to a current key actor—either positive or negative.

Strategies to enhance the link between intention and behavior:

1. Enhance perceived relevance of behavior.
2. Encourage anticipation of feelings.
3. Induce feelings of hypocrisy.

This approach to organizational change is useful for helping workers acquire new or improved skills in their work with consumers. It is also useful at other levels of the organization. One of the major challenges for program managers is influencing change of others in the organization. Sometimes these are people at the same organizational level and sometimes they are people in administrative levels to which the program manager reports. The approach to change presented here is effective in all of these situations. This approach is also useful for fostering change in the community where the program operates. Our intention is for social administrators to learn and practice these skills with any change that the manager has reason to believe will enhance performance. In each chapter we provide examples of how these strategies can be used with a variety of audiences.

Chapter 3

An Analytic Framework
for Social Program Management

A social program is the aggregate of actions of people directed toward accomplishing a single consumer outcome goal. It is through the social program that people are helped. Workers find satisfying and fulfilling work by achieving results with consumers through their role as specified by the social program. It is by managing within the framework of the social program that social administrators achieve results with consumers. Finally, social programs manifest society's desire to assist some of its members.

This chapter starts the development of an analytic program framework that provides managers with the information they need to administer effective programs and implement the principles of consumer-centered social administration. The framework will be developed in the next three chapters. In addition, each chapter concludes with a section on how the program components can be used on a daily basis to manage consumer outcomes and how the change skills (Chapter 2) can be used to influence people to enhance results.

Program Framework Learning Objectives—Part 1

- *Identify the ways that the program framework assists a manager to implement consumer-centered management principles.*
- *Identify research-based links between management behavior and organizational characteristics that affect consumer outcomes.*
- *Describe how to blend social problem analysis with social work values for a social problem.*
- *Describe the importance of obtaining information about consumers, social problems, and effective interventions to elements of the program framework.*

Textbook of Social Administration: The Consumer-Centered Approach
© 2007 by The Haworth Press, Inc. All rights reserved.
doi:10.1300/5802_04

- *Identify the importance of developing interventions at multiple levels.*
- *Write a social problem analysis.*
- *Identify the direct beneficiaries of a social program.*
- *Identify the way to use the problem and population analysis in management as it relates to acquiring and using information, acquiring and directing staff, acquiring and using resources other than staff, and facilitating change by using persuasion.*

PRINCIPLES OF CONSUMER-CENTERED MANAGEMENT AND SOCIAL PROGRAM SPECIFICATIONS

Careful consideration of each of the multiple aspects of the social program is one of the ways that social administrators apply the client-centered principle of *venerating the people called clients/consumers.* Workers and consumers engaged in activities that produce the desired outcome are influenced by other factors including key individuals in the community, the method of helping, and the energy and focus brought to the transaction by the worker. The consumer-centered administrator takes the responsibility to create the conditions that maximize the probability that this transaction will have the intended benefit.

What the social worker does when engaging with consumers makes a difference. Social workers come to this helping transaction with values, knowledge, and skills acquired through social work education and experience. Their behavior is also influenced by other factors including community values, social policy, and agency climate. These factors can draw the workers' time and attention away from consumers. It is through attention to critical program elements that the social administrator *creates and maintains the focus.* Reminding workers of critical consumer outcomes that lead to achieving desired results, enlisting key individuals to play a role in assisting consumers achieve, and creating an environment that maintains everyone's attention on consumer results are just three ways by which administrators use the program framework to create and maintain the focus.

Social administrators demonstrate *a healthy disrespect for the impossible* when they tirelessly alter program components to increase the positive impact on consumers. Although a document that includes specifications for all of the program components appears to be a finished document, the consumer-centered manager knows that the specifications are not adequate in that the program will not be successful with every consumer. Within the boundaries of program specifications consumer-centered managers remain flexible and inventive in the pursuit of improved consumer results.

The fact that no program no matter how well specified is 100 percent successful keeps consumer-centered managers *learning for a living.* New research may suggest altering the nature of the worker/consumer transaction; new policy initiatives at the local, state, or national level may require altering program objectives or change the mix of key community individuals needed to produce consumer benefits. New consumer challenges require rethinking program goals and objectives. These are just a few examples of the continual learning required to keep a social program responding effectively to a changing environment.

The use of program specifications requires repeated interactions with people over time. In the case of program specifications, the change skills (Chapter 2) are employed in consistent interactions with workers, key community individuals needed to achieve consumer goals, and policymakers at all levels, in order to help align behaviors with program specifications and to increase the impact on consumer outcomes. These are just a few examples of ways that managers use the program framework to produce benefits to consumers.

RESEARCH THAT SUPPORTS THE SOCIAL PROGRAM ANALYTIC FRAMEWORK

It is the social program analytic framework that identifies the elements that social administrators use to intervene so that the consumer/worker interaction is as effective as possible. This position is beginning to be supported by research. Only recently has the relationship between program, agency, and administrative characteristics been linked to outcomes for consumers. This research base is not strong because the relationship between program elements and consumers' outcomes has not been the focus of much study. Chapter 1 reviewed this research in detail. Program elements have been found to make a difference by Littell and Tajima (2000) who found that a child welfare program's characteristics accounted for a small but statistically significant amount of variance in consumer outcomes. Sosin (1986) found that when supervisors reminded workers that child welfare case reviews were needed, fewer children were in care for long periods. Harkness and Hensley (1991) found that when supervisors asked mental health counselors questions about client outcomes and interventions related to outcomes, adult outpatients reported greater satisfaction with counseling. In a related study, Harkness (1997) found that this type of supervision was positively associated with client's goal attainment. These are just some of the findings that support the idea that the program characteristics and behavior of the manager make a difference to consumers.

As the research is beginning to demonstrate that program characteristics make a positive difference for consumers, most of us also have seen examples of poorly designed programs. Some of the research is demonstrating that some program elements can even have a negative impact on consumers. For example, Barnoski and Aos (2004) found that when a program called Functional Family Therapy was implemented as intended with juvenile offenders, there was a 38 percent reduction in felony recidivism. However, when the program was not implemented as intended, there was a 17 percent increase in this outcome. This clearly argues for a more thoughtfully designed and managed program. Following are a few bad examples that we have seen.

- Workers and consumers are not clear as to what is expected of them.
- Other agencies, professionals, consumers, and the public are not clear as to the purpose of the program, thereby leading to conflicts and lack of support.
- Funding sources do not know what it takes to do the job, thereby producing unrealistic expectations.
- Workers are asked to do too much with too little.
- Meetings and paperwork proliferate because of a lack of clear expectations.
- Crisis orientation or other modes in which much energy is expended are implemented, but there is no improvement of performance.
- The latest "hot idea" is selected for program interventions, thereby avoiding a careful exploration of potentially more powerful alternatives.
- Child welfare workers are asked to manage a caseload of thirty-five children in foster care, make frequent contact with each child and parent, as well as make certain that children regularly visit their parents, regularly report to the court, and so on.
- Mental health case managers indiscriminately use community services, such as arranging individual psychotherapy or day hospital attendance, for virtually all cases.
- Child welfare workers arrange counseling and homemaker services regardless of case specifics.

Still another problem is the dearth of resources for the most troublesome cases. In part, some agencies cream off the most desirable and easiest consumers. These agencies seek to increase the number of consumer referrals by keeping the eligibility criteria vague and widening the resources for referrals. This allows them to take the best available consumers. Consumers deemed inappropriate are left with few options.

Another problem related to programs is the lack of supportive behavior by external constituencies such as the court systems or hospitals. For community mental health programs to be successful, a variety of key players must consistently perform in certain ways. Maintaining people with psychiatric disabilities in the community is virtually impossible with a judge who refuses to consider community alternatives for treatment of commitment cases. Similarly, in child welfare, permanency for children cannot be accomplished with a juvenile court judge who refuses to return children to their homes or who will not terminate parental rights.

All of these problems have negative consequences, including the lack of job satisfaction of so many employees. Staff are asked daily to intervene in the most difficult and complex human situations with too few supports and resources, and sometimes with too little guidance. Few mechanisms are in place to systematically show them the results of their efforts or to celebrate their successes.

The following case highlights the consequences of incorrect program design. The program seemed to be operating well. In fact, the program devoted virtually all of its efforts and resources to teaching skills that the consumers already knew how to do. The program needed outreach, case management, and in vivo support but had no such capacity. The design flaws could be the wrong target population, or the wrong sets of service technologies.

The Northeast Mental Health and Guidance Center operates a day treatment program for about thirty people with psychiatric disabilities. The program operates from nine to five, five days a week, and includes activities focused on recreation and socialization, health, daily living skills, prevocational skills, arts and crafts, stress management, meal planning, cooking, music, and interpersonal relations. Counseling services and a medication clinic are a part of the program. The staff is also concerned with the degree to which consumers are satisfied with the program and how well the clients are doing when not at the center. The staff is warm, caring, and works diligently. The only data collected is on rehospitalization and symptomatology. Program staff were asked to evaluate the vocational and daily living skills of a sample of consumers in terms of whether they had the ability to use the skills and to what degree they used the skills when in the community. Each consumer was assessed as being able to perform at least 90 percent of the fifty-two skills included in the inventory. However, fewer than half of the consumers performed these same skills in the community although the skills were in their repertoire.

Most of the aforementioned program flaws can be attenuated, if not solved, by thoughtful consideration of specific program elements. A carefully designed and managed program offers the promise of improving outcomes for consumers, increasing efficiency, producing higher levels of job satisfaction, reducing conflict, and eliciting more support from constituencies. Program design is one set of management strategies that can improve the performance of the organization.

WHAT YOU NEED TO KNOW
TO BEGIN PROGRAM ANALYSIS

Program management is similar to continuous quality improvement in that it is a process in constant revision. Program elements are revised as you learn more about the consumers, their successes and their problems as well as your intervention. As some elements are revised, it is necessary to reconsider others. Although the presentation of the program elements in this text is necessarily linear, the social administrator must keep the nonlinear and iterative nature of this work in mind.

The design framework requires managers to consider and reconsider all of the design elements relative to the final result. In program design, the final result is the achievement of consumer outcome goals. Analysis, decision, and evaluation are all anchored in the outcomes one seeks to achieve with consumers. This is in contrast to a common design approach that starts with an "attractive intervention idea" and then builds the other necessary elements around it, including goals, objectives, and target populations.

There are three additional overarching considerations that managers attend to while working through the program elements. These are (1) the blending of social programs with social work values, (2) the continuous need for information, and (3) the use of multiple levels of intervention.

Overarching Considerations When Managing Programs

- *Blending social problem analysis with social work values*
- *Obtaining the needed information on*
  - *consumers;*
  - *problems; and*
  - *effective interventions.*
- *Intervening at multiple levels*

Blending Social Problem Analysis and Social Work Values

Social work theories come from social problem analysis. The problem analysis necessarily includes the harmful factors that contribute to the social problem. The analysis usually includes a host of individual and environmental toxins. Unfortunately this can lead to simplistic and victim-blaming conclusions.

- The substance-abusing mother is told to stop using drugs if she wants her children returned home.
- The youth is leaving foster care because she has reached the age of majority. She has limited life skills but is told she needs classes in budgeting.
- The person with a psychiatric disability needs daily living skills training or psychotherapy.
- The unemployed welfare mother needs vocational training.

In our society, which places such a high value on self reliance, many people jump from the presenting problem to these simplistic solutions. It is relatively easy to gather support and sanction for these kinds of interventions. Although dated, this statement by Fairweather (1972) is still relevant, "Thus it appears to be axiomatic that an intervention is acceptable to a society in direct proportion to the degree that the innovation does not require a change in the roles or social organization of that society" (p. 7).

Others choose to blame the environment. Poverty, lack of intellectual stimuli, hostile community attitudes, depressed local economies, poor housing, and lack of recreational and socialization opportunities have been thought to be the cause of social problems. The "blaming-the-environments" ideology is derived from a similar thought process. This ideology looks for differences in the environmental circumstances of two groups or two individuals and identifies the differences as the cause of a problem.

These blaming perspectives are both right and wrong at the same time. By the time a person reaches a human service agency both sets of factors have contributed to the consumer's situation. Cause becomes less relevant than what is going on now and what is to be done to work with the person to obtain the desired results.

Community integration is also a highly regarded social work value. Many programs are based on principles such as promoting the most normal and family-like environment, maintaining vulnerable populations in their own home, or returning them to their community. Clearly the design of the day treatment program mentioned earlier did not recognize the underlying value of community integration prior to selecting the response.

A thorough critical analysis of the social problem is critical to the management of an effective program. The values recognized by the social administrator prior to the design phase do make a difference. When recognized and addressed, values help frame the problem and the solutions that arise become coherent and consistent with the problem.

Information Needs

The information needed to specify the elements of an effective social program is considerable. This includes information and data on the social problem, description and extent of people confronting the social problem, and the past performance of alternative interventions. Sources of information range from census data and government statistical publications to the professional literature and the collective practice wisdom of agency personnel.

The qualitative research on consumers' experiences with the social problem is particularly useful for gaining insights on how people experience problems from being homeless to living with a major mental illness to maintaining sobriety. Some of these insights are in the popular literature; rather than being research based they powerfully communicate experiences of consumers . Still another method for gaining consumers' insights is to involve them in the program in a variety of ways. For example, focus groups of consumers can be a powerful method for gaining insight into what should be included in the various program elements.

The selection of an intervention is particularly demanding in terms of information. The designer confronts four obstacles. First, social work helping theories need to be based on the latest available knowledge, but the research is not always adequate. Sometimes it is a lack of relevant research. Sometimes it is that the research reports contain little information on the intervention being evaluated; that makes replication impossible. Sometimes the research is based on pilot programs that have had considerably more resources than your organization will have access to.

Second, there is a tendency to select an intervention on the basis of popular trends or ideas, or the reputation of a particular program, rather than on evidence of its efficacy. Case examples about successful consumers are frequently taken as evidence of the success of a program. A program may have a positive reputation based on the charisma or forcefulness of an administrator. Interventions may become popular because of an article in a professional journal, which, although reporting positive results, has used a flawed evaluation methodology. This predilection is unsound. Popularity is a poor surrogate for evidence of effectiveness.

Third, there is a natural inclination to apply current agency methods to new problems or new target groups. For example, in many places skills training remains a principal intervention for people with psychiatric disabilities seeking a richer community life. It may be packaged as case management, day treatment, or even as a vocational program, but the basic intervention is the same with rather disappointing results.

However, the central constraint confronting the manager is access to what is known. Few managers have the time to be familiar with the most recent research. Fortunately, there is an increasing number of articles that review evidence-based practices (Thomlison, 2003; Mueser et al., 2002). There are also organizations that prepare research summaries on intervention effectiveness. The Cochrane Collaboration and the Campbell Collaboration are two sources for this type of information. One of the values of these collaborations is that their reviews examine the research evidence for a program and report the results, whether they are positive or negative. For example, the Cochrane review of Scared Straight finds that this program has harmful results. This is critically important information. These reviews, although not as timely as most managers would like, are easily checked for evidence of the efficacy of existing popular program ideas.

The Cochrane Collaboration is an international organization that coordinates the efforts of health care professionals and researchers around the world to prepare, maintain, and disseminate systematic reviews of health care research. Although heavily oriented toward interventions in physical health, they produce reviews of interest to social work. Some examples of their reviews of interest to social workers are as follows:

- "Scared Straight" and other juvenile awareness programs for preventing juvenile delinquency
- Parent-training programs for improving maternal psychosocial health
- Interventions for learning disabled sex offenders
- Home-based social support for socially disadvantaged mothers
- Family and parenting interventions in children and adolescents with conduct disorder and delinquency aged ten to seventeen
- Vocational rehabilitation for people with severe mental illness

The International Campbell Collaboration is a nonprofit organization that aims to help people make well-informed decisions about the effects of interventions in the social, behavioral, and educational arenas (www.campbellcollaboration.org). The Campbell Collaboration is a more recent endeavor and consequently most of the following examples of review titles downloaded in January 2004 were not completed. Regularly visiting their Web site will be useful for staying updated on the latest results.

- *Systematic review of the impact of welfare reform on family structure*
- *Cognitive-behavioral interventions for sexually abused children*
- *Effectiveness of the Families and Schools Together (FAST) program*
- *Individual and group based parenting for improving psychosocial outcomes for teenage parents and their children*
- *Cognitive-behavioral training interventions designed to assist foster carers in the management of difficult behavior*
- *Home based support for socially disadvantaged mothers*
- *Supported housing for the seriously mentally ill*
- *Family and parenting interventions in children and adolescents with conduct disorder and delinquency aged 10 to 17*
- *Group based parent-training programme for improving emotional and behavioral adjustment in 0 to 3-year-old children*

Levels of Intervention

An ecological perspective suggests that consumers achieve results through interventions directed at a variety of levels: individual, group, family, organizational, institutional, community, and societal (Bronfenbrenner, 1995b). The relationships within and between levels can comprise a given social work theory at any moment in time. A sample of interventions organized by level for three human service fields is shown in Table 3.1. It should be noted that an intervention directed at any single level can have impact on other levels that are not the direct targets of intervention.

At each level, several strategies will be available. Unfortunately, many of our past efforts have been narrowly focused on the level of the individual and usually have involved only one strategy. The complexity of the problems we face usually demands multiple-level interventions in order to have a reasonable chance of success. For example, a program that wants to achieve and maintain employment for consumers with psychiatric disabilities must have job development with employers, job coaches, integrated teams with vocational rehabilitation, and mental health providers; must work with the consumer to identify desirable directions for job search and confidence-building activities; and must have the provision of follow-along supports (Becker & Drake, 2003). In fact, employment will probably not be maintained unless there are socialization and housing resources associated with the program. As a general rule, interventions focused on multiple levels are more likely to produce benefits with consumers and achieve program goals.

TABLE 3.1. Sample Interventions

Level of Intervention	Community Mental Health	Child Welfare	Elderly
Individual	Case Management Psychotherapy Pharmacological treatment One-to-one volunteer match with consumer Individual vocational Rehabilitation	Counseling for child Counseling for mother/father Individual parent Education Parent education Material Parent advocate/ child advocate	Case management Consumer education Advocacy
Family	Family therapy Family support group Respite care Psychoeducational workshops	Family therapy Family contracting Homemaker services Home visitors	Caregiver support programs Family problem-solving meetings Consumer education
Group	Group therapy Medication monitoring groups Support groups Skills development groups	Substance abuse treatment group Parent education classes Batterer groups Parent support groups Sexual abuse victim groups	Caregivers support Adult day care Community advocacy Silver-haired legislature
Community/ neighborhood	Drop-in center Mobile crisis unit Emergency shelter	Child care exchanges Juvenile court case review systems Parent center	Mutual help neighborhood organizations Older citizens centers
Institutional	Change criteria for Hospitalization Change criteria for Discharge	Change child placement criteria Institute school-based life skills programs	Reform guardianship rules or program Create ombudsman within program
	Change criteria for involuntary hospitalization Make the consumer the director of the service Create consumer ombudsman	Change definition of which children can become state wards	Consumer protection legislation
Societal	Increase funding for community support services	Increase post-care funding for children aging out of care Universal provision of parenting education	Improved division of assets legislation Improved elder abuse legislation

Principles for Intervention Selection

- *The social work perspective (bioecological) is a useful way of viewing a social problem and stimulating interventions.*
- *Care must be exercised in avoiding blaming interventions.*
- *Consideration of individual and environmental strengths should be included.*
- *Interventions need to blend consumer and societal desires.*
- *Multiple-level interventions are more promising.*

THE ELEMENTS OF THE PROGRAM FRAMEWORK

The program framework has its roots in the work of Taber and Finnegan (1980). We have modified it based upon our experiences over the last twenty years. It is our position that when social administrators use the framework elements to think critically about a program and to support the worker/consumer transaction, a program will have increased chances of success in producing the desired outcomes for consumers. The program framework includes the following components:

- Analyze the social problem.
- Determine who the direct beneficiary of the program is to be.
- Determine the social work theory of helping.
- Identify the key persons required to produce benefits to consumers.
- Specify the helping environment.
- Describe actual helping behaviors.
- Identify emotions and responses.

In this and the next chapter, we describe each of these components and provide specific guidelines for making decisions about each program element. Since textbooks are by nature linear, we present the components in the order given in the aforementioned list. However, we emphasize that in real life the use of this framework is nonlinear and iterative. Taken together, however, what follows is a specific analytic framework for the management of social programs.

PROGRAM ELEMENT:
SOCIAL PROBLEM ANALYSIS

The first step in program design is an analysis of the social problem that the program will address. The social problem analysis is the basis for establishing the program goal. Inadequate understanding of the social problem and inappropriate goal setting are major flaws in our social programs and act as a wedge between consumers and managers, and consumers and the organization.

There are several common problems with program goals.

1. They are usually vague (e.g., stimulating social interaction, improving the quality of life).
2. They are overly ambitious (e.g., prevent domestic violence, eliminate poverty).
3. They describe the helping process rather than the consumer outcome that should be produced (e.g., to provide services, to develop a program, to teach).

One of our favorite goal statements exemplifies all of these problems: "Develop and establish a system for identifying and referring technical and professional resources to coordinate and enhance staff expertise of organizations, assisting persons to make informed career decisions, develop new careers, or successfully achieve mid-life career changes." What does this mean?

Inadequate goal setting makes it difficult, if not impossible, to manage a program and keep it on course. Inadequate goal setting opens us up to criticism and attack for being ineffective, self-serving, and wasteful. Inadequate goal setting frustrates employees who do not see their efforts pay off. This leads to the "activity trap." Work expands to fill the time available for its completion. In short, we cannot get where we want to go if we do not know where we want to go. To gain acceptance and yield the desired outcomes, a program must come from an analysis of the particular social problem.

If as a program manager I know that our goal is for a child in foster care to achieve a safe permanent home as quickly as possible, either by returning home, being adopted, or having someone assume guardianship of the child, then my job is much easier. I can keep program staff on target by reminding them that this goal is our primary purpose, not necessarily satisfying the juvenile judge. I have an improved chance of obtaining community support by reminding people that this is what we do. I have a better chance of influencing the juvenile judge by reminding him or her that this is what we are all trying to achieve.

Defining the Problem

A social problem exists when a cultural group or some segment of society identifies a deviation from a social standard that is believed necessary for the maintenance of cultural life. When society recognizes a problem, it seeks redress through a social policy and programs. The importance or severity of the social problem is based on the degree of perceived threat to the integrity of cultural life and the size or status of those people who are labeling it as a social problem. Human service managers do not create social problems. However, they play an important role in helping society recognize a problem. They are also critical in forming the program response once society or the community has identified a social problem.

Since human service programs are solutions or part of a solution to an identified social problem, it is important to think through a careful yet pragmatic analysis of the social problem. As Taber and Finnegan (1980) stated in their original description of the framework: "A clear description of the problem for society and for individuals lays the groundwork for establishing goals and justifying the need for the problem's amelioration" (p. 6). Incomplete problem analysis inevitably leads to vague or overly ambitious goals, misguided intervention strategies, and imprecise targeting of services.

Yet even the best analysis is likely to be incomplet,e requiring a manager to continually learn and modify the program accordingly. One example was the creation of a new substance abuse treatment program for substance-abusing mothers with children in state custody. A high incidence of substance abuse among mothers was recognized as a barrier to reunifying children with their families in a timely manner. Prior failed treatment approaches were examined and it was found that although these mothers were being referred for treatment, they were not receiving these services because they did not consistently show up. At the same time, the agency had the results of a study that suggested that many substance-abusing mothers eventually did have their children reunified. It just took longer for this reunification to occur than for non-substance-abusing mothers with children in state custody. Review of the treatment literature and consultation with substance abuse treatment professionals resulted in the recommendation that each mother who was assessed as having a substance abuse problem at the time of juvenile court adjudication of her case be assigned a recovery coach who would accompany her to the treatment program, have frequent and consistent contact with her, and help remove barriers to participation in treatment. The ideal recovery coach was a woman who had a history of substance abuse and was in recovery for several years. After two years of piloting this program it was found that it did not have the desired result of increasing family reunification. A sample of cases was examined more closely to try to determine why this program had failed. In this review it was found that the mothers who became the consumers of this program had many more years of substance abuse history than the "usual" substance-abusing mother and in many cases termination of parental rights was being pursued.

In this example, a great deal of time and attention went into the analysis of the social problem. Yet due to a lack of information about some features of the problem, inappropriate conclusions were reached. Incomplete information and unintended consequences are part of the program management process. The social administrator in this situation was wise to use consumer outcome information to test the social problem analysis. Social problems confronted by social programs are exceedingly complex and many times it is only through examining the success or failure of outcomes for consumers that we learn about the adequacy or inadequacy of our problem analysis.

In Chapter 1, we introduced the notion that human service managers are responsible for blending the agendas of a variety of groups, such as consumers and the larger society. Social problem analysis provides one opportunity for doing this because such an analysis requires the dual obligation to individuals (e.g., consumers, their families) and to the larger society. Each program must be justified along both dimensions for the program to have a reasonable chance for adequate support (e.g., funding and community goodwill) and success.

In the example of substance-abusing mothers, the administrator was attempting to respond to society's interest in achieving permanency for children in a timely manner as dictated by the Adoption and Safe Families Act. On the other hand, the administrator felt an obligation to the mother to make extraordinary efforts to help her begin recovery and have her children returned. One of the most difficult child welfare challenges is to balance the needs and interests of parents, children, and society.

Typology for Social Problem Analysis

The complexity of social problems has led to a variety of frameworks for analysis. For the busy human service manager, however, the problem analysis task must be more modest. Minimally, it needs to identify and organize the key factors that will guide the critical decisions involved in the program design. The following typology (Taber & Finnegan, 1980; Taber, 1987) identifies the three elements of a social problem analysis and the relevant dimensions of each.

Typology for Social Problem Analysis

1. A social condition is a problem for society because

    a. it is a resource cost;
    b. it is a threat to the health and safety; and
    c. it is a threat to societal values.

2. A social condition is a problem for individuals because

    a. it is a deprivation of a minimal standard of health and decency;
    b. it is threat of abuse or exploitation; and
    c. it is a barrier to full social participation.

3. Factors contributing to the problem's existence or prevalence

Biological/physical	*Individual*
Behavioral	*Familial*
Social	*Community*
Psychological	*Societal*
Economic	*Historical*
	Political

    This typology presents the major rationale for a social condition to garner sufficient support to become a social problem and, therefore, be worthy of the allocation of societal resources. A social problem framed such that the consequences to society and the individual are vividly demonstrated makes a powerful argument for supporting the resulting program. Identifying the multiple factors that are known or thought to contribute to or maintain the problem helps provide a more realistic view of the complexity of the problem. Since the social program will target some of these contributing factors, it also provides a check against simplistic solutions. Clearly a program that addresses one factor (e.g., individual) will be instantly recognized as being too simplistic.

Alert

Avoid lack of services as a contributing factor. Lack of services does not cause the problem but rather lessens the chance of solving it.

Conducting the Problem Analysis

First, in the center of a large blackboard or piece of paper, write the phrase that captures the problem. Here are some examples:

- Multiple rehospitalizations (recidivism) of people with psychiatric disabilities.
- Children in state custody returning to care within a year of being re-unified with their family.
- Social isolation of older poor people.
- Older youth in foster care not acquiring work experience.

This first step is not trivial. The phrase that goes into the center makes a difference. Different starting points generate different analysis and different programs. There is no formula directing you where to start. We have found that the more specific you can be the more useful the product. For example, sexual abuse of young girls is more useful than child abuse. We have also found that a certain amount of trial and error is useful. Reframe the problem if the initial framing of the problem does not seem to work.

Second, on the top right side of the phrase, list how the situation is a problem for society. Use the three dimensions under this category to help provoke thinking. Society is a broad term that can refer to any grouping or subgrouping of people who experience the problem but who are not the individuals of concern. For example, drug abuse can lead to an increase in crime that affects members of the community in terms of fear, increased expenses for police, and so on.

Third, on the bottom right side of the phrase, list how the situation is a problem for the individual. Refer to the aforementioned typology to help develop this. The individual is almost always the consumer but sometimes may include others such as the consumer's family.

Fourth, on the left side of the phrase, list the factors that contribute to the problem's existence or prevalence. The main sources of such information come from practice experience and the relevant research literature. The goal here is to generate as many factors as possible. It is not unusual to produce lists of ten to twenty-five factors. For clarity, you should group them in some fashion.

Table 3.2 contains a sample problem analysis using the problem of truancy. The example demonstrates how each cluster of contributing factors and consequences is made up of many sub-factors. In fact the reader may

TABLE 3.2. Example Problem Analysis

Contributing Factors	Problem	Consequences

Stressful home situation
  Abuse parent(s)
  Low socioeconomic status
  Unemployment
  Illness in family
  Need to care for young
    children at home
		Societal consequences
		  Loss of educational funds
		  Vandalism and property damage
		  School becomes controller
		    rather than educator
		  Loss of contribution as an adult
		  Court and correctional system
		    costs

Parenting skills
  Low level of education
  Acceptance of abuse
  Lack of supervision
	Truancy	

Child's experience, attitudes,
and beliefs
  Academic failure
  Rebellious attitude
  Low self-confidence
  Drug use
  Peer group influences
  Learning disability
  Physical limitations
    (auditory, visual)
  Boredom
  Social isolation
  Difficulties with law
    enforcement
		Individual consequences
		  Decreased academic functioning
		  Negative label
		  Leads to delinquent acts
		  Drug use
		  Risk of exploitation
		  Negative attitude toward adult
		    responsibilities
		  Learn avoidance
		  Decreased earning capacity

School, community and society
  Racial conflict
  Inconsistent reporting of
    attendance
  Relevance of curriculum
  Transitions between grades
  Suspension policies
  Expulsion policies
  Unconcerned teachers
    and other staff		

know of other clusters of factors and/or sub-factors as well as types of consequences. It is useful to make the problem analysis as complete as possible.

This demonstrates the complexity of our social problems. What at first may seem like a relatively simple problem for a child is actually embedded in a complex set of family, school, and community factors that when considered provides a more realistic view of the problem. This also demonstrates the limits of many of our helping strategies. Many interventions are aimed at one of the sub-factors of a cluster of contributing factors. These are unlikely to have much of an effect. We strive to select evidence-based interventions that have an effect on several contributing factors. At the same time we recognize that even with an intervention strategy that may have a positive effect on several factors, there are serious limits to our ability to "solve" any social problem.

Translation of Table 3.2 into a narrative problem statement becomes a powerful means of communication with a variety of constituents. The description of the problem and its consequences for the individual and society is a vivid portrayal of the problem. The lengthy list of contributing factors clearly communicates the complexity of the problem. The list of consequences not only for the individual but also for society makes a strong case for community support in addressing the problem.

At this point you generally have a good idea of your goal for the program. Write it down in draft form, identifying the consumer group and focus on the benefit(s) that they will accrue. More specific direction and criteria for goal statements will follow. However, for now, the goal statement should take the following form:

The (consumer group) will (achieve or obtain what benefit).

For the example in Table 3.2, the draft goal statement could be: For youth with school attendance problems, the goal is to increase the number of days that they are in school.

PROGRAM ELEMENT: IDENTIFY THE DIRECT BENEFICIARY OF THE PROGRAM

A critical question in designing social programs is "who benefits?" Yet many human service managers abrogate their responsibility and authority by only vaguely answering this question and implying that all people who can be thus described can be served and helped by the program. One can imagine that some of this tendency for vague definitions of who is eligible for services arises from difficulties of precisely defining the population or the desire not to label consumers. After all, who wants to be identified as "poor," "abused," "seriously emotionally disturbed," and so on? However, given that society seems unwilling to provide services to any population in a universal and unconditional manner, vague definitions may actually be more harmful than labels.

The result of imprecise specification of who is eligible for a given service means that critical decisions are made by frontline professionals often in highly idiosyncratic ways. Imprecise definition of the people to be served is also a major source of interagency and agency-public conflict. Creaming and denial of services or benefits becomes more likely. People who are denied service often view the decision as arbitrary and capricious. Referral sources, for example, a juvenile court or hospital, sometimes request service for "inappropriate" consumers—those that the program is not designed to serve. In some agencies these referrals consume a great deal of time to process before a decision "not to accept" is made. This is a waste of precious resources that could be devoted to serving "appropriate" consumers. These problems would be avoidable if clear specifications were formulated.

Another problem caused by inadequate definition of the target population is reduced benefits for consumers. Deciding who will and will not be served must be done thoughtfully and analytically, and with consideration given to consumers' needs, program theory, and critical constituents, such as legislators and governing boards. Identification of who will benefit (and who will not) cannot be an area of wide discretion and arbitrariness. The case study of the Mental Health and Guidance Center cited earlier is a good example. One view of the story is that the program had the correct goals and was employing a strong intervention technology but that it was just serving the wrong clientele. In other words, the day treatment program would be justified and would offer considerable promise for helping if it served only individuals with psychiatric disabilities who did not have vocational and daily living skills in their repertoire.

Another example is a residential treatment program for children that received 296 referrals in a 27-month period and accepted 61 youth or 20 percent of the referrals. The paperwork, the meetings, and the travel costs associated with the 236 children who were not accepted is unconscionable. These valuable resources could have been used to benefit consumers. This has also led some state agencies to include "no reject" provisions in their contracts that require contractors to accept all referrals.

Still another example demonstrates some of the complexity involved in developing precise definitions. In one state, the mental health system will provide services to seriously emotionally disturbed (SED) child and youth. However, the definition of a seriously emotionally disturbed child is vague and only the mental system is sanctioned to make that determination. This has led some child advocates and parents to charge that a mental health provider will only identify a child as seriously mentally disturbed if they have the resources to provide services to the child. Some of these parents then have to resort to the child welfare system to obtain assistance. This means that parents must try to work with a system that is designed to respond to abuse and neglect rather than mental illness and this opens the possibility of a parent being required to give custody of their child to the state to obtain services.

This example is particularly useful because given the state of our knowledge of children's mental illnesses, it is extremely difficult to arrive at a definition of a seriously emotionally disturbed child that can be used for determining eligibility for services. The following definition is provided as a concrete example. It was originally developed in 1985 but sadly continues to be relevant. Stroul and Freidman (1994) continue to include the following as a useful example:

For a child to be considered seriously emotionally disturbed, the child's behavior must exhibit one or more of the following characteristics:

- The behaviors shall have occurred with sufficient frequency to be considered a pattern of responses or to be so intense that the consequences led to severe measures of control by the environment (seclusion, restraints, hospitalization, chemical intervention, etc.)
- The behaviors, although possibly provoked, are judged to be extreme or out of control of proportion to the provocation or an inappropriate age reaction.
- The behaviors have been judged sufficiently disruptive to lead to exclusion form school, home, therapeutic, or recreational settings.
- The behaviors shall be sufficiently intense or severe to be considered seriously detrimental to the child's growth, development, or welfare, or to the safety or welfare of others. (p. 8)

This definition, although attempting to be precise, is vague in much of its wording. Each of the four points is intended to help identify a specific group of children but each allows multiple interpretations; so to know exactly which child is "eligible" to be identified as SED is a potential point of conflict. The fact that this definition was formed prior to 1985 but continues to be presented as a positive example is testament to the persistent difficulty of arriving at a precise definition.

Both managers and frontline professionals must answer the question, "Who benefits?" A casework program for teenage parents had established its target population as those youth in their first or second trimester. A pregnant teen in her third trimester was denied service because "good" casework practice cannot be performed so late in the pregnancy. This decision was made despite the fact that there were no other services available. Is this a decision for the caseworker, the manager, or both? Identification of who will and will not benefit cannot be an area of wide discretion and arbitrariness.

This presentation of the importance of precisely defining the consumer population and the implications of poor choices may lead the reader to the conclusion that although this is critically important, it cannot be done. It is not our intent to render the social administrator powerless by raising awareness of the pitfalls and many negative examples. The next section assists the social administrator to make the important decision regarding who will become a consumer of the program.

To Identify the Direct Beneficiary of the Program, the Social Administrator Needs to

1. *be keenly aware of the need to be as precise as possible;*
2. *continue to learn as much as possible about potential consumers so that definitions can be continually revised;*
3. *engage key actors in discussions of the adequacy of these definitions and their application to specific cases so that the best possible decisions can be made for consumers;*
4. *recognize that some conflict situations arise from disputes about who is eligible or can benefit from services rather than other negative motivations;*
5. *be directly involved in these decisions to settle disputes and learn more about who is benefiting from the program.*

Consumer Population Analysis: The First Set of Decisions

Deciding who will benefit from the program is a complex process involving a set of decisions that constantly require revision. The process is complex because although there may be a limited number of decisions, the interaction between them multiplies the possibilities. This requires that all decisions be considered tentative. Once a decision is made it will likely need revision based upon the next decision. All decisions will also need revision based upon learning more about the problem, community, and potential consumers.

The first set of decisions includes the following:

- Which social problem will be the addressed?
- What evidence-based interventions are available to address the problem?
- What resources are or appear to be available to sustain the program?
- What geographic area will be the focus of attention?

Although the previous problem analysis may make the answer to the first question obvious, the process of learning about the problem may lead to revisiting the tentative decision made at the first stage in favor of a more specific or slightly different problem. For example, it is not uncommon to start the program design process by identifying the problem as child abuse or neglect. Once the problem analysis is completed, it is obvious that this is a very large category with many subtypes. Consequently, a decision may be made to narrow the problem of concern to neglect (still a large category) or physical abuse or sexual abuse.

The discussion of levels of intervention and evidence-based practices, to be revisited in the next chapter, are also factors to be considered when deciding who will ultimately benefit from the program. A well-tested intervention strategy that addresses multiple factors is ideal but may not be available. However, a well-tested intervention may be available for a single or small number of factors that may be worth augmenting with ideas for intervening at additional levels. This may lead to a decision to start with a small program to test the new intervention ideas.

By now the reader is also thinking about the limitations on the program scope based upon available resources. If there is strong evidence for a particular intervention, the resource requirements of the program can be easily determined. A judgment about the potential scope of the program can be made based upon the perceived cost of the program and the available resources. There may be a tendency when balancing these concerns to think of ways to cut costs while delivering the evidence-based program. One should know that alterations to well-tested programs are likely to result in ineffective interventions. Implementation of interventions and modifications based upon cost cutting are likely to destroy tested results.

The fine balance between social problem, available interventions, and available resources may be accomplished by considering a larger or smaller geographic area. A low incidence problem may require a larger geographic area to produce a sufficient number of consumers to justify the program. Conversely a high incidence problem or few financial resources may require a focus on one small part of a community.

Step 1: Consumer Population Analysis Questions

- *Which social problem will be the addressed?*
- *What evidence-based interventions are available to address the problem?*
- *What resources are or appear to be available to sustain the program?*
- *What geographic area will be the focus of attention?*

The Population Experiencing the Problem or Likely To

The decisions tentatively made during the previous analysis result in some general idea of who will be served. This includes subgroups of people who are either experiencing the problem or are particularly vulnerable to it. Those who are vulnerable to the problem are considered to be at-risk of experiencing the problem.

A description of the subgroup to be potentially considered as consumers requires deciding the following:

- Will people experiencing the problem *or* those likely to experience it be the target of intervention?
- Will all people experiencing the problem or at risk for it be the target of intervention, or just those with certain characteristics (e.g., most or least severe instances of the problem or more or fewer risk factors)?

If the decision is made to focus the program on people experiencing the problem, then it is useful to describe the characteristics of these people. It is important here to recognize the wide variation in the ways that people experience any social problem. Severity is one way to describe these situations. Some people experience few symptoms or experience them relatively infrequently; others experience the problem intensely and almost continually. Common co-occurring problems are also important to recognize. For example, some people experience depression and substance abuse at the same time. It is important to recognize this complexity when selecting a relevant intervention. Identifying the probable number of individuals at various levels of severity of the problem or with co-occurring problem is also important for deciding who will ultimately benefit from the program.

If the decision is made to focus on those at-risk, a similar description of this group is warranted. Populations vary widely in terms of how they experience the complex set of risk factors that were identified in the problem analysis. They also vary widely in the number of risk factors to which they might be vulnerable. Identification of the probable number of people in these groups is important to making good decisions on who will become consumers.

Step 2: Consumer Population Analysis Questions

- *Will people experiencing the problem or those likely to experience it be the target of intervention?*
- *Will all people experiencing the problem or at risk for it be the target of intervention, or just those with certain characteristics (e.g., most or least severe instances of the problem or more or fewer risk factors)?*

The Target Population

The target population is that subset of people who are eligible for the program. It is probable that not all of the poor youth who are at risk of poor academic performance will be the focus of a particular intervention. The previous analysis makes it obvious that it is unlikely that a single program in a single agency could do it all. The program theory and the agency auspice are the two primary sets of factors that establish limits for the target population.

A prevention program necessarily casts a wider target population net than a treatment program. It may, therefore, exclude individuals who are already experiencing the problem. On the other hand, a treatment program may require the problem to be in evidence. Alcohol abuse prevention and treatment programs are good examples. A particular helping theory may limit the at-risk population because it requires a relatively homogeneous population of consumers. Certainly parenting an infant versus an adolescent requires very different parenting education and consequently a very different target population even though both parents may be at risk of abusing their child.

The helping theory contains expectations of consumers that also limit the target population. It is not reasonable to include at-risk individuals within the target population if they clearly cannot meet expectations. A parent education program requiring an eighth-grade reading ability probably cannot be targeted to mothers who do not read at this level.

Program auspice, or who is running the program, may also limit the targeted population. Courts, schools, or mental health centers have very different constraints placed on them. In the case of maintaining youth within the community, each of these entities may include a slightly different population. Legal mandates included in state or national legislation may also limit the target population, as will funding policies.

Step 3: Consumer Population Analysis Questions

- *How does the program theory effect the population to be served?*
- *How do agency auspices effect the population to be served?*

The Consumer Population

The consumer population is that subgroup of the target population who will become beneficiaries of the service. We know that only a portion of people eligible for a program will in fact receive service. The key question for the manager is who from the target population will receive services and who will not. Three sets of limiting factors usually come into play:

Pragmatic Considerations

The most common pragmatic consideration is program capacity. Although the resource question has been raised in the previous sections, it is of sufficient importance to raise again. That is, at any one point in time, program resources are available to serve x amount of eligible people. Too often programs have been rendered impotent because these tough decisions have not been made and caseloads have ballooned, workers have been unable to do their jobs, and consumers and the public are frustrated by the results. If limits must be set, the manager must decide which cases will take priority. Will individuals be served on a first-come-first served basis with a waiting list? Once an opening occurs how will it be filled? The point is that these decisions can and should be made by the manager, not by frontline workers at an affiliated service location or by other decision makers such as judges and influential community members.

Ethical Considerations

A person may be eligible for a program but may not want to receive services. For many programs, consumers must be voluntary, at least in the sense that they make themselves available to receive services.

Capabilities of Consumers

To benefit from the programs, consumers must exhibit certain abilities or possess certain resources. Alternatively the program must be designed to take these into account. Individuals in the target population may need transportation to participate; they may need to be available at certain times of the day; they may need to be willing and able to participate in a group. The question for the manager is what minimum capabilities a consumer must possess to have a reasonable chance of benefiting from the program. For an example of a population analysis, refer to the example included in Chapter 5.

Step 3: Consumer Population Analysis Questions

- *What pragmatic concerns limit the population to be served?*
- *What ethical concerns limit the population to be served?*
- *Are there capabilities of consumers that limit the population to be served?*

SOCIAL ADMINISTRATORS' USE
OF THE PROBLEM AND POPULATION ANALYSIS

The problem and population analysis may appear to be something that a manager does in the process of writing a program proposal to obtain funding for the program. It is very useful for these purposes. It is also so much more than that. It is a hypothesis that states: "This is how I understand the problem and based upon this understanding I will select interventions that will improve the situation for those experiencing the problem." The problem and population analysis contain a great number of assumptions that the program manager must continually evaluate. The problem analysis includes the latest knowledge about the consequences of the problem and the contributing factors. However, that knowledge is never complete and always evolving. The population analysis includes the latest knowledge of the local community and the fit between the program and the community. These are also hypotheses that may prove true now but may be false next month or next year as the community and program continue to evolve. In addition to the social administrator continually testing program assumptions against experience, these program elements are useful for determining resource requirements and targets for change efforts. Consequently, administrative use of social problem and target population analysis is organized according to the skills of

- acquiring and using information;
- acquiring and directing staff;
- acquiring and using resources other than staff; and
- facilitating change through the use of persuasion.

Acquiring and Using Information

It is apparent that the problem and population analysis are information intense (Exhibit 3.1). The program manager requires information on the specific consequences of the social problem for consumers and society. The factors that are said to explain or maintain any social problem are many and the interactions between factors are complex. Knowledge about the importance of any single factor or the interactions between factors emerges over time. All of this requires managers to continually learn and revise their understanding of the social problem as information becomes available.

The key questions regarding information asked by the social administrator are as follows:

- What information do I need?
- How does the manager acquire this information?
- Who needs this information?
- How is the information used?

EXHIBIT 3.1. Managers' Information Needs About the Social Problem and Population Analysis

Managers need the latest information on

> the factors that are said to explain or maintain the problem;
> the consequences of the problem for the community; and
> the consequences of the problem for consumers.

This information is acquired through

- research literature;
- informal sensing within the agency and community; and
- interactions with consumers.

Who needs information about the problem and population?

- program manager;
- program staff; and
- key people in the community, including those who have control of resources such as funds and consumer.

This information is used to

- direct program staff;
- influence key people in the community.

One way to begin this information analysis is to list the various people who need information about the social problem and the population to be served. This includes the following:

- The program manager
- Program staff
- Key people in the community, including those who have control of needed resources such as funds and consumers.

The social administrator builds and manages the program based upon the best current understanding of the problem and the population. This understanding is always incomplete and many times inaccurate. Only information can confirm or disconfirm current understandings.

For example, Alice takes over a program for older youth in foster care, which is intended to assist them to make the transition to adulthood and become productive members of the community. A major component of the program is the teaching of "independent living" skills through classes that are taught in the evening and on Saturdays. Among other things, there are classes on obtaining a job, budgeting, and staying safe while living alone. Staff have taught these classes for more than two years and are proud of their efforts and the results of tests taken by the youth at the end of each class.

Alice has read extensively about how adolescents learn and has had considerable experience working with them. The literature and her experience have demonstrated that youth best acquire these important skills through real-life practice rather than in the classroom. She has found that this is particularly true for youth that have not had the best success with formal education. She realizes that her workers need better information about consumers of the program and how they acquire new skills.

This example demonstrates one type of information needed about the problem and population analysis to keep the program as effective as possible. In general, managers need information regarding the following:

- Factors said to contribute to or maintain the problem
- Consequences of the social problem for the community
- Consequences of the social problem for consumers

The research literature is one important place to acquire needed information. Program managers also acquire needed information from informal sensing. For example, a manager attends a community meeting and hears that the homeless mentally ill tend to spend time near certain stores and that this results in consumers avoiding these businesses. This is a critically important source of information about the consequences of the problem for the community.

The best way to really understand the consequences of the problem for consumers is to spend time with them. This can be easily done by visiting with consumers in a waiting room or going with a worker to a meeting with a consumer. A focus group of consumers is an important way to gather information on their experience with the problem and also with the program. The largest obstacle to managers acquiring this type of information is TIME. With the multitude of demands on a program mangers time, it is difficult to regularly allocate time with consumers. This takes a conscious and continuous effort on the part of the administrator.

Acquiring and Directing Staff

It is our belief that program staff with the latest knowledge, skills, and values consistent with the problem and population analysis will be more effective with consumers. The social administrator's task is to use her or his understanding of the problem and population as part of the staff selection process. This requires identification of the desired knowledge, skills, and values that are important for staff to have and to determine ways that this information is used to select the best people to do the job (more on staff selection in Chapter 8).

Like the program manager, it is important for staff to understand that knowledge of those factors that are said to contribute to the problem is evolving, as are consequences to society and the consumer. Program staff who believe that there is one factor that caused the problem and that this must be changed are unlikely to respond positively to program changes based upon new understandings of these factors and their interactions. Similarly, a person who focuses narrowly on selected consequences of the problem for the community and the consumer is unlikely to hear the community, when a new troubling consequence comes to its attention, or the consumer who related his or her personal experiences.

Using the problem and population analysis in directing staff requires helping staff stay current with the latest understandings. This involves the usual dissemination of new knowledge as it becomes available. It also involves encouraging staff to maintain contact with Web sites and listservs that continually update information on the social problem and its consequences. In addition, social administrators regularly reward staff for bringing new information about the problem and its consequences to the attention of the work team.

Acquiring and Using Resources Other Than Staff

As the social administrator thinks about the factors said to contribute to or maintain the social problem, she or he begins to gain insights into the type of helping technology that is required to make a difference for consumers. This in turn begins to identify the other resources required for program success.

For example, the factors said to contribute to the problem of socially isolated elderly in the community include several aspects concerning mobility. These include older people beginning to have more physical conditions that limit mobility, poor elderly not being able to afford to maintain an automobile, and the community not seeing itself as having sufficient resources to maintain an adequate level of public transportation. If the program manager wants to increase the social interaction of poor elderly with others in the community, the intervention will need to include creating opportunities that are neighborhood focused so that transportation is not a factor or create a program that relies on moving people. Although the answer to this problem may not be clear, the consequences for selecting the helping technology and the related resource requirements are apparent.

The population analysis also contributes to the identification of required funds in that it identifies the number of consumers in the community likely to benefit from the program. The combination of the desired caseload size and number of potential consumers indicates the number of staff required to address the problem at the community level. Frequently, the resources available to address the problem are less than needed so that the program can only address a part of the problem. However, a good population analysis may also indicate that the number of potential consumers is small. The parent education example is relevant here. The narrow target population identified for this program results in the conclusion that thirty-five families are likely to benefit. This may be an ideal situation in that the resources for this size group are sufficient to meet the projected need. It could also be a problem in that a funding source may be reluctant to support such a small program.

As these examples demonstrate, the relationship between the social problem and population analysis and the program's resource needs is complex. The essential questions that guide the administrators thinking in this area are as follows:

- Given the social problem analysis, what types of helping technologies seem to be indicated as a needed part of the program?
- What are the potential consequences of applying these technologies for staff time and caseloads?

- What are the implications of these choices for the program budget?
- How does this match the need identified in the community by the population analysis?
- How does this fit with the resources available in the community?

Facilitating Change By Using Persuasion:
The Problem and Population Analysis

The previous sections focused on the program managers' use of the social problem and population analysis in relation to information, staff, and other resources. This section gives examples of the application of the change skills identified in Chapter 2 in relation to these two program elements. The change model used in this book is based upon a well-researched model of persuasion. Exhibit 3.2 is a reminder of the major components of this change model

The examples presented in this section are chosen to demonstrate the use of selected skills with workers, others in the agency, and those in the community. Recall that any change effort starts with the identification of the person to be influenced and the behavior desired of that person. In the press of everyday business, it is sometimes easy to overlook this important first step. The following examples will begin by identifying who the target of the change effort is and the behavior desired of this person. For clarity, this is highlighted in the examples as are elements of the change model and selected strategies.

Worker Example

George is a program manager supervising a team of nine workers. Through his normal process of case readings, he notices that John does not regularly complete the multifaceted consumer assessment that is part of the

---

EXHIBIT 3.2. Theory of Behavioral Intention

The current research on exercising influence indicates that a person is more likely to exhibit a behavior when they

- perceive that they have behavioral control;
- have a positive attitude toward the behavior;
- feel that the behavior is normative; and
- have the intention to perform the behavior.

program specifications and is based upon the multiple factors that have been found to contribute to or maintain the problem. George has noticed that in staff meetings, John makes comments that indicate that he thinks that the problem has a single cause and that if consumers simply change that part of their life, they will achieve positive outcomes.

George decides that he will spend some time over the next couple of weeks to attempt to have John *(person*)* regularly complete the multifaceted consumer assessment *(behavior)*. George realizes that he could simply tell John that the program guidelines say that the multifaceted consumer assessment must be done with each consumer. However, he also knows that compliance will be low unless John has the intention to perform the behavior where this intention is based upon his belief that he can complete the assessment *(behavioral control)*, his feeling that the assessment is expected *(normative)*, and he feels positively *(attitude)* toward completing the assessment. George knows that John has the skills to complete the assessment because he was required to successfully complete the assessment in training. George has also seen John conduct the assessment during a visit with a consumer.

George decides to focus on John's attitude by *adding a reason to think positively* about the assessment. He also decides to emphasize that completion of the assessment is the *norm* in the work unit as he knows that almost all workers regularly complete the assessment. George blends these two strategies together by having part of a staff meeting devoted to a brief discussion about the assessment. He wants staff to share their experiences with the assessment and its relationship to outcomes for consumers. As workers share their experiences, he intends to draw out examples of cases where a variety of factors were identified as targets for change and how this has been a positive experience for consumers. This process will reinforce for John that completion of the assessment is the norm within the team and will also give him concrete examples where factors other than the one that he thinks is important were useful. George will also follow up the meeting by examining John's next new case to see whether the assessment has been completed.

Agency Staff Example

This example uses the previously mentioned program for older youth in foster care learning independent living skills by teaching classes. Alice wants the information staff to learn about how adolescents learn and develop to translate to changes that will be specified through other components of the program framework. Among the many steps she identifies as

---

*Italics is used to remind the reader of key elements of the change model described in Chapter 2.

part of this change effort, one step is to influence program staff *(people)* to say that they agree that the classes they have been conducting may not be the best way to get the youth to learn and then to agree to implement a new program model *(behavior)*.

Alice realizes that to get to the point where staff will want to try a new program model *(intention to perform the behavior),* they will need to feel that a different approach is more effective *(feel that the behavior is normative)*. She decides to start the learning process by arranging for her staff to acquire information on how adolescents learn by having an expert in adolescent development *(linking messages to new important people)* make a presentation. She also asks three youth who are currently participating in the program *(increasing the importance of an existing key actor)* to present at the same time on their learning experiences and how they learn best. She also has several articles available for staff who may wish to obtain this information in this way.

Community Example

Alex manages a program for people who do not have shelter in Midtown. Recently, there has been considerable news coverage of some of his consumers who previously lived in other communities. From these reports many people in Midtown are getting the impression that the community is becoming a magnet for people who need housing because of its "generous" shelters and other programs.

A recent study conducted in Midtown found that there were 400 homeless individuals in the community. A similar study in a community that is 50 percent larger and near Midtown found 1,000 homeless individuals. If Midtown "attracted" the homeless at the same rate as the other community, there would be at least 500 individuals needing shelter. Clearly, Midtown is not a "magnet."

Alex decides to meet with a local reporter *(person)* to influence him to write an article comparing the number of homeless in the two communities *(behavior)*. Alex decides to try to increase the reporter's attitude about writing the article. Alex draws upon the influence strategy of citing proven results *(weight of the evidence)*. He makes copies of the two studies (and notes in the margins) that were conducted using the same methodology by people not associated with shelter programs in either community . He prepares a table of the latest population figures for each community along with the results of the two studies. He includes in this table estimates of the rate of homeless individuals from state and national studies that show that the number of people in Midtown requiring shelter is as expected.

SUMMARY

This is the first of three chapters that identify elements of the program management framework used in this text. These elements form the basis for important management decisions as well as targets for intervention to improve outcomes for consumers. The use of these elements in management change is illustrated by using the model presented in Chapter 2. Chapters 4 and 5 will present the other program framework elements that are necessary to complete the program.

Chapter 4

Specifying and Managing
the Social Work Theory of Helping

Every social program is based upon ideas about how social workers and consumers can work together to achieve desired outcomes. This chapter makes this theory of helping explicit through the program goal, objectives, and mutual expectations. The uses of this program design element are also described using the structure of acquiring and using information, acquiring and directing staff, acquiring and using resources other than staff, and facilitating change.

Program Framework Learning Objectives—Part 2

- *Identify the components of a program's theory of helping.*
- *Select an evidence-based intervention based upon the latest research literature, your knowledge of the population to be served, and an ecological approach that recognizes that most interventions need to incorporate strategies at multiple levels.*
- *Write a consumer outcome program goal that meets specified criteria.*
- *Write consumer outcome program objectives that meet specified criteria.*
- *Write minimal expectations of consumers and workers that will achieve the consumer outcome program objectives.*
- *Identify ways to use the program theory to acquire and use information, acquire and direct staff, acquire and use resources. other than staff and facilitating change by using persuasion.*

Textbook of Social Administration: The Consumer-Centered Approach
© 2007 by The Haworth Press, Inc. All rights reserved.
doi:10.1300/5802_05

WHAT IS A THEORY OF HELPING?

A recent check of Social Work abstracts indicated that from 1977 through 2003, there were 3,240 abstracts that included the word theory and 634 that used theory in the title. Clearly theory has an important place in social work. However, it is not always clear what an author means by the use of the word. The Internet site www.dictionary.com lists the following six definitions for theory.

1. A set of statements or principles devised to explain a group of facts or phenomena, especially one that has been repeatedly tested or is widely accepted and can be used to make predictions about natural phenomena.
2. The branch of a science or art consisting of its explanatory statements, accepted principles, and methods of analysis, as opposed to practice: *a fine musician who had never studied theory.*
3. A set of theorems that constitute a systematic view of a branch of mathematics.
4. Abstract reasoning, speculation: *a decision based on experience rather than theory.*
5. A belief or principle that guides action or assists comprehension or judgment: *staked out the house on the theory that criminals usually return to the scene of the crime.*
6. An assumption based on limited information or knowledge; a conjecture.

Notice the range of definitions. Definition's 2 and 4 contrast theory with experience and practice. This sense of theory is that it is something quite different from practice. Social workers who emphasize learning from their practice might subscribe to this definition. One can imagine someone in the field saying that it is possible to be a fine social worker without every studying theory just like the musician mentioned in the definition. Similarly, basing decisions on experience rather than theory is common.

In this text, we use the word theory in the sense of the first definition. We use theory to mean a set of statements that explain results for consumers. This is consistent with ideas about using evidence-based practices. The statements that comprise the theory would ideally have passed the rigorous tests required to be identified as an evidence-based practice.

In simple terms, evidence-based practice models are those that are shown to be effective through controlled experiments like those used to prove the efficacy of medications. There is increasing discussion of evidence-based practice and its application to social work practice with much of this focused on the ethical obligation to practice with tested interventions (Gibbs and Gambrill, 2002; Howard and Jenson, 1999; Gambrill, 1999; Thyer, 1995). Macdonald (1998) states, "When we intervene in the lives of others we should do so on the basis of the best evidence available regarding the likely consequences of that intervention."

A recent evaluation of programs working with juvenile offenders provides an example. Barnoski and Aos (2004) found that when a program called Functional Family Therapy was implemented in a competent manner with juvenile offenders, there was a 38 percent reduction in felony recidivism. However, when the program was not implemented as intended there was a 17 percent increase in recidivism. In mental health, strong positive correlations have been found between evidence-based supported employment practice fidelity and outcomes (Becker, Smith, Tanzman, Drake, & Tremblay, 2001; Becker, Xie, McHugo, Halliday, & Martinez, 2006; McGrew & Griss, 2005), and between fidelity of assertive community treatment and client outcomes (Bond & Salyers, 2004; McHugo, Drake, Teague, & Xie, 1999). Yet, research suggests that the implementation of evidence-based practices is the exception not the rule (President's New Freedom Commission, 2003; Lehman, Steinwachs et al., 1998).

Sackett, Straus, and Richardson (1997) provide a slightly different definition of evidence-based practice. Their definition is the conscientious, explicit, and judicious use of current best evidence in making decisions about individuals. The use of the term current best evidence is important. If our interventions were restricted to those that have been demonstrated to be effective through controlled experiments, there would be many situations in which we would not intervene. The term best evidence here is very much like the phrase widely accepted in the definition of theory. When results of randomized controlled experiments are not available, intervention is directed by best evidence or the best body of research that exists.

The definition of theory includes the words "repeatedly tested." Although a randomized controlled experiment is a powerful research design that can establish a cause-and-effect relationship, scientists have learned that the result of a single experiment is insufficient. If several experiments with the same intervention all produce similar results, we have much more confidence in the efficacy of the intervention. This type of evidence is brought together in a meta-analysis. Meta-analyses are the summarization of randomized controlled studies using statistical analysis to quantify the degree of effect that can be expected from the intervention. Where experiments are not available, the best evidence is summarized in systematic reviews. Systematic reviews are the synthesis of research studies in which the researchers outline their methodology and sources of biases.

Many reviewers of interventions develop levels of evidence that help guide the selection of interventions. For example, Thomlison (2003) used the following four levels of evidence for child maltreatment interventions.

>   Level 1: Well-supported, efficacious treatment with positive evidence from more than two randomized clinical trials.
>
>   Level 2: Supported and probably efficacious treatment with positive evidence from two or more quasiexperimental studies, or where researchers found positive evidence from only one randomized clinical trial.
>
>   Level 3: Supported and acceptable treatment with positive evidence from comparative studies, correlations studies, and case control studies: one nonrandomized study: or any type of quasiexperimental study.
>
>   Level 4: Promising and acceptable treatment with evidence from experts or clinical experience of respected authority or both. (p. 544)

In mental health, the following scheme of levels of evidence (Cook, Toprac, & Shore, 2004) is often used:

>   Level 1: The least five published studies with scientifically rigorous designs (randomized clinical trials, well-controlled quasi-experimental designs) using a variety of meaningful outcome measures.
>
>   Level 2: Less than five published scientifically rigorous studies and/or studies using single outcome measures or less rigorous dependent variables.
>
>   Level 3: Published studies of less rigorous design (e.g., pre/post designs with no control group, client self-report of perceived changes following receipt of services).
>
>   Level 4: Multiple organizational "case studies" with reported outcomes published in peer-reviewed journals.
>
>   Level 5: Expert panel recommendations based on empirical research evidence but NOT including expert consensus (e.g., based on "surveys" of expert clinicians, surveys of consumer preferences, unpublished program evaluations, etc.). (p. 310)

Although the specific definitions of the levels are debatable, this provides a useful example for discussion. For example, are two randomized clinical trials sufficient for an intervention to be defined as "well-supported"? The answer to this might depend, in part, on the field of practice.

This implies that social workers must be knowledgeable about the existing research, the level of evidence, and the strengths and limitations of the methodologies that are employed. Studies using secondary data-analysis and statistical analyses such as causal modeling are not as powerful as controlled experiments, but these methodologies answer important questions that may not yet be testable by randomized controlled trials. Also, qualitative studies play an important role in that they provide a wealth of information concerning peoples' experiences. In mental health, meta-analyses of the many first-person accounts of recovery have identified the elements critical to recovery (Rapp & Goscha, 2006) and the processes undertaken by consumers (Ridgway, 2001). These are important to understanding consumers' thoughts, emotions, and experiences with their situations as well as planned interventions.

In the program framework of this text, the service transaction or what social workers do when they work with consumers is one of the most important considerations. This transaction is built upon an evolving understanding of the problem and the program's consumers. The problem analysis provided an initial understanding of the problem through identification of the multiple factors that contribute to or maintain the problem and its consequences for the person and society. The population analysis identified the consumer.

In Chapter 3, we introduced levels of intervention and suggested that given the complexity of social problems, multiple interventions directed at multiple levels are indicated. In fact, many of the practices that have the greatest empirical support are consonant with this idea (e.g., assertive community treatment, supported employment, integrated dual diagnosis treatment, and strengths model case management). Each of these include interventions at individual and community levels, individual, family, and group, and most contain requirements for institutional-level interventions focused on structural features of the service.

The theory of helping is influenced by the levels of intervention to be used for the program. It is especially critical when defining expectations of consumers and workers. For example, an employment program that includes direct work with employers would necessarily require certain workers' behaviors (e.g., frequency of contact) and consumer behavior (e.g., willingness to allow workers to intervene, which may require disclosure of disability). In contrast, a program that only helped a client prepare a résumé would have a different set of minimum expectations.

The theory of helping is the specific evidence-based intervention that the social administrator believes will assist the consumer achieve mutually desirably goals. It consists of

- The consumer outcome goal
- Consumer outcome objectives
- Expectations (behaviors) of workers
- Expectations (behaviors) of consumers

This is a theory in the sense that we believe that if workers and consumers do their work as expected, then the consumer outcome objectives will be achieved. If the objectives are achieved then the goal will be achieved. There are other program framework elements that one could argue for inclusion here. For example, all social workers know that the environment influences behaviors of workers and consumers. This is a program element that is included in Chapter 5, which arguably could be discussed here. Our reasons for not including other elements here is simply pragmatic. We have found that including too many elements in the theory of helping becomes confusing.

Social Work Theory of Helping

- *The consumer outcome goal*
- *Consumer outcome objectives*
- *Expectations or behaviors of workers*
- *Expectations or behaviors of consumers*

The diagram in Exhibit 4.1 demonstrates a theory of helping using a juvenile justice example. The framework requirements for expectations, objectives, and goals are not provided in detail. However, this simplified model demonstrates the basic idea that if the worker and youth live up to their expectations then the objectives will be achieved, and if these are achieved then the goal will be obtained.

This model of the social work transaction has several advantages. One is that it provides a framework for a detailed specification of the intervention. Interventions are seldom described in this type of detail. Even evidence-based practices are not always specified to the level of behavior and the links between behavior and outcomes. For example, Henggeler, Schoenwald, Borduin, Rowland, and Cunningham (1998) identify their book titled

EXHIBIT 4.1. Example Theory of Helping

Worker Expectations (Behaviors) Concerning:	Youth Expectations (Behaviors) Concerning:
Youth	Worker
Family	Family
School	School

Consumer Objectives

Youth increases activities with positive peers.
Youth increases activities with parents.
Youth improves school performance.

Consumer Goal

Youth who have been adjudicated as juvenile offenders remain living with his or her family and remain free of criminal activity.

Multisystemic Treatment of Antisocial Behavior in Children and Adolescents as a treatment manual for practitioners; Chapter 3 in the book includes a section on assessing family functioning.* The process that practitioners are to use includes developing hypotheses, gathering evidence, implementing interventions, observing these interventions, identifying barriers to success, and designing interventions to overcome these barriers. Although this is accompanied with case examples and is a clearer definition of worker behavior than many other manuals, it is still not quite behavior. On the other hand, if every behavior is included, the list gets too long to be useful. This is pointed out to suggest the need for specificity while recognizing the accompanying problem. Later we make some suggestions as to how social administrators might deal with this dilemma.

Second, this framework helps keep in mind the connections between behaviors, objectives, and goals. The example provided in Exhibit 4.1 suggests that if youth increase their activities with positive peers and parents, as well as improve school performance, they are more likely to remain free of criminal activity. These connections are more often than not implied in our work with consumers. This framework makes it explicit and testable on an on-going basis.

---

*While the research base for *Multisystemic Treatment of Antisocial Behavior in Children and Adolescents* is being debated, we use this example because of its well-developed treatment and training manuals.

Third, this model allows social administrators to manage for improved consumer outcomes by testing each element as well as relationships between elements. For example, if consumer goals are not being achieved it is possible to examine the link between objectives and the goal. It may be that some objectives need to be deleted, added, or changed. The difficulty may be that workers or consumers may not be meeting expectations. This could happen for a variety of reasons including not being aware of the expectations, not having the skill or ability to perform the expectation, or the expectations may simply be the wrong ones to achieve the objectives.

FRAMEWORK REQUIREMENTS FOR GOALS

A program theory comes directly from the problem analysis. Goals address the desirable outcome for the consumer. The objectives and expectations come from a selection of contributory factors for which technologies exist to produce positive change. Most programs have but one goal, and (as will be seen later) multiple objectives. Every goal should meet all of the following criteria:

The Goal Must Be Related to the Social Problem Analysis.

The goal statement should be directly derived from the problem statement. Since most social problems are complex, involving a host of contributing factors, any single program usually seeks to influence but a few. In fact, many factors are well beyond the ability of current social work interventions to produce positive change. To insure the problem–goal relationship, the manager should return to the list of factors contributing to the existence or maintenance of the social problem, and circle those factors that his or her program seeks to influence or change. It is these factors that provide the substance for the program goals. The goal derived from the problem analysis described in Exhibit 4.1 is for the youth who have been adjudicated as juvenile offenders to remain living with their family and free of criminal activity.

The Goal Must Be Outcome Oriented.

The goal statement should be written for consumers and not for the agency. For example, program goals *should never* be phrased in terms of "the program will provide." This is what the agency is going to do, but it does not specify the desired outcome. Rather than stating that "the agency will provide prevocational training and job placement," the goal should be something like "consumers will obtain employment."

The Goal Must Be Realistic.

The goals must be fiscally, technologically, ethically, and legally possible. The child abuse prevention research can illustrate these criteria.

Fiscal Realism

Child abuse prevention efforts are costly. The only program that has demonstrated efficacy is the nurse home visitor program developed by David Olds (Olds, 2002). This program, like most prevention programs, requires that the entire population of a geographic area be included in the program. In this case, every pregnant mother in the target area is visited at the beginning and during the second trimester and this is followed until the child is two years of age. Yet the amount of funding available for child abuse prevention is rarely sufficient for such a program.

Interest in child abuse prevention grew as Ray Helfer's concept of child abuse prevention trust funds became popular. Originally funds for child abuse prevention would be generated from a surcharge on marriage licenses, birth certificates, and divorce decrees (Martin, Scott, Pierron, & Bauerle, 1984). This concept has been broadened to include revenues from other sources such as donating money by checking a box on your state income tax check form and special license plate fees. However, it is unlikely that this type of funding source can provide sufficient funds for many home visitor programs. In Illinois for example, this type of revenue generation yielded $16 million in the 2002 state fiscal year. This might seem like a lot of money until you consider both the size of the state (over 12 million) and that these funds are also to be used for all forms of interpersonal violence (State of Illinois Office of the Auditor General, 2002). Child abuse trust funds are just not large enough to fund the currently most effective child abuse prevention program.

Technological Realism

Child abuse prevention became popular before the work of David Olds when little was known about prevention of child abuse. Most of the early programs were based on simplistic ideas such as if parents had parenting education, or social support, or respite from taking care of a child then they would not abuse their children. Although some of these ideas may be true for some parents, they have not been proven to be effective child abuse prevention strategies.

Ethical and Legal Realism

Child abuse prevention efforts must balance community interest with individual freedoms. Efforts to reach out to parents cannot legally or ethically include intrusion into the home. States are allowed to intrude into the home when there is a report of abuse or neglect but not prior to that as might be thought desirable for a prevention program.

The Goal Must Be Clearly Stated.

The goal statements should be understandable to most people. They should be devoid of agency or professional jargon, adjectives, and adverbs (e.g., "appropriate," "stabilized"). We have an obligation to communicate clearly with our consumers and communities and not just with other professionals.

The Goal Must Refer to the Consumer Population.

The goal statement needs to specify the target or consumer population (e.g., frail elderly aged 75 and over, pregnant teenagers). This population has been explicitly defined in the first program design step. In most cases it is most effective to have the goal statement start by identifying the consumer. For example, youth who are exiting foster care due to age will have a job, a medical card, and sufficient savings to cover start-up costs (deposits), and one-month living expenses.

The Goal Must Be Precise.

The goal statement should be observable and measurable or at least it strongly implies this quality. Many child welfare advocates argue that child and family well-being are desirable child welfare outcomes. Although this is difficult to argue against, a goal statement that identified either of these as an outcome would suffer from being imprecise. There is little or no consensus on definitions and measurement of well-being. However, the previous example for the youth exiting foster care due to age is measurable.

The Goal Must Be Positive.

Goal statements should be written in terms of what will be accomplished rather than in terms of the absence of something (e.g., increase employment versus reduce unemployment). At times, attempts to make a goal statement

positive will do injustice to precision and clarity. In these cases, it can be negative. Some would argue that "to reduce hospitalizations" is more precise than "to increase tenure in the community." In most cases, beginning a goal with "to increase . . . " will propel the program designer in the right direction.

Requirements of Program Goals

- *Related to the social problem analysis*
- *Identify the consumer outcome*
- *Realistic*
- *Clear*
- *Identify the consumer*
- *Precise*
- *Positive*

FRAMEWORK REQUIREMENTS FOR OBJECTIVES

Objectives are statements that specify the outcomes that are necessary for the goal to be achieved by consumers. Objectives decompose the goal into the specific benefits that are to accrue to the clients. These consumer outcome objectives are not the only ones required. Programs also need to acquire resources and produce service events. However, for the purposes of the theory of intervention, only the consumer outcome objectives are included here. Objectives require problem analyses and information about the consumer population, key players, and other components of program design. This is an interactive process, requiring the administrator to consider many design aspects simultaneously.

There are eight criteria for an adequate objectives statement. Four of these are identical to those discussed for goal setting: Objectives must be *consumer outcome oriented, clear, positive,* and *realistic.* The four additional criteria for objectives are as follows.

The Objective Is Related to the Goal.

The objectives decompose the program goal into statements of specific benefits. In the theory of helping the consumer outcome specified in the goal statement are consequences of other changes. For example, a youth having difficulty staying in school (the goal) is likely to achieve this end as a result of other changes related to his or her relations with peer, relations with teachers, and the learning environment and behavior in school. These changes are the consumer outcome objectives.

The Objective Must Set a Single Standard.

Each objective should have a number or percentage or rate that defines *adequate* performance. Rarely will any objective be reached for all consumers, nor does the manager ever want to be in the position of implying such. For example, an objective may state that 75 percent of all consumers will be employed for a minimum of ten hours a week. The figure set should be based on the manager's assessment that it is attainable and that performance below this figure would be disappointing. The single standard is a powerful way of building realism into the program. (Chapter 6 contains a fuller discussion of setting standards.)

The Objective Is Measurable.

Every objective should be directly measurable and observable. It should be unambiguous.

The Objective Has Time Parameters.

Time limitations should be stated. Common time parameters are fiscal year, program year, calendar year, or quarterly.

Criteria for Consumer Outcome Objectives

- *Related to the goal*
- *Identify a consumer outcome*
- *Clear*
- *Positive*
- *Realistic*
- *Measurable*
- *Set a single standard*
- *Include a time parameter*

To illustrate the establishment of objectives, consider the example of a program to reduce antisocial behavior in adolescents. The objectives are derived from the problem analysis and the research literature. Henggeler, Schoenwald, Borduin, Rowland, and Cunningham (1998) conducted an extensive literature review and found the following to be associated with antisocial behavior.

1. An association with deviant peers is virtually always a powerful direct predictor of antisocial behavior.
2. Family relations predict antisocial behavior either directly or indirectly by predicting association with deviant peers.
3. School difficulties predict association with deviant peers.
4. Neighborhood and community support characteristics add small portions of unique variance or indirectly predict antisocial behavior by, for example, affecting family, peer, or school behavior. (p. 8)

Consequently, example objectives for this type of program would establish an objective for each of the findings and be similar to the following:

1. Ninety percent of the youth in the program will participate in after school sports and clubs, community-based sports and service organizations, church groups, recreational center activities, after school volunteer, or paid employment within one month of enrolling in the program.
2. Ninety percent of the youth in the program will have in person contact with a parent and a positive peer (friend) at least three times per week within two months of enrolling in the program.
3. Seventy-five percent of the youth in the program will have teachers report improved school performance within six weeks of enrolling in the program.

Check these objectives against the criteria. They are offered as examples that meet the stated criteria. A particular program may have more, fewer, or different objectives. The objectives may have different standards or time frames. Although the example is drawn from the *Multisystemic Treatment Manual,* it does not necessarily constitute a full set of consumer objectives for such a program.

FRAMEWORK REQUIREMENTS FOR EXPECTATIONS

Specifying the reciprocal obligations of consumers and social workers completes the theory of helping. In our society, certain role behaviors are widely known and accepted. One learns how to be a patient, how to be a parent, how to be a student. We all master these roles and have a keen understanding of what we can expect from the people in the opposite role—the doctor, the child, the teacher. Without precise knowledge of legitimate expectations there will be breakdowns of communication and strong feelings of resentment at being "let down." Here is an example. A friend says her psychiatrist did not help her. Discussion of the visit with the psychiatrist revealed that my friend was passive and uncommunicative. I explained that the intervention was predicated on her active verbal involvement. Several months later, she reported the psychiatrist as being much more helpful.

The role of consumers of social services is not as well understood. There is the unfortunate stereotype of "client in denial" or "dependent person." The consumer–psychotherapist relationship is becoming better understood, especially in upper middle-class circles. Literary portrayals have popularized the therapist–patient role. Many literary allusions to social worker–consumer relations portray the reciprocal roles as dominant–submissive, manipulative–helpless. Since the social worker–consumer role is so little understood, it is not surprising that many cases used for teaching social work involve extended discussion about clarifying acceptable behaviors and mutual obligations.

Identification of legitimate reciprocal obligations recognizes the mutual, interacting, and reciprocal nature of social work. The "powers and duties" that each person carries when acting toward the other becomes clear. It is important here to specify the minimum expectations the consumer can hold toward the worker and those the worker can hold toward the consumer. Neither the consumer nor the worker should be set up for failure due to unreasonable expectations. At the same time both must be challenged to learn and grow.

In the example of the friend of one of the authors and the psychiatrist, an expectation of verbal involvement was established. When the friend asked what she should talk about it was suggested she leave directing the conversation to the professional but that she talk about anything that came to mind. These minimum expectations were sufficient to significantly alter the helping transaction.

Expectations are derived from several sources. Evidence-based practices are the most obvious source but the descriptions of these interventions seldom have sufficient detail to identify expectations. In addition, agency policy and professional obligations should be thought about. Table 4.1 lists some of the factors to consider along with examples of expectations.

Another set of decisions is the consequence of an expectation not being met. Can a consumer appeal, and if so, how? Will service be terminated? Will certain reports or records be made? Will failure to meet expectations lead to certain decisions?

TABLE 4.1. Consumer and Worker Expectations

Factor	Possible Expectation
1. Professional or agency ethics	Confidentiality—the worker should only share information about the consumers' situation with their written permission or in compliance with law.
2. Consumer needs	Sessions will be held in the consumer's home.
3. Nature of intervention	Sessions will be held only when all family members are in attendance.
4. Agency policy	Failure to attend activities for a one-month period will result in inactive status and this required reapplication for services.
5. Professional commitments	No action will be taken on behalf of the consumer without the consumer's explicit approval.
6. State statutes	A written plan will be completed within three weeks.
7. Custom	Consumers and workers will review their contract every three months.

In most social work programs, a program description cannot list all possible sets of expectations. As is true of so many management areas, the goal is to identify those behaviors that are critical to consumer success that if left unspecified are less likely to occur. This implies a continual process of learning and revision. Clearly language is also a problem. For example, an expectation might be that the worker contacts the consumer at least once a week. However, what defines a contact? Is a phone call sufficient or is a face-to-face meeting intended? The difficulties and importance of language will be addressed more completely in Chapter 8. For now it is important to state expectations as behaviorally as possible and define terms carefully.

SOCIAL ADMINISTRATORS' USE
OF THE THEORY OF HELPING

Specification of the theory of helping is an important component of the success of a program in helping consumers to achieve their goals. This program element also has a great deal of utility as an administrative tool. Administrative use of this program element is organized according to the skills of

- acquiring and using information;
- acquiring and directing staff;
- acquiring and using resources other than staff; and
- facilitating change through the use of persuasion.

Acquiring and Using Information and the Theory of Helping

There are two important questions for the social administrator regarding the theory of helping that require information. These are as follows:

- How do I know that the theory is being carried out?
- How do I know that the theory is effective?

The first question requires several different types of information. The theory posits that if the expectations or behaviors are carried out, then the consumer outcome objectives will be achieved and the goal will be obtained. To answer the first question requires the social administrator to have information about performance of the expectations.

Informal Sensing of Program Fidelity

A social administrator can acquire information through formal or informal sensing. By formal sensing we mean measurement with some type of instrument. By informal sensing we mean the normal interactions with staff and consumers.

Informal sensing of worker expectations occurs when the social administrator interacts with consumers and talks with them about their work with staff. The social administrator listens carefully to what consumers say to determine what is occurring in the service transaction, what consumers expect, and what they would like to see done differently. The social administrator probes consumers' general statements for behavioral specifics. With each consumer having a unique perspective it is necessary for the social administrator to interact with as many consumers as possible. Patterns in consumers' reactions are noted and worker behavior that is reported is checked against the list of expectations of workers. Since consumers and the service transaction change over time, it is important for the social administrator to interact with consumers as frequently as possible.

Informal Sensing of Worker Expectations

- *Talk with consumers.*
- *Listen for behavior and consumers' desires.*
- *Probe general statements to identify behavior.*
- *Identify patterns in consumers' responses.*
- *Compare these patterns to staff expectations in the theory of helping.*
- *Interact with consumers as frequently as possible over time.*

Informal sensing of consumer expectations also occurs through the social administrators interactions with staff. This is very much like the interactions with consumers in terms of listening, probing, and talking with staff about consumers on an ongoing basis. The social administrator also gains insight into worker behavior by asking about worker reactions to consumer behavior. This can be especially useful with consumer behavior that a worker finds particularly difficult. By asking what the worker does in response to this behavior, it is possible to identify worker expectations that might not be adequately addressed in the theory of helping. This is also an important time to ask the worker for ideas on how he or she could have responded differently.

A particularly important source of sensing occurs as part of field mentoring where the supervisor accompanies the case manager on visits with people or meeting with particular community resources. The supervisor can observe the case manager and provide feedback on their skills. Here is one example. Employment staff at a mental health center involved in the implementation of supported employment had been struggling with developing their skills in the area of job development. In fact, many of the staff had avoided going out to contact employers because of their fears and lack of skills. The staff involved in the project had been through training in job development and had some time to practice and role-play skills in training and team meetings. The employment staff's supervisor began to go out with her staff to observe how they were doing job development. The supervisor soon realized that her staff did not have the skills or the confidence to adequately engage and work with employers in order to help people obtain employment. The supervisor aggressively set a goal to spend 40 percent of her time for three months going out with her staff with the purpose to model skills, give feedback on skills, and build confidence. Six months later, one of the employment staff talked about the experience.

> After our training in job development, our supervisor set the expectation that we should be doing job development and set a certain number of contacts that we should be having with employers each month. I didn't really do it. I didn't like to do job development and did not feel comfortable doing it. I wasn't even sure about how to do it so I wasn't doing much. Later, my supervisor said she wanted to help us be more effective with our job development and would be going out regularly with us to talk with employers. At first, I was really upset and did not want to do it. After a while, though, I realized that I was feeling more comfortable with talking with employers and that my supervisor was really helping me do it better. I really liked it when I started getting clients jobs through my contact with employers. I realize now how helpful it was and how much better I am at job development.

Informal Sensing of Consumer Expectations

* *Talk with staff.*
* *Listen for behavior and consumers' desires.*
* *Probe general statements to identify behavior.*
* *Identify patterns in staff responses.*
* *Listen for consumer behavior that the worker is having difficulty responding to.*
* *Brainstorm with staff about other ways to respond to this behavior.*
* *Compare these patterns to expectations in the theory of helping.*
* *Interact with staff as frequently as possible over time.*
* *Field mentoring.*

Formal Sensing of Program Fidelity

Formal sensing of the expectations occurs when instruments are completed by consumers and staff that report on behavior. Two existing types of instruments that can be used for this purpose are client satisfaction and fidelity instruments. Data from these instruments are used in very much the same way as detailed for informal sensing.

Client satisfaction instruments are one way to get a formal reading on consumer perceptions of worker behavior. Although there are a variety of client-satisfaction instruments in the literature, those that have consumers report on the frequency of worker behavior are what is needed for the purposes of sensing worker fulfillment of expectations. Exhibit 4.2 includes sample satisfaction items drawn from an instrument that was designed for parents with children in foster care. The items were developed from parents and are behavioral. In use, parents respond to these items on a scale that indicates the frequency of the behavior.

Fidelity instruments are a recent development that assesses the degree to which an evidence-based intervention is being implemented as intended. Fidelity instruments were developed because it was found that although an intervention might be demonstrated to be effective, when the intervention is transported to another agency or setting, it may not have the intended effects due to incomplete implementation. The developers of Multisystemic Therapy (MST) have developed several fidelity instruments including a supervisor adherence measure (SAM) (more on that later) and a therapist adherence measure (TAM). The TAM is designed for consumers to report on their experience with their work with therapists. Sample items are included in Exhibit 4.3.

EXHIBIT 4.2. Sample Client Satisfaction Items for Parent with Children in Foster Care

- My caseworker encourages me to discuss when things were better in my family.
- When my caseworker makes a mistake, she or he admits it and tries to correct the situation.
- My caseworker tells me what she plans to say in court about my family and me—both negative and positive.
- My caseworker explains to me what will happen in court.

Source: Harris, G., Poertner, J., & Joe, S. (2000). The parents with children in foster care satisfaction scale. *Administration in Social Work 24* (2), 15-27.

EXHIBIT 4.3. Sample Items from the Therapist Adherence Measure (TAM)

- The therapist recommended that family members do specific things to solve our problems.
- Family members and the therapist agreed on the goals of the session.
- There were awkward silences and pauses during the session
- The therapist's recommendation required family members to work on their problems almost every day.

Source: Henggler, S. W., Schoenwald, S. K., Liao, J. G., Ketourneau, E. J., & Edwards, D. L. (2002). Transporting efficacious treatments to field settings: The link between supervisory practices and therapist fidelity in MST programs. *Journal of Clinical Child Psychology, 31*(2), 155-167.

In adult mental health, fidelity scales have been developed for each of the six evidence-based practices that were targeted for adoption in the National Evidence-Based Practice Implementation Project: supported employment, integrated dual diagnosis treatment, assertive community treatment, family psycho-education, illness management and recovery, and medication algorithms (Drake et al., 2001; Torrey, Finnerty, Evans, & Wyzik, 2003). These instruments were developed based on the strong research base that each practice enjoys. The items in these instruments are a mixture of structural elements (e.g., caseload size, organization of teams) and clinical elements (e.g., motivational interviewing, individualized treatment). Each item is rated on a five-point scale. The ratings are based on case record reviews, observations of practice, and interviews with staff, consumers, families, and agency leaders. An example of a fidelity item is located in Exhibit 4.4. Copies of these instruments can be downloaded from http://mentalhealth.samhsa.gov/cmhs/communitysupport/toolkits/illness/. A fidelity scale for strengths model case management has also been developed and is obtainable through the University of Kansas School of Social Welfare, Office of Mental Health Research and Training. There is also a scale, the State Health Authority Yardstick (SHAY), which measures the efforts of state mental health authorities to facilitate the implementation of evidence-based practices (EBPs) in provider agencies. It includes ratings of planning, funding, training, leadership, and policy supports. The General Organization Index (GOI) measures twelve facilitative conditions within an agency for EBP implementation, including program philosophy, penetration, assessment and treatment planning protocols, supervision, process and outcomes monitoring systems, and quality assurance.

Obtaining information on the service transaction is difficult and costly regardless of the method used to collect the data and none of the methods is perfect. People completing a questionnaire might answer in a way that they think is socially acceptable rather than reflecting their real experiences. Consumers might think that negative responses might influence decisions about the service they receive. Despite the costs and shortcomings, this type of information is useful to the social administrator for managing the program so that it produces the intended results.

Data on Consumer Outcomes—Goal and Objectives

How the social administrator knows if the theory is effective is determined from data on the consumer outcomes that are specified by the goal and objectives. Recall that the criteria for the goal and the objectives included the provision that they be measurable. Consequently the information system for the program must include collection of data on these outcomes. Measurement of consumer outcomes will be discussed in more detail in Chapters 6 and 7 as will formatting of outcome reports so that they have a positive impact on staff. What is important here is what the social administrator does with this information.

Keep in mind that the basic concept of the theory of helping is that if the consumer and worker fulfill the expectations of the theory, then the consumer outcome objectives will be achieved and the goal is achieved. There-

EXHIBIT 4.4. Sample Fidelity Scale Item

Motivational Interventions	20 percent of interactions with clients are based on motivational approaches	21 to 40 percent of interactions with clients are based on motivational approaches	41 to 60 percent of interactions with clients are based on motivational approaches	51 to 80 percent of interactions with clients are based on motivational approaches	>80 percent of interactions with clients are based on motivational approaches
	1	2	3	4	5

Definition

All interactions with dual disorder clients are based on motivational interviewing that include

1. Expressing empathy
2. Developing discrepancy between goals and continued use
3. Avoiding argumentation
4. Rolling with resistance
5. Instilling self-efficacy and hope

Rationale

Motivational interviewing involves helping the client identify his or her own goals and to recognize, through a systematic examination of the individual's ambivalence, that not managing one's illnesses interferes with attaining those goals. Research has demonstrated that clients with developmental disabilities (DD) who are unmotivated can be readily identified and effectively helped with motivational interventions.

fore, one use of the data is to check on the theory. Ideally, all of the data would show that the theory is working as intended and the social administrator keeps the program functioning as intended. However, it is likely that one or more elements of the theory are not achieving the desired result. In this case the social administrator needs to examine the elements (e.g., goals, objectives) of the theory that the data demonstrate are not being achieved and makes corrections. This may mean changes in the expectations, objectives, or even the goal.

Improvement or maintenance of consumer outcomes is accomplished with staff through the helping transaction. It is staff that interacts with consumers who need encouragement, rewards, and incentives to improve. The ways that the social administrator uses outcome data for these purposes is critical. First, staff should be rewarded for positive performance. This can be done in a variety of ways including but not limited to the following:

- Post the data and congratulate the staff on their good work.
- Talk about the data in a meeting and verbally reward staff for their efforts.
- Send out a reward memo to all staff.
- Invite consumers to a meeting to share their success stories.
- Stop by and say thanks to each worker in the unit.
- Send an individualized reward memo to selected staff.

Second, outcome data are used for problem sensing and solving. This is done by creating opportunities for staff to brainstorm ideas for program improvement. This can be done in a variety of ways including but not limited to the following:

- An agenda item in a staff meeting that seeks creative ideas for program improvement. Ideas are simply collected without any positive or negative evaluation.
- Send an email asking staff to take five minutes and share three to five ideas on how to improve performance on a selected consumer outcome.
- Go to the work space of selected workers and brainstorm with them on ways to improve a consumer outcome.
- Conduct a focus group of consumers and ask them what they think would help.
- Have a lunch called "improve consumer results" where the only requirement is to bring an idea and the agency provides the food.

Acquiring and Directing Staff and the Theory of Helping

The use of the theory of helping in acquiring staff is done by using the expectations of staff and consumers as a basis for hiring. The expectations are behaviors of staff and consumers. Consequently, the social administrator seeks to hire staff who can and want to work with consumers of the program using the intended behaviors. The expectations of staff should form a major part of the job description that is used to advertise the position and to conduct the interview. There are additional elements in the job description and in recruitment of personnel that are important and these are discussed in Chapter 8.

The expected behaviors are also useful for selecting staff by using them in the job interview. The best staff are those who have the behavioral skills to do the job and can demonstrate these skills in a variety of situations. The interview can be used to ask job candidates to explain situations where they have performed the types of identified tasks. Candidates can also be asked to demonstrate the behaviors by role-playing an interaction with a consumer or another member of the staff.

Some uses of the theory of helping in directing staff have been identified in the section on use of information. Collecting data on expectations and outcomes and then using this information for rewarding staff and problem solving are essential elements for directing staff. Another mechanism for directing staff is case review. As Harkness and Hensley (1991) found, when supervisors asked mental health counselors questions about consumer outcomes and interventions related to outcomes, they reported improved outcomes. The link between the theory of helping and case review is the outcomes identified in the goal and objectives. Discussing individual cases with staff provides a powerful opportunity to talk about consumer progress toward each of the outcomes identified in the goal and objectives. Talking about what each person needs to do to achieve a particular outcome is an ideal time to reinforce expectations as well as to listen for what is currently occurring in the service transaction.

An important and seldom considered element of personnel management is keeping staff hopeful. Although much attention has been given to burnout, perhaps it would be more useful to attend to the concept of hope. A person is exhibiting hopeful behavior when they can think of several ways to get out of a difficult situation, and they typically pursue their goals with energy. Synder (1994, 2000) has conducted considerable research on the concept of hope and has developed a model that consists of goal-directed determination and of planning ways to meet the goals. The interactions that workers have with clients are necessarily emotional and sometimes difficult.

Consumers frequently need to work on achieving a goal for an extended period of time and may need several attempts before they are successful. A program manager understands this and connects the consumer outcomes with worker goals. When a worker is having difficulty helping a consumer achieve a particular outcome, the manager can help brainstorm a variety of ways to make progress. This coupled with reminding the worker of past successes in similar situations reinforces the two elements of hope.

Finally, managers need to help staff stay updated with the latest knowledge in the field. The consumer outcome objectives provide the connection to this part of directing staff. Our knowledge of effective interventions continues to grow albeit not as quickly as most of us would like. A management task is to stay updated on the latest research regarding what is working in the field and to use this information for program improvement. When a program is finding that the achievement of a particular outcome objective is not as good as desired and an effective intervention to achieve this outcome is identified, the manager facilitates workers who are acquiring the skills to carry out the new intervention and monitors the effect on the attainment of outcome objectives.

The Use of the Theory of Helping and Acquiring and Directing Staff

- *Expectations of staff are included in the job description.*
- *Expectations of staff and consumers are used in the job interview.*
- *Case review is used to talk about consumer progress toward achievement of outcomes.*
- *Case review is used to talk about what each person needs to do to achieve a particular outcome.*
- *Consumer outcomes identified in the program objectives are used to keep staff hopeful by brainstorming various ways to assist a consumer to achieve a particular outcome and by reminding staff of past successes.*
- *The social administrator continually looks for more effective interventions related to consumer outcomes and helps staff to acquire the needed skills.*

Acquiring and Using Resources Other Than Staff and the Theory of Helping

There are many types of resources that are required to operate a program. However, in this section we are concerned with those resources that focus on the transaction between the consumer and the worker. Perhaps the three most important resources in this regard are as follows:

1. Consumers who will benefit from the program.
2. Workers with the skills to perform as expected (discussed in the previous section).
3. Time for consumers and workers to do the work.

It may at first seem strange to think of consumers as a resource. However, without consumers or with consumers who cannot benefit from the service transaction, the program will not succeed. For example, consider a program that is created to help older youth in foster care to acquire skills to function in the community with the time parameters in the objectives established for youth of average intelligence. As long as this type of youth become consumers of the program, it has a reasonable chance of being successful. However, if the program experiences an influx of youth who are severely developmentally disabled, it is likely that the time parameters will not be met. There are a variety of actions that the administrator can take at this point. For example, she can change the time parameters, develop separate programs for these youth, or influence the referral sources to assure the program of youth who can benefit from the program. Each of these actions has consequences that the administrator must consider. For example, if the time parameters were changed, the program may require additional funds to serve each youth longer. If a separate program is established, the staff will require additional training. If the referral source is targeted to identify the most appropriate youth, how will the youth with developmental disabilities acquire the needed skills? The point here is not to evaluate the possible actions, their consequences, or trade-offs. The social administrator simply needs to keep in touch with consumers as resources, ensure that those who can benefit from the program are served, and take action when consumers change in ways that were not anticipated by the program.

The most important resource for achieving the desired results with consumers may be time. The youth in the previous example will acquire the skills needed to function in the community if they have the opportunity to perform the behavior as many times as required under the guidance of a knowledgeable and compassionate person. This takes time. If the program dictates that this learning takes place under the direction of a worker, then the worker needs to have the time to devote to the youth. This is obvious yet there are many demands on workers time. Staff meetings, paperwork, court appearances, training are just a few examples. Caseload sizes may be too large to allow the amount of time needed for each client.

It is the administrator's responsibility to assure that workers have the time to spend with consumers to achieve the desired outcomes. Worker time is a finite and precious resource. Typically workers only have about 37 hours per week to devote to their job. This means that all requests for meetings, training, paperwork, and so on should be evaluated by the administrator in terms of the time these activities will take away from consumers. It also means that administrators must be knowledgeable about the current demands on workers' time. Structuring the agency and its work so that workers have the time that they need with consumers is an important administrative task.

Facilitating Change By Using Persuasion and the Theory of Helping

It is easy to see from the outline of administrator responsibilities for acquiring and using information, acquiring and directing staff, acquiring and using resources other than staff that there are many opportunities to exercise influence to assure that the service transaction functions as intended. This section will present just a few examples to demonstrate ways of using the skills identified in Chapter 2. The examples are chosen to demonstrate the use of selected skills with workers, others in the agency, and those in the community. Recall that any change effort starts with the identification of the *person* to be influenced and the *behavior* desired of that person. In the press of everyday business, it is sometimes difficult to remember key concepts. Also recall that the change model used in this text is based on the idea that learning and growth occurs through consistent interactions between people. In other words, it is unlikely that any change will occur in a single meeting. Change requires persistence. The following examples will begin by identifying who the target of the change effort is and the behavior desired of this person.

Theory of Behavioral Intention

The current research on exercising influence indicates that a person is more likely to exhibit a behavior when

- *they perceive that they have behavioral control;*
- *they have a positive attitude toward the behavior;*
- *they feel that the behavior is normative; and*
- *they have the intention to perform the behavior.*

Worker Example

For the first example, consider the need for a worker to acquire a new skill to use with a consumer. The independent living program that has been mentioned finds that many youth require mental health services but are not using them despite the fact that they have financial access to services through Medicaid. The administrator discovers from informal sensing that staff are not comfortable talking with the youth about their potential need for mental health services. Consequently, workers *(person)* talking with youth about their need for mental health services *(behavior)* is the desired change. One reaction to this may be to send staff to training and in some situations this may be appropriate. However, in general, training is not sufficient and may be wasteful if the skills do not transfer to the job.

Chapter 2 identified four elements of exercising influence along with several strategies that can be used for each element. For the purposes of the examples presented here we will identify the person, the behavior, and selected strategies for each of these elements.

Enhanced perceived behavioral control, in this example, is the workers' belief that they can perform the behavior. Consequently, *behavioral rehearsal* and *modeling* are useful strategies. Whether these are done in a formal training event, a staff meeting, individual supervision, or most forcefully in the field, the desired behavior can be modeled by having someone with the skill role-play the desired conversation with the youth. This is followed by a discussion of the behavior that was demonstrated. *Behavioral rehearsal* can then follow by having each staff member practice the behavior. This practice is most effective when the worker receives feedback on their performance with verbal rewards for performing a behavior as intended and suggestions for how to do it differently the next time when the need for refinement of worker behavior is noted.

Enhancing the workers' attitude toward the behavior may be accomplished by talking with workers about *the advantages and rewards* to the youth for having the desired conversation. The realization that youth receiving needed services have fewer episodes of depression may lead workers to value the targeted behavior. *Enhancing this behavior as a norm* may be accomplished by having a youth who has been successful in acquiring this type of help speak with workers about the role of the worker in helping him or her acquire mental health services and the effect it has had on his or her life. This is the strategy identified as *linking the message to an important person.* Finally, helping the worker move from intention to behavior might be accomplished in a fairly straightforward manner by *enhancing the perceived relevance of the behavior* with statements such as "I know how much you want these youth to reach their goals and not having to deal with so many bouts of depression will really help them in their normal activities in the community."

This example may seem rather elaborate and complicated. It may be that in some contexts only a few of these strategies may be needed. However, in other contexts it is likely that all of these will be required. The key is sensing the degree to which staff require influence strategies and use the minimum necessary to produce the desired result. This requires administrators to know what is important to staff and to periodically check whether the desired behavior is occurring.

Agency Staff Example

For the agency example, consider that the director of the agency has weekly staff meetings for the purpose of reminding staff of important events that have occurred during the previous week. It is your judgment that these meetings are taking valuable time away from workers' interactions with consumers and that the information could be shared in a different manner. Consequently, the desired change is for the agency director *(person)* to distribute necessary information in a different manner and to cancel these meetings *(behavior)*.

Recall that strategies used to influence the director follow a four-prong approach. The idea of *perceived behavioral control* may be slightly different in this example. Recall that the research on persuasion defines this element as the belief that something exists that will make the behavior more or less difficult to perform. In the case of the worker trying out a new skill, the barrier may be the workers' perception of their ability to perform the task. In this case modeling and behavioral rehearsal may be the answer. In this case, the administrator may not know exactly what the director believes exists that would make canceling the meetings difficult. Consequently, the administrator may select the strategy *of removing obstacles* by meeting with the director and seeking clarification of the purposes of the meeting and brainstorming other ways to accomplish the director's goals.

The director's *attitude toward the new behavior* (canceling the meetings) is likely to be an important factor in his decision. The administrator may select the strategy of *adding a new reason to think positively about the behavior.* To carry this out the administrator will *emphasize the advantages and rewards* for canceling the meetings including workers spending more time with consumers, consumers being more satisfied with their time with workers, and consumers achieving more of their goals. The administrator will also *show compatibility of values* by reminding the director that consumers are more likely to achieve their goals when they spend time with workers and consumer goal attainment has always been something that the director has valued.

To address the *normative component,* the administrator might try *linking the message to an important person* by talking about the importance of consumer goal attainment to the funding agency. Finally, to help *move from intention to behavior* the administrator might *remind the director of previous support* for the importance of workers' time with consumers. The implication here that may not need to be stated is that not canceling the meeting would be inconsistent with this previously stated value. Recall from Chapter 2 that when using *cognitive dissonance* you only want to offer enough incentive to induce compliance and let dissonance reduction do the rest.

This example, like the first one, may seem overly complicated. It was developed to follow what is known about persuasion as presented in Chapter 2. When learning techniques of persuasion, it is important to think about each element and the accompanying strategies. As one becomes more comfortable with these types of interactions, the selection and use of strategies becomes more natural. In this example, it is possible that all or most of the strategies will be used in a single meeting with the director and will not be presented in the discrete linear fashion presented here. They will simply all become part of the conversation.

Community Example

For the community example, consider the independent living program example where there are an increasing number of youth coming to the program with severe developmental disabilities. The change is directed at the child welfare agency director *(person)* and having him agree to continue to refer youth who are not developmentally disabled or agree to fund a program for this special population *(behavior).*

Similar to the example with the agency director, it is unlikely that the administrator knows enough about the child welfare agency director to use a strategy such as modeling for *enhancing perceived behavioral control.* So *obstacle removal* is chosen as a useful strategy for at least the initial meeting. This meeting will be devoted to identifying the obstacles to referring youth who can benefit from the program and brainstorming with the child welfare director about ways to remove these obstacles. *Inducements and rewards* may also play a role. When an idea that appears to be promising is generated for removing obstacles, the administrator can remind the child welfare director of the rewards for adopting this approach and possibly provide an inducement by volunteering to do some of the required work. For example, perhaps one of the ideas for removing an obstacle is to involve the agency responsible for funding programs for people with developmental disabilities in conversations about their responsibility for these youth. The administrator may volunteer to locate the best person in the agency and initiate the call to set up the meeting.

To enhance the child welfare director's *attitude toward changing* the pattern of referrals the administrator might *add a reason to think positively about the behavior* by *citing proven results* and *showing compatibility of values*. The proven results in this case are the outcomes for those youth who have been involved in the administrator's program. The need for information about outcomes for consumers as identified in the program's goals and objectives has been discussed and here is another use for this information. Showing compatibility of values may be as simple as reminding the child welfare director that you both highly value the goal of youth exiting the child welfare system with the skills needed to function in the community.

Changing or reinforcing the *normative component* in this example is *linking the message to a new important person*. The administrator has developed a relationship with an advocate for persons with developmental disabilities, who is widely respected within the community. In meetings with the child welfare director, the administrator reminds him or her that this advocate knows about this particular problem and is very interested in being of assistance. Finally, to help *move from intention to behavior,* the administrator uses the strategy of *encouraging anticipation of feelings*. In this case, this means reminding the child welfare director of how good it will feel to know that all youth, including those with developmental disabilities, are acquiring the necessary skills. Do not forget the role of persistence. This problem is not likely to be solved quickly or easily. The accomplishment of the desired change will require multiple interactions with the child welfare director over time.

SUMMARY

This chapter presented the theory of helping as the "heart" of the program framework. The theory of helping consists of the consumer outcome goal, the accompanying consumer outcome objectives, and the expectations of those involved in the helping transaction (workers and consumers). There are specific criteria for each component of the theory that results in a consistent and coherent explanation of how consumers are to benefit from the program. The link between the theory of helping and management behavior was presented through consideration of acquiring and using information, acquiring and using staff and other resources. Finally, application of the change model in Chapter 2 is used to demonstrate how managers can use it to improve outcomes for consumers.

Chapter 5

Program Framework:
The Rest of the Story

Chapters 3 and 4 have identified elements of the social program framework along with examples of how managers use them to maximize benefits
for consumers. First we considered the social problem and its consequences
to society and to consumers. This was followed by an analysis of who
would become the intended beneficiary of the program. Chapter 4 described the theory of intention. This includes the consumer outcome goal of
the program, the consumer outcome objectives that are said to lead to the
goal being achieved, and the expectations of workers and consumers that
will result in the objectives being achieved. That is only part of the story.
This chapter presents the remaining elements of the program management
framework and examples of how these are used by social administrators. The
program framework elements are as follows:

- The stages of helping
- Key actors required for the consumer benefit
- The helping environment
- Emotional responses
- Actual helping behaviors

Program Framework Learning Objectives—Part 3

- *Identify the stages of the helping transaction and describe them for an example program.*
- *Identify the key actors required for the success of consumers and their minimal
  behavioral requirements and apply this to an example program.*

Textbook of Social Administration: The Consumer-Centered Approach
© 2007 by The Haworth Press, Inc. All rights reserved.
doi:10.1300/5802_06

- *Describe the environmental characteristics of the helping transaction that contribute to consumer success.*
- *Describe the emotional responses of consumers that are most likely and the appropriate worker response.*
- *Describe the emotional responses of workers that are most likely and the appropriate responses by co-workers and supervisors.*
- *Write a rich multilayered description of the helping transaction.*
- *Identify ways to use the program elements presented in this chapter to acquire and use information, to acquire and direct staff, to acquire and use resources other than staff and to facilitate change by using persuasion.*

STAGES OF HELPING

Many services can be seen as progressing through a sequence of steps. The sequence is influenced by administrative rules and regulations, professional training, the client experience, and the nature and design of the intervention. In some service sectors, regulations greatly influence the steps. For example, under most state Medicaid plans, a treatment plan must be completed within thirty days of a mental health client being admitted for service. Most states child welfare policy requires that a permanency planning goal for children under care must be established within a certain number of days.

Many interventions prescribe the nature of events, timing, and sequence. It is likely that evidence-based interventions specify the key events and their sequencing in their manuals. For example, the Individual Placement and Support Model (IPS) of supported employment requires a highly focused assessment, then quickly moves to job development and employer contact within thirty days of intake (Becker & Drake, 2003). The client experience often shapes the rhythm of services. Services for homeless individuals often require extended periods of engagement activities to overcome the alienation and lack of trust that many of these individuals possess.

Failure to follow the stages of helping has led to ineffectiveness and, at times, harm to clients. In mental health, transitional employment programs (TEP) were designed so that a person with psychiatric disabilities would work at a job with a job coach for up to six months. At that time, the consumer was to move to a regular competitive job. Often, however, the persons would be deemed "not ready" or the persons themselves became so comfortable in the TEP job that they were allowed to continue (sometimes for multiple times). Most of these people never moved to competitive employment, the goal of the program.

Day programs for people with psychiatric disabilities were designed to teach skills needed to live in communities and to provide opportunities for socialization. Day programs were to be transitional. Yet many consumers of these programs would spend years (and in some cases the better part of their lives) in these daily activities. The research suggests that day treatment programs rarely contribute to employment, community integration, or recovery.

The stages of helping section describes the "usual" or anticipated process for a complete episode of service. Every helping transaction has a beginning, middle, and end. Although much of the real-world service delivery is not linear, this process assists managers, workers, and consumers to stay focused on their goal. A description of a service stage usually includes key activities for each helping phase, the length of the phases, the result of each phase, and key decision points. The most common and generic formulation is assessment, case or intervention planning or contracting (including goal settings), intervention, and evaluation. Unfortunately, this breakdown is not very descriptive of any specific service, and the categories, especially intervention, are probably too broad. The manager should use labels that are tailored to his or her service. Some examples of stages of helping are included in Exhibit 5.1.

EXHIBIT 5.1. Examples of Stages of Helping

Strength Model Case Management

  Engagement: Beginning the Partnership
  Strength Assessment: Amplifying the Well Part of the Individual
  Personal Planning: Creating the Achievement Agenda
  Resource Acquisition: Putting Community Back into Community
    Mental Health
  Graduated Disengagement (Rapp & Goscha, 2006)

Harm Reduction Program for People with HIV Who Abuse Drugs:

  Getting to Know Each Other (engagement and assessment)
  Consciousness Raising (pre-contemplation)
  Decision-making Phase (contemplation)
  Preparation Phase
  Implementation (action)
  Maintenance (gradual disengagement)

Victim–Offender Mediation Program

  Screening Session
  Victim–Offender Conference and Mediation Phase
  Establishment of Mutual Contract
  Contract Compliance Monitoring
  Contract Completion

It is important to define a result or culminating event for each stage so that both worker and client will know when they are ready to move on. Results could be a signed contract, a decision (e.g., a psychosocial club member takes an in-house work position), a completed assessment report, a client's satisfactory performance level, or a time limit (e.g., after three months, contract renegotiation will occur).

KEY PEOPLE REQUIRED FOR THE CONSUMER TO BENEFIT: WHO NEEDS TO DO WHAT?

The emphasis in this book has been on the transaction between the worker and the consumer. This service transaction is viewed as the most important interaction in the agency or program. Yet any experienced social worker understands that there are many people who contribute to the success or failure of the consumer. Consider the following examples.

A consumer with a psychiatric disability works with a social worker to obtain a part time job. Occasionally this consumer has brief periods of anxiety that make it impossible for him to concentrate. He has learned that if he can be allowed to take a break and perform some type of physical exercise, the anxiety is reduced and he can return to work. The social worker goes with the consumer to job interviews and assists in explaining this type of accommodation. For the consumer to be successful in keeping a job the employer needs to agree to allow him to work off the anxiety attacks. In return the consumer will tell his supervisor when he needs to leave the job and when he returns.

A child welfare caseworker is working with a mother who is in recovery from substance abuse. The worker and mother have agreed that it is time for her children to return home for an extended trial visit. The worker and the mother are concerned that the stress of caring for the children might trigger a relapse episode. The mother has agreed to attend daily sessions at the treatment program for at least two weeks to discuss with staff the stress of parenting and appropriate responses. Treatment staff agreed to call the caseworker immediately if the mother missed an appointment or needed relief from parenting.

A school social worker and a chronically truant thirteen-year-old girl have a goal of increasing daily attendance. As part of the plan a retired social worker in the girl's neighborhood has agreed to go to the girl's house every morning for a month and walk with her to school. The volunteer has agreed to talk with the girl about some of the positive things that the girl is doing including school attendance. The volunteer has agreed to call the school social worker immediately if the girl refuses to go to school.

It is clear from these examples that the success of many consumers is linked to other people who are central to the service transaction. These people must know their role and willingly perform it for the consumer to have a chance at success. Although this is widely recognized in practice, it is seldom an explicit element of program management. The program framework calls for recognition of these key actors and the behavior required of them to contribute to consumer success. It is simply impossible for managers to influence action that produces outcomes without knowledge of that behavior.

In this area the manager must answer the following three questions.

1. Who are the people other than the worker and the consumer who are required for successful outcome attainment?
2. What is the minimum set of behaviors that each of these people must consistently perform for the consumer to achieve desired outcomes?
3. How will these behaviors be elicited and maintained?

Who Are the People Other Than the Worker Who Are Required for Successful Outcome Attainment?

In the examples at the beginning of this section the key actors are obvious. For the mental health consumer to maintain a job, the employer is a key person. For the recovering mother, the substance abuse counselor is essential, and for the chronic truant it is the volunteer. These examples are not meant to be all encompassing, so these are not likely to be the only key actors. However, it is easy to see the connection between the consumer outcome and the behavior of other people.

For a particular consumer and a particular outcome there is likely to be a key actor who cannot be foreseen in a program framework. However, most key actors are obvious with patterns of similar actors across consumers of a program. These are the key actors to be identified and are of concern to management. Many of these key actors can be identified through evidence-based interventions. Another way to think about this is to take each outcome objective and consider who might be required to assure that consumers will achieve that outcome. Another way to identify key actors is to think about the systems that the consumer is involved with, including their friends, family, and community contacts. In addition, think about key actors who may be within the program agency and those in the broader community.

One danger with this exercise is the tendency to list more people than absolutely necessary. So now that you have identified a list of key actors, prune it to only those who are *absolutely necessary.*

For example, Henggeler, Schoenwald, Borduin, Rowland, and Cunningham (1998) identify seven overlapping ecological environments that are important to include when implementing Multisystemic Treatment (MST) for maintaining children and adolescents with antisocial behavior safely within the community. These begin with the child's caregiver and siblings and move out to extended family, peers, neighborhoods, school, provider agency, and community (p. 14). For the children involved in this program to be successful, key people within each of these environments must be included in the intervention. Key actors within the school are likely to be the teacher, principal, and social worker. There are other people within the school who may be useful to the worker and/or child, but the three identified as key actors are absolutely necessary.

MST is a complex and inclusive program but then so are the lives and challenges of these children. Other program models are likely to have fewer key actors. However, the explicit recognition of the seven ecological environments is a useful tool for other programs.

Identifying Key Actors

- *Check evidence-based practice manuals.*
- *Examine each program objective and think about who is required to participate with the consumer to assure successful attainment of the outcomes.*
- *Think about the consumers' social systems including friends, family, and other community contacts.*
- *Think about people with the program agency who are required for consumer success.*
- *Think about community agencies and systems and people within them who are required to assure successful consumers.*
- *Eliminate from the list all of those who are not absolutely necessary to assure consumer success.*

What Is the Minimum Set of Behaviors That Each of These People Must Consistently Perform for the Consumer to Achieve Desired Outcomes?

The examples at the beginning of this section demonstrate minimum behaviors for each of the key actors. The employer is asked to agree to allow the consumer to leave his job and work off the energy associated with increased anxiety. The volunteer who is going to walk the thirteen-year-old girl to school is asked to do just that: talk with her about school successes and call the school social worker if she refuses to go to school. The substance abuse counselor is asked to do a bit more, in that daily sessions are thought to be necessary for a two-week period. In addition, the counselor is asked to call the caseworker if the mother does not show up for an appointment. In each case it is not difficult to identify additional behaviors that might be helpful. However, are they absolutely necessary? It is sufficiently difficult for social workers to elicit the behavior of key actors without making the job more difficult by extending the list.

Behavior of Key Actors

What behavior is necessary for the consumer to achieve the outcome?
Is this behavior absolutely necessary for the consumer to achieve the desired outcome?

An example of the key actors together with the required behavior and ways to elicit this behavior for a case management program designed to prevent elderly from entering nursing home care is presented in Table 5.1. Notice how extensive the list becomes for what might otherwise be thought of as a fairly simple program. The last column of the table identifies ideas for eliciting the desired behavior. The consumer goal is not likely to be achieved unless everyone plays a role. Workers and supervisors need to know what that role (behavior) is and how to help everyone accomplish it. Consequently, managers need to consider how they might elicit the desired behavior from key actors.

How Will Key Actor Minimum Behaviors Be Elicited and Maintained?

The first two steps of identifying the key actors and the specific behaviors are starting points for eliciting and maintaining these behaviors. It is likely that some of the behavior of key actors will occur without prompting or encouragement. In many cases it may only be necessary to talk to a key actor about what is expected (behaviorally) of them. There are some formal

TABLE 5.1. Key Actors, Required Behavior, and Ideas for Eliciting the Behavior

Key Actors	Behavior Required	How to Elicit Behavior
Area Agency on Aging Employees (AAA)		
1. Information and Referral Workers 2. Congregate and Home Delivered Meals Workers 3. Senior Center Workers	1. Refer clients to program 2. Encourage and counsel clients 3. Deliver nutritionist meals on a timely basis 4. Furnish recreational, education, social events 5. Accept referrals from program	1. Educate and inform workers about program 2. Give out written materials about program 3. Initiate and maintain contact with program supervisors in writing, in person, phone calls, and interagency meetings.
Social and Rehabilitation Services (SRS) Employees		
1. Social Workers 2. Income Maintenance 3. Administrators	1. Help clients receive financial assistance for food, medical insurance, and home health, respite 2. Deliver homemaker, personal care attendant 3. Accept referrals for income eligible clients	1. Maintain continual contact in writing, through phone, in person, and interagency meetings 2. Inform them of client's needs 3. Bargain and negotiate on behalf of client
Home Health/Hospice Workers		
1. Nurses 2. Occupational 3. Physical Therapists 4. Nutritionist 5. Social Workers	1. Refer clients to program 2. Inform and discuss client status, progress 3. Recommend changes needed in services for clients 4. Accept referrals for program	1. Set monthly meetings to discuss shared clients, potential new clients 2. Record meetings 3. At interagency meetings plan, write and implement recommendations that address service problems at local, state, federal levels
Hospitals		
1. Doctors 2. Medical Professionals 3. Social Workers	1. Encourage clients to pursue program 2. Report patient progress with Coordinator 3. Help patients live in a non-medical facility through home-based technology, education, medicines	1. Educate doctors and discharge planners about program 2. Maintain contact with resident's medical professionals 3. Work with medical professionals making the home adaptable to medical needs.
Homemakers/Personal Care Attendants/Respite Workers/Volunteers		
1. AAA 2. SRA 3. Home Health Agencies 4. Private 5. Nonprofits	1. Report changes in behavior, emotions, and physical health 2. Demonstrate a caring, respectful attitude 3. Deliver services as agreed upon in contract	1. Request monthly feedback regarding their observations of resident 2. Periodically observe and/or participate in person with duties of contracted parties 3. Invite participation in the interagency meetings

administrative mechanisms for identifying and eliciting the behavior. These include

- interagency agreements;
- a purchase of service contract;
- joint training of staff; and
- a pilot test of a new program.

In some cases influencing a key actor to elicit the behavior may require a carefully planned effort using the model of persuasion identified in Chapter 2. The key actor is the person and the behavior is the desired response. Recall that the model suggests that action *(key actor behavior)* is preceded by intention to act, which is linked to perceived behavioral control, attitude, and norms. Whether the key actor behavior is elicited by the worker or the manager, either directly or through one of the administrative mechanisms, change strategies need to be selected to target each of these elements.

For example, the child welfare program manager has foreseen the need for brief periods of intensive contact between recovering mothers and substance abuse counselors at the time of trial home placement of children. The child welfare program manager approaches the administrator of the substance abuse agency with a request for an interagency agreement that includes the provision of intensive services for a four-week period following trial reunification of children with recovering mothers. The manager prepares for a series of meetings regarding the agreement by identifying persuasion strategies to enhance behavioral control, increase the administrators positive attitude toward the behavior, enhance the normative importance of the behavior, and move from attitude to behavior.

Behavioral control is not seen as a large consideration since the substance abuse administrator's desired behavior is not complex. However, the child welfare manager reminds herself not to use high-pressure tactics and to attempt to use inducements and rewards to the substance abuse agency for signing this agreement. Since her budget is limited, the child welfare manager cannot offer to pay for the services and decides to emphasize the rewards that will come to the substance abuse agency from the community's recognition of their role in helping reunite children and recovering parents.

The child welfare manager decides to place a great deal of emphasis on increasing the substance abuse program administrator's attitude toward the behavior. The administrator is known for his commitment toward recovering people leading normal lives in the community, so the manager thinks that she only needs to remind him of the advantages of participating in the agreement, show how this is compatible with his values, and identify the positive consequences of signing the agreement. The manager is also prepared to increase the normative component by telling the administrator that the juvenile judge thinks it is important for recovering mothers to have intensive services for a brief period following trial reunification. Lastly, the child welfare manager decides to use encouragement of anticipation of feelings as a means to increase the administrator's move from intention to behavior. This is a short example of a potentially long and involved process. Recall that change requires persistence and the use of multiple strategies.

THE HELPING ENVIRONMENT

Social work has long recognized the importance of the environment to the behavior and functioning of people. Notice your behavior when you enter a classroom. Where you sit and what you do while in this environment is the product of many similar events that have taken place over your lifetime. In child welfare, there is a great deal of emphasis on parents (usually mothers) visiting with their children who are placed in foster care. Think about this visit in different environments and the difference it might make to the mother and the child. How might the parent and child's behavior be different if the visit took place in the child welfare office, the foster family's home, the parents' home, the park, or at the school that the child attends?

From the bioecological perspective people learn, change, and grow through regular interactions over time with other people, objects, and symbols in a particular environment (Bronfenbrenner, 1995a). The social work theory of helping specifies the expectations of consumers and workers including the frequency of their interactions. Specifying the helping environment includes the other people, objects, and symbols that are a part of the helping transaction and facilitate learning and growth for consumers and workers.

The description of the setting specifies those characteristics that will enhance accessibility and/or the reciprocal interaction between consumers and workers that ultimately leads to the client outcome. A service setting is the typical situation, both physical and social, in which interactions take place. The physical situation may be the counselor's office, a street corner, or the client's apartment for case management; a work site for job training; or the offices of a community agency for an advocacy service. Particular requirements for space, privacy, or comfort for people with disabilities are clearly indicated. For recreational/socialization programs, it is considered important to have an environment that offers materials to stimulate participation and interaction. Privacy is essential for some programs, but openness and accessibility may be equally essential for others. Organizing tenants in a low-income neighborhood, or a social activity program for people with psychiatric disabilities, are examples.

The social aspects of the service setting are as important as the physical aspects. How many people are usually present? What is the symbolic value of the location or the situation for different participants? Is it desirable that the setting be the client's "turf" or the worker's? Setting the stage for client–worker interaction includes defining values, goals, or purposes as much as adjusting the lights or closing the door.

Special features of the program that facilitate access should also be described. Will transportation be provided? What times and days will the service be available? Will child care arrangements be offered? Access is influenced by these physical factors and by social factors. Will the workers be of the same racial or ethnic group as the consumer? How will consumers in a waiting room be made comfortable? In small rural areas, people may be embarrassed to be seen entering a mental health clinic or a child welfare office. Could there be an entrance that is not visible from the street? Could the service be offered in a different setting, such as a library?

Some service events might take place in an office, some in another agency, some in a courthouse, and some in the home of the consumer. Environments affect behavior, so it is worth the time and effort to try to create the best conditions for the consumer in these settings. For example, if a social worker sees the need for a child friendly room in the courthouse to minimize the stress to children who need to be present, discussion of this with the juvenile judge may produce a positive result. Here again is a perfect place to use the skills of change and influence to create the best possible environments.

Another environment is the community. Outreach modes of service delivery offer notable benefits and downsides. The benefits include easier access for clients and higher probabilities of clients continuing in service. The research on Assertive Community Treatment has found a retention rate of over 80 percent for a year. In contrast, traditional (site-based services) seldom exceed 50 percent retention rate for even six months (Axelrod & Wetzler, 1989; Bond, McGrew, & Fekete, 1995).

Assessment is often enhanced when it occurs in the places where clients spend their lives (e.g., home, classroom, work). In an office setting, the worker's sources of information are limited to what the client says, how he or she behaves, and perhaps what is contained in the case record. Since a client's behavior in an office is likely to be different than behavior in other settings, it may not be a good reflection of relevant client behavior. A worker can learn much from experiencing a person's home, and this knowledge can provide leads to effective helping.

After a few months, a case manager was invited to meet with a client in the client's home. When the case manager was invited into the homes, he noticed right away a large bookcase in the living room had hunks of dried mud and rocks on every shelf. The case manager asked the consumer, "Jim," to tell him about the items on the bookcase. Jim explained he enjoyed going to the river and finding rocks and fossils. The case manager listened and learned about Jim's interest while observing that Jim became more animated as he talked about the rocks and fossils. The case manager asked Jim how he knew so much about the subject. Jim replied he'd picked it up by spending time at the river and remembering what he had learned in a high school science class. The case manager asked Jim if he would be interested in finding out more about this interest. Jim replied, "Yes." The community Jim lived in had a university. The case manager assisted Jim in securing a scholarship to take a geology class. Jim enjoyed the class immensely and signed up for more classes on geology. Eventually Jim was hired by the university to classify rocks and minerals. (Rapp and Goscha, 2006, p. 108)

Another strength of an outreach mode of service delivery concerns effectiveness of teaching skills. People often have difficulty transferring skills learned from one setting to another. For example, parents who learn noncorporal forms of discipline in a classroom are often challenged to implement those procedures in their home. People with developmental disabilities who are learning how to cook spaghetti for four people on an electric stove may find it perplexing to prepare spaghetti for one on a gas stove. Teaching skills in the environment and under the conditions in which people have to perform them is more effective.

Although these are powerful reasons to consider an outreach mode of service delivery, there are some downsides. People's homes can be wrought with distractions, including television, children, visitors, and so on. A quiet place to do work may be difficult to find. If the worker uses a vehicle emblazoned with the agency's name, the client could feel embarrassed and stigmatized. Worker safety becomes a major concern. Lastly, outreach can be more expensive for the agency, especially in sparsely populated rural areas.

___

Key Questions for Specifying the Helping Environment

1. *What will occur in the environment that supports the consumer outcome objectives?*
2. *What are the various environments where service transactions will take place?*

3. What is the probable symbolic impact of each environment on consumers' behavior?
4. What characteristics of the environments, both physical and symbolic, need to be present or absent to make it accessible and comfortable for consumers?
5. Who needs to be present or absent from the helping transaction?
6. What objects are essential to include in the environments to facilitate the helping transaction?
7. What symbols should be included in the environments to facilitate the helping transaction?

EMOTIONAL RESPONSES

Every social worker has experienced emotional reactions while working with a consumer. Many of these responses are predictable and are a normal part of these highly charged situations. Both workers and consumers experience emotional reactions. Most workers have experienced responding emotionally in ways that help the client and in ways that do not. In other words, most of us make mistakes. Yet this emotional component of the helping transaction is seldom considered by those who develop or manage social programs.

The emotional responses of consumers and workers are crucial to the achievement of outcome objectives. Although we do not know of any research that explicitly links emotional reactions to a particular consumer outcome, this is probably due to lack of research attention rather than lack of impact. It is difficult to imagine a child welfare worker being successful in returning a child home to his or her parent without explicitly talking about the emotions that were part of the separation and return. It is difficult to imagine a mental health worker successfully working with a person with a psychiatric disability without talking about the emotions that accompany auditory hallucinations. Community support program work requires intensive personal involvement on the part of both consumers and workers. Consumers can become frustrated in their efforts to survive in a complex social and work environment with limited adaptive skills. Workers often face the disappointment of slow progress or regression.

The tasks here are first to identify the emotions that are most likely to be experienced by consumers and specify the most helpful response by the worker to these emotions. Second, one needs to identify the emotions likely to be experienced by the worker and the accompanying response. How will the worker respond to the identified emotions? What provisions will be made to help workers—supervision, team interventions, support groups, training? A few examples from actual program descriptions should make the point clear. A more complete example is included in the program description at the end of this chapter.

In socialization training for severely physically handicapped children workers need to be hopeful and firm with reasonable expectations. Feelings of pity should not play a part in working with these children. Handicapped children, it would seem, cannot possibly incorporate acceptable performance standards unless they experience the existence of these standards, and their own experience in meeting them again and again.

In family counseling where social workers are seeing several family members together and there is severe family conflict, it is not reasonable to expect that a series of emotional sessions could be held without affecting everyone involved. It might be important that workers make clear both before the session begins and during it, the nature of these emotional reactions and the appropriate response by everyone who is part of the sessions. It is also important for the worker to have specific guidance on handling her/his emotions both during and after these sessions.

Another example is from a program for severely disabled or terminally ill clients. Social workers, especially those who have not had to come to terms with their own mortality and frailty, find it threatening and disabling to talk frankly with consumers about death. Elderly terminally ill clients often talk in detail about the arrangements for their funeral or how their personal goods should be distributed among children. The worker may find this discussion sad and feel that the consumers should not discuss their own impending death in such fashion because it is "giving up."

Key Questions for Specifying Emotional Responses

- *What are the most common emotional reactions of consumers?*
- *What has been found to be the most effective worker responses to these emotions?*
- *What are the most common emotional responses of workers to the helping transaction?*
- *What has been found to be the most effective way to help workers with these emotions?*

THE ACTUAL HELPING BEHAVIORS

Complete description of any complex phenomenon is impossible. However, we can examine a phenomenon from a variety of perspectives, thus increasing our insight and understanding. Imagine a large Victorian house sitting in the middle of a city block, obscured by a tall fence. The grandeur and intricacy of the house cannot be seen from any one perspective. By approaching the fence and viewing the house from each available knot hole or break in the fence, however, one obtains a variety of views of the house. A rather complete description is obtained from the totality of the perspectives. A social program is equally complex. Specifying the various elements of the program framework gives multiple and partial views of the intervention. Although we specified behaviors when we identified expectations, this was a minimal list of behaviors. This final component of the program framework takes another look at the helping transaction and attempts to describe in more detail the richness of the endeavor. This normally includes representative and observable behaviors of both workers and clients. This rich narrative description of the most essential elements of the service transaction provides workers and others with a virtual movie of these events that may come alive in ways that specifying behaviors and outcomes does not.

Although a behavioral description is difficult, certain patterns of communication, of conduct, and typical actions can be identified. The frequent use of examples of interactions may be the most efficient means of describing these behaviors. The worker in a day treatment facility may physically restrain a client who is violent so that neither may be injured. The client in a sheltered workshop will become better groomed, will report promptly for work, and will perform assigned tasks. The group therapist may shout and show anger in repudiating antisocial activities. The caseworker with a rape victim will listen closely to her; will exhibit warm, supportive behavior; will be factual; and will not destroy evidence. A staff member working with a mental hospital resident who is preparing to go into the community will sit next to the resident at lunch and provide prompts and feedback when the person habitually rearranges food on a plate before eating.

Just as in the case of identifying key actors, the program manager must think about the behaviors that are essential to the success of the consumer and the program. Those behaviors should be summarized, outlined, or illustrated by an example. The following is an example of a parent education class that is part of a child welfare intervention.

This example focuses on the session that explores the communication skills of exploring alternatives, problem ownership, and I-messages—all of which are important skills for parents to master in order to use positive behavior management. By this point in the series of classes, the participants will be accustomed to the routine of the classes, and they should be seeing some changes in their own and their children's behavior.

Dinner is over and the two child care volunteers for the evening have arrived. The Parent Educator, with the help of one of the mothers and her eleven-year-old daughter, moves the dining tables out of the way and arranges fifteen chairs in a circle with the flip-chart placed just outside the circle. The participants begin to arrive in the dining room, bringing their workbooks, pads, and pens. Several of the participants carry coffee cups, which they fill on their way to take seats. The Parent Educator greets each participant by name and chats informally with various members of the class. By 7:00 p.m., all of the participants have taken seats.

The format for the class will be a few minutes of checking in with participants to see if there are pressing parenting concerns that the Parent Educator needs to incorporate into the presentation and discussion; a discussion of the previous week's homework to reinforce the concepts learned last time; presentation of new material through discussion and role-play; discussion of the practice exercises for the coming week; and a summary of the content presented.

The Parent Educator begins the session by greeting the group and referring to the flip-chart on which are listed the main topic and objectives for the evening. She opens the discussion by asking participants how parenting has gone for them since the last class. Since all of the participants have experience with the self-disclosure that is demanded by treatment for substance abuse, participants are open to participating in the group by sharing their personal experiences. Several participants briefly describe problems they encountered with their children and one participant tells of a positive experience she had with trying something discussed the week before. The Parent Educator listens reflectively to the participants' concerns and describes how each of them illustrates a concept from an earlier class or may be related to the topics for the evening. It is important that the Parent Educator blends participants' immediate parenting needs with the material she plans to present and that she lets participants know their concerns will be addressed further. Participants who share during this time receive positive feedback from the Parent Educator for their efforts and for contributing to the group.

Next the Parent Educator asks what experiences participants had with the homework assignment from the week before, which helped to practice reflective listening. Again, several participants discuss their experiences and the Parent Educator praises them for their efforts. When participants ask questions during this portion of the class, the Parent Educator refrains from putting herself in the position of expert but instead asks the group for solutions. This reinforces that the members of the group have a great deal of knowledge and experience in parenting themselves. When solutions to problems come from the group itself, participants see their peers and themselves as more capable.

In introducing the new material for the evening, the Parent Educator uses a variety of techniques. First she asks the group what they think exploring alternatives might mean. Some of the participants may have read the material in their workbooks prior to the class, although there is no expectation that they will have, and they may volunteer what is meant by exploring alternatives. The Parent Educator develops the idea of exploring alternatives, explains how to use the method, and offers examples. To stimulate discussion, she asks the group questions, such as why a parent would want to use exploring alternatives.

After having explained the concepts the session focuses on, the teacher leads the group through exercises in exploring alternatives, using I-messages, and determining who owns a problem. The Parent Educator structures activities taking into account that individuals in the group have different learning styles, choosing exercises that involve participants in hearing, speaking, reading, and writing. The Parent Educator role-plays several situations with different participants, each time asking the other participants to watch for certain behaviors. Following each role-play, the Parent Educator asks those who had roles to describe what it felt like to be that person in that situation. Frequently throughout the presentation, the Parent Educator invites participants to ask questions.

When all new material has been presented, the Parent Educator summarizes the major points of the material, then turns the group's attention to the homework exercise. The Parent Educator reads aloud and explains the instructions for the exercise and asks participants to think about a particular time they will try the exercise with their children.

The session ends on time and the Parent Educator thanks all participants for their participation and hard work. Some of the mothers linger and talk for a few minutes, while others go get their children from the playroom. By 9:15, all of the mothers have taken their children from the playroom. The Parent Educator thanks the child care volunteers and asks them how the evening went for them. It is important that the Parent Educator give the volunteers positive feedback for their work with the children and that she make sure the volunteers feel they can handle the children. If there are situations that the volunteers feel they are unable to handle, the Parent Educator will schedule a training session to improve the volunteers' skills and confidence. (modified from Rapp & Poertner, 1992, pp. 84-85)

CREATING ATTRACTIVE PROGRAMS

We have now completed the elements of the program framework. A concern that cuts across all elements of the program is its attractiveness to consumers. Many of our social programs are perceived by many of the people they are designed to aid as unattractive; something to shun or avoid. The reasons are complex. Anger, fear, and embarrassment are easy to see in social services that restrict freedom and choice such as child protective services, parole services, and various total care services such as nursing homes, psychiatric hospitals, or residential treatment. The stigma that accompanies receipt of many social services can be a powerful deterrent.

People we seek to serve often lack hope or self-confidence. The oppression of their lives causes a fatalism that would make service receipt a waste of time and effort. The people live in fear. Attribution of "failure" is often directed to personal deficiency of a generalized and enduring nature: "I am weak," "I am sick."

Professional practice can be hope inducing but can also be spirit breaking. For example, people with psychiatric disabilities confront a life replete with macro- and micro-aggressions to the human spirit. Macro-aggressions include the use of restraints and isolation rooms, or being forced into a police car for transport to the hospital or jail, or the use of payeeships. These are similar to the methods used by repressive governments to break the spirit of political dissidents. Micro-aggression refers to the messages covered in the myriad of interactions that people who receive services have with providers and others. In so many ways, the mental health system has institutionalized low expectations and blame for failure. Although micro-aggressions are more subtle than macro-aggressions, they are as powerful and pernicious in breaking the human spirit.

At times, our programs are not aligned with the goals of our clients. A person who wants a job working with animals is forced to devote several weeks to "vocational testing" to identify the type of job they would be "good at." A person with psychiatric disabilities wants to be a "better mother" but is prescribed excessive amounts of medication that saps her energy and makes her only want to sleep. An elderly person wants to remain at home with the necessary assistance but instead efforts are made to place her in a nursing home because the assistance is not obviously available. A homeless person with a serious substance abuse problem wants a place to live but is told he must stop using substance first or get into a program.

There are other reasons including that the program is inconvenient (time, place, etc.), or language and ethnic barriers. Social programs should be designed to be as attractive as possible to the clients we seek to serve. Programs should be *convenient* as to location, time, and sensitive to transportation. The *environment* should be welcoming and comfortable. Services should maximize *client choice* by expanding options and the client's authority to choose among the options. Services should seek to minimize unwanted intrusiveness. The services should be *respectful* of cultural difference and seek to be compatible with the client's culture. Clients should be given *roles in improving* the services. This could involve client focus groups and program evaluation, members of governing or advisory boards, assuming staff roles, or acting as role models and mentors for current clients. The *staff* is the most important dimension. They need to be courteous, respectful, compassionate, and competent; always putting the client first and seeking to improve their own skills.

Creating Attractive Programs

- *Consider convenience as to*
  Location
  Time
  Transportation
- *Consider the environment*
  Welcoming
  Comfortable
- *Consider consumer choice*
  Expand options
  Roles for consumers within the program
- *Consider cultural differences*
- *Consider staff*
  Courteous and respectful
  Compassionate
  Competent
  Consumer first orientation
  Learning for a living

EXAMPLES OF SOCIAL ADMINISTRATORS' USE OF PROGRAM ELEMENTS TO ENHANCE CONSUMER BENEFITS

Some applications of the change model to the program elements included in this chapter are obvious. Some examples were included as the program framework elements were presented in the chapter (i.e., key actors). This section will present selected examples from the four program framework elements defined in this chapter. Consistent with Chapters 3 and 4 and this text's management model, we present examples of the use of these design elements linked to the management areas that are essential skill areas for social administrators.

- Acquiring and using information
- Acquiring and directing staff
- Acquiring and using resources other than staff

Acquiring and Using Information and Key People Required to Produce Consumer Benefits

The key questions regarding information remain as follows:

- How do I know that the behavior of key actors is being carried out?
- How do I know that the behavior is producing the desired outcome?

It is unlikely that the information system can accommodate measures of key actor behavior. These important data are acquired through informal sensing. Social administrators use their interactions with workers and consumers to ask whether key actors are performing the required behavior. Program managers also use their community contacts to obtain data on key actors' behavior. Using normal contacts with service providers in the community presents an opportunity to directly ask about their interactions with staff and consumers and listen for cues about desired behavior.

Informal Sensing of Key Actors' Behavior

- *Ask workers whether key actors are performing the required behavior.*
- *Ask key actors about their interactions with your staff and consumers.*

Data regarding the second question of knowing whether the behavior is having the desired results are the same as that of Chapter 4. The test for every aspect of the program framework is outcomes for consumers. Are the consumer outcomes identified in the program objectives and goal attained? The program information system must include data on all of the consumer outcomes identified in the objectives and the program goal.

Acquiring and Directing Staff and Emotional Responses

This component of the program framework requires staff to have the following skills:

- Identification of consumers most likely emotional responses
- Responding appropriately to consumers emotional responses
- Identification of their own most likely emotional responses
- Responding appropriately to their emotional responses

These skills can be assessed during recruitment of staff by asking candidates to provide examples in each of the four categories. Job candidates can also be asked to role-play an interaction with a consumer to demonstrate identification of and responding to expected emotional responses.

These same skills need to be the subject of ongoing training and staff development. Training tends to focus on policies, procedures, and worker behavior with scant attention to expected emotional responses. In the hectic and emotionally charged world of direct service, it is easy to forget to pay attention to emotional responses. We are reminded of a worker who experienced the death of a child on her caseload. At the staff meeting the next day there was no mention of this tragic event. This led the worker to become emotional and tell her colleagues that she needed them to recognize this death and her grief. This could have been done in a more normal manner if everyone had remembered the importance of attending to workers' emotional responses and responding as indicated in the program specifications.

Acquiring and Using Resources Other Than Staff and the Helping Environment

Recognition that the helping environment needs to include certain characteristics for the benefit of the consumer is acknowledgment of the need for resources. In this context these resources consist of whatever is required to produce the required environment. As discussed earlier this includes space, people, objects, and symbols. Decisions about these elements of the environment also have implications for other resource requirements. For example, if the service event is to occur in the home of the consumer, then worker's time for travel and having a sufficiently small caseload to assure that the service events occur as specified are important considerations.

Frequently, obtaining necessary environmental resources involves collaboration with other agencies. Alter (2000) identifies three types of collaborative forms for social agencies. Obligational partnerships are partnerships whose purpose is to exchange resources. They tend to be informal, relationship dependent, and based on reciprocity. This emphasizes the importance of the social administrator developing and maintaining relationships with other service providers in the community. The principle of reciprocity requires thinking in terms of what the administrator or others in the agency can do for others in the community. An example of obtaining environmental resources through this type of partnership might be a church voluntarily allowing a room to be used during the week for supervised visits between parents and their children in foster care.

The second collaborative form is the promotional partnership that seeks to accomplish a goal that no single agency could accomplish. These partnerships are formal and are designed to enable managers to pool their resources. An example of this type of partnership that is relevant to obtaining environmental resources might be some form of colocation of staff. Using a child welfare example, it may be determined that it is critical for a substance abuse assessment professional to be present during the first meeting with a parent after court action to place a child into foster care. The child welfare administrator approaches the local substance abuse treatment agency administrator and works out a formal agreement that a substance abuse professional will be at the courthouse in a specified conference room each morning when there is a child abuse or neglect custody hearing.

The third collaborative form identified by Alter is the systemic partnership. This is the most formal type and is characterized by integration of staff and resources. A totally integrated service system building would be an environmental. For example, a community mental health center might create a drop in center for homeless with staff from several agencies such as disability determination, substance abuse treatment, and employment and training, where their respective functions are so well integrated that the consumer is unaware which staff work for which agency.

Finally, we are presenting an example of a social administrator's use of resources for program management that is not linked to the helping environment. So far the discussion of resources has assumed that they exist within the community and it is our belief that communities are resource-rich environments. One can easily imagine situations where this is not the case. For example, many people question the provision of the Adoption and Safe Families Act (ASFA) that calls for states to seek termination of parental rights and adoption for most children who have been in care fifteen of the most recent twenty-two months. Do substance abuse treatment programs exist that result in a substance-abusing parent being sufficiently into the recovery process to have children returned in less than two years? At the same time that an administrator might be using her or his advocacy skills to alter this provision of the ASFA, he or she might pursue collaborative development of a pilot program to test the feasibility of early reunification in situations where the parent has a history of substance abuse. The social administrator might contact a university substance abuse researcher about writing a literature review that identifies effective elements of substance abuse treatment. A partnership between a substance abuse treatment program, the child welfare agency, and the university could result in a proposal to test a pilot program to serve this important population.

It may be that the social administrator spends the largest amount of her or his time acquiring the resources needed to produce desired outcomes for consumers. This means that a great deal of attention must be paid to the resource demands of every element of the program management framework. The social administrator continually practices persuasion and change skills to acquire needed resources and seeks out collaborative partnerships to benefit consumers.

*EXAMPLE PROGRAM SPECIFICATIONS: THE APPLICATION OF THE WRAPAROUND APPROACH TO SCHOOL-BASED MENTAL HEALTH SERVICES**

The following example of program description is presented so that the reader has a more complete understanding of the various elements. This is not presented as a "perfect" example. It is unlikely that there is such a thing. Such program descriptions are dynamic documents that are continually subject of revision based upon increased understanding of consumers and interventions.

I stepped into the classroom for the first time when I was just five years old. Everything was huge; there was so much noise, so many kids, and so much to do. It was impossible to concentrate. It did not take long before I hated this place, so many expectations and I just could not do it. I could not sit still that long, I did not "get" everything as fast as the other kids. I remember the first time I was asked to leave to go to a "special" reading class. This was for the retarded kids and everyone knew it. When I would return to my regular class everyone would make fun of me for being stupid. I do not know, eventually I just agreed with them. As I got older, my fear and hatred for school just increased. I would do anything not to have to go. I made it through eighth grade before I finally got kicked out. It was not until I was twenty that I came to the Community Mental Health Center; I was just tired of living. I could not find a job; I had been in and out of prison for the last couple of years for different petty stuff. Finally the drugs and the alcohol just wore me out.

The Problem of Severely Emotionally Disordered Children Obtaining an Education

In America today, we are failing an ever-growing population of children, those children who have been diagnosed with Severe Emotional Disorders

---

*These program specifications were written by Erik Van Allen of the Kansas Department of Social and Rehabilitation Services. Reprinted with permission.

(SED). Examples like the one given earlier are not difficult to find. For various reasons, this number of children has grown and continues to be under-identified. The schools define these children as having internal or external behavior problems that impede their learning at school. In addition to this, the state, through the community mental centers, defines these children as being between the ages of four and eighteen who have an axis one diagnosis, meet certain diagnostic criteria on the Child Behavior Checklist (CBCL) and Child and Adolescent Functioning Assessment Scale (CAFAS) assessments, and who are having significant impairments in either school, home, or the community. The failings of the school to educate these children can be seen in their significant underachievement in an educational setting. These children consistently receive lower grades, lower scores on achievement testing, have high rates of truancy, do not graduate or receive certificates of completion as often as a non-SED child, and tend to drop out of school at a much higher rate than other special education students and non-SED students.

Consequences of the Problem for Society

This can lead to numerous problems for society and these children. Failure in school leads to lower earning jobs. The inability to find a "good" job that pays well and that has benefits leads to increases in poverty and an increased reliance on the social welfare systems and public insurance such as Medicaid. Failure in school also leads to increased rates of truancy and dropouts. This has been seen to have a significant impact on school day crime, increases in deviant behavior, and increased early contact with the juvenile justice system. Finally, failure in school leads to a low sense of worth and self-esteem. Children who have failed at school internalize this failure. The result of this could be an increased reliance on drugs and alcohol, and increased rates of continued severe and persistent mental illness as an adult.

Consequences of the Problem for the Children

Problems for the child are similar in nature to the problems for society, but are felt in a much more personal nature. These children often feel stigmatized and labeled by both their peers and adults. Being called stupid, retarded, and so on, becomes internalized and the children begin to believe this about themselves. Internalizing this language leads to dramatic decreases in self-esteem and self-worth. These decreases lead to social isolation and a lack of peer supports. In addition, the consequences regarding increased use of alcohol and drugs, and increased mental illness are the same as what is mentioned earlier. Oftentimes these children have legal troubles as a result of truancy and dropouts from school. They are unable to find quality jobs, are forced to rely on welfare and other institutionalized supports, and are unable to participate in a postsecondary education.

Factors Contributing to the Problem

The reasons schools and communities often fail these children are varied, but can be broken into two basic categories. The first, obstacles that these children bring into a school setting, can sometimes be changed, but for the most part are going to remain an integral part of the youths' lives. For example, the psychiatric problems that these children bring are associated with a variety of diagnosis. These can include but are not limited to Attention Deficit Hyperactivity Disorder, Reactivity Attachment Disorder, Obsessive Compulsive Disorder, and Oppositional Defiant Disorder. Some reasons for onset include simple problems with the hard wiring of the brain that may be managed through the use of medication. Other times, it may be environmental stressors such as divorce, death, or other traumatic experiences in the child's life. In addition, oftentimes these children come into the classroom with learning disabilities that compound their difficulties in working with teachers.

Whatever the causes, schools and teachers are having a difficult time finding ways in which to teach these children. Today, schools still have trouble accepting children with these disorders. They are labeled by everyone as "problem" children. They are assigned a paraprofessional, who is supposed to support them, but is usually undertrained and underpaid. When this does not work, the next solution is to put them into classrooms that are separated from the regular education student body. Here these children stay until they either leave school on their own, or are kicked out because of behavior. Other problems at school include little communication with the parents, and almost no collaboration with other community organizations that are working with the same children (the community mental health center, the courts, the juvenile justice system).

Population Analysis

The following population analysis is for students in the Wayne School District who are at risk of an alternative school placement and out of home placement. These students have a higher risk of not achieving their full academic potential due to emotional disturbances. These emotional disturbances hinder their academic progress leading to increases in truancy and dropouts, and a decrease in the rate at which they graduate from high school with a diploma. The program design to follow will examine ways to increase the level of achievement in schools of children who are diagnosed with a severe emotional disturbance.

General Population

The general population consists of all students who currently attend the Wayne School District (n = 5,298). These students all fall within the catchment area of Community Mental Health Services, allowing them to be served by this organization. There are currently ten schools within the Wayne School District. They include eight elementary schools, two middle schools, and one high school that is located on two separate campuses. The elementary schools have a total enrollment of 2,539 students in grades K through 6. The middle schools have a total enrollment of 857 students in grades 7 and 8. Finally, the high school has a total enrollment of 1,899 students in grades 9 through 12. Grade 9 is located on a separate campus with an enrollment of 727 students. The school district is located in a small Midwestern city with a population of approximately 45,000 and a large university. The district is predominately white with 80 percent of all students falling in this racial/ ethnic category. Following this, 9 percent of all students are black, 5 percent are Asian, 4 percent are Hispanic, and 1.5 percent falls into the other racial/ ethnic category. Of all students, 29 percent qualify for free or reduced lunches.

At-Risk Population

The at-risk population of students includes most of the students that have individual education plans (IEPs) or 504 plans and is served through special education programming. In the Wayne School District, 906 students are served through special education. The largest percentage of these comprises gifted students with 29 percent of all special education students in this group. Following this, 28 percent of students being served are classified as learning disabled, 24 percent as speech/language impaired, 7 percent as other health impaired, 6 percent as emotionally disturbed, and 3 percent are classified as other (autism, developmental delay, early childhood, hearing impaired, severely multiple handicapped, and visually impaired). Excluding the gifted who receive no other services, these students tend to have lower grades, lower scores on standardized tests, increased rates of truancy, and a decreased rate of graduation. Many of these students have multiple labels and approximately 650 are at risk of not achieving their full academic potential.

Target Population

The target population consists of students attending the Wayne School District who are receiving special education services and are classified as emotionally disturbed (ED) or have a primary classification other than ED and a secondary classification of ED. These students are at the greatest risk of failing to achieve their academic potential. This fact is made more apparent when ED is combined with other impairments. In the Wayne School District, these students are suspended more frequently and have a higher incidence of acts of violence. There are currently 56 students with a primary classification of ED. It is estimated that another 44 students meet the definition of ED but have a more severe disability in another category. Therefore, the total target population for this program is approximately 100 students.

Consumer Population

The students who are consumers of this program attend the Wayne School District, are receiving special education services, and are classified as emotionally disturbed (ED) or have a primary classification other than E D and a secondary classification of ED. These students will have completed an intake at Community Mental Health Services and meet the definition of severe emotional disturbance (SED). This definition is specific to children who are having severe and persistent difficulties at home, school, or within the community. These children also must have an Axis I diagnosis and fall within the clinical range on the CBCL (between 30 and 70) and the CAFAS (over 100). In addition, these children must be experiencing severe impaired functioning in one of three life domains (school, home, community). Finally, these students will be seeking the appropriate mental health services from an approved list of mental health providers within the community and be referred to community-based services provided by Community Mental Health Services. This is a requirement of the program for two reasons. It allows the mental health staff to maintain confidentiality within the classroom and it limits the liability to both the school and the community mental health center. These students have been seen to have persistent difficulties maintaining their behavior within the school setting, leading to suspension, expulsion, or a referral to a contained classroom due to their behavior; or the student is seen as entering the district from a state hospital or a level 6 residential treatment facility. As a condition of entering the program, families are required to seek mental health services. Also, the student must meet both the schools definition of ED and the state definition of SED. These conditions will limit the number of families who can choose to participate. The estimated number of students likely to become consumers is twenty-five. Services will be provided to all children and families who meet the aforementioned requirements based on the date of referral to the program. Consumers will be served on a first-come-first-serve basis. An assessment of the student's severity of need will be used to determine the least restrictive environment that would maintain the student's behavior.

State of the Evidence: Review of the Research

The Effectiveness of School-Based Mental Health Services for Children, a ten-year research review by Hoagwood and Erwin (1997), is a meta-analysis of research that used random assignment, a control group, and standardized outcomes. Of the 5,046 articles reviewed, the researchers found 16 that met the aforementioned criteria. The meta-analysis found three types of interventions that had empirical support for their effectiveness. These interventions included cognitive-behavioral therapy, social skills training, and teacher consultation. Cognitive-behavioral therapy includes individual psychotherapy and group psychotherapy used as a tool for behavioral modification. Social skills training included case management and psychosocial groups that emphasized and practiced appropriate behaviors. Finally, teacher consultation included continuing education and consulting provided to schools and mental health professionals' support to teachers who have SED children in their classrooms. As compared to other interventions including residential treatment, specialized classes, and day treatments, these interventions were seen to have targeted outcomes that had a greater frequency of functioning and symptom reduction.

In *Education's Role in Systems of Care* (Eber and Rolf, 1998), the wraparound approach used in Illinois was evaluated over three years for student and family outcomes. The researchers found that the wraparound services in these school districts made a positive impact on the internalizing domain scores of the CBCL for the children served. In addition, the researchers found that if wraparound services were in place there was a significant decrease for the need of extra academic assistance between years one and two. Less than a quarter of these students needed to leave their home school and 33 percent of these students moved to a more restrictive environment.

Cheney and Osher (1997) evaluated two school-based mental health programs, the Positive Education Program (PEP), and a school-based wraparound initiative in Illinois (LADSE-WRAP). They found that PEP, which involves the parents at many levels of its program, had high parent satisfaction rates and transitions by students to more restrictive placements less than 25 percent of the time. LADSE-WRAP, which also involves parents to a high degree, has shown a marked decrease in out-of-home placements and hospitalizations for students, and an increase in child and family functioning.

The aforementioned reports demonstrated an increase in positive outcomes with the involvement of parents to a high degree and the use of a wraparound approach to service delivery. Adding support to this argument was a study by Johnson, Morriss, and McElhiney (1998) that evaluated the impact on student outcomes with the support of a parent liaison. The study compared behavioral indicators of students whose families had either high contact (N > 12) or low contact (N < 11) with the parent liaison and the satisfaction of their performance as reported by parents. If a parent liaison was present and had high contact with the parents, results suggested a positive impact on the student by a decrease on the scores of the behavioral indicator and an increase in parent satisfaction.

Oestman (1996) described the use of the Behavioral Skills Program (BSP) in the Lincoln Public Schools. The program was described as a collaborative effort between the Lancaster Child Guidance Center and the Public Schools system that combined intensive therapeutic services (individual counseling, case management, etc.) and educational services at a self-contained site for students identified as having a behavior disorder (BD) and having a history of psychiatric hospitalization. The study used pre- and post-measure CBCL scores and Kaufman tests for academic achievement. When students were provided a treatment environment that provided for academic success, rewarded pro-social behavior, facilitated positive relationships with adults, and had a strengths and adjustments focus, there was a significant increase in academic scores and improvement in internalized problem scores. This program was most effective for elementary-level students.

Rones and Hoagwood (2000) provided a review of research on school-based mental health services. The results of this review suggest that there is a group of school-based mental health programs with empirical evidence of impact across a range of educational and emotional/behavioral problems. The researcher found that implementation of the programs were similar in inclusion of parents, teacher, and peers (the wraparound approach), the use of multiple modalities (interacting at different levels), integration of the program into the general classroom, and developmentally appropriate program components (tailoring the education curriculum to the development of the child versus the age of the child). The article focused on several specific programs. The first, PATHS (Promoting Alternative Thinking Strategies), aims to increase children's ability to discuss and understand emotions. Within one month of implementation of the PATHS program, participants were associated with significantly higher emotional vocabularies, greater ease of discussing emotions, and a greater understanding of others' feelings. The ACHIEVE program attempts to intervene on multiple levels through modification of school policy, implementation of classroom management strategies, development of curriculum changes, and facilitation of parent–school communication. The implementation of project ACHIEVE has shown to reduce child disciplinary problems and promote students achievement.

Selected Interventions

Based on the research, the following interventions were selected for implementation in the program:

1. The use of the wraparound process using existing school-based mental health models: the wraparound process will intervene at several levels at the same time. The wraparound process is based on the involvement of the family in the decision-making process. In addition, creative solutions can be developed to meet the need of the individual students through the use of community resources and with all parties involved in the process.
2. Increasing family involvement is essential to the achievement of educational and social/emotional goals and outcomes. The program will use a parent support worker to increase contact with parents. In addition, parents should be included on all committees, boards, and in evaluations to ensure that services are planned and delivered in accordance with the families needs.
3. Increase in staff education, training, and staff development: this would include the practice of LMHTs in the place of typical paraeducators. The systematic training of all staff will provide consistent engagement with students. Finally, the program will increase the collateral contact with regular education teachers and administration and will provide training and consultation as needed.
4. Mental health counseling services will be provided to the youth employing a mixture of cognitive-behavioral therapy and social skills training.

Program Theory

Program Goal

To increase the level of academic achievement* in schools of children who are diagnosed with having a severe emotional disturbance (SED).

Program Objectives

Consumer Outcome
1. Sixty percent of students will be working at or above grade level in all subjects as measured by standardized testing.
2. Twenty percent of students will exit into full-time mainstream classes.
3. The amount of time for school suspensions among all program participants will decrease by 50 percent.
4. Sixty percent of program participants will be able to attend school functions including dances and sporting events.
5. Thirty percent of program participants will have the opportunity to participate in extra-curricular activities.

Other Objectives
1. All students will attend school 80 percent of the time.
2. Eighty percent of students will be attending mainstream classes 50 percent of the time.

Mutual Expectations and Consequences

In order to achieve the intervention goals and objectives, several people have responsibilities that must be carried out. These responsibilities are as follows:

Student
• The student will know about the transition goal and criteria for entrance back into the mainstream classes from the day he or she enters the program.
• The student will be involved in all plans and meeting as much as possible.
• The student will be listened to.

---

*Improved grades, improved scores on standardized and achievement tests, decreased truancy and dropout rates, and increased graduation rates.

- The student will be made aware of and follow clear and predictable procedures and expectations in the classroom.
- The student will attend school on a regular basis.
- The student will take all medication as prescribed.
- The student will work on assigned curriculum throughout the school day.
- The student will meet with an individual therapist, case manager, and participate in group therapy as determined by the wraparound team.

Family
- The family is involved in all planning decisions and attends all planning meetings.
- The family will be listened to.
- The family will have a liaison or advocate provided to them for support.
- The family will meet all school staff, will know their names and phone numbers, and will have contact with classroom staff on a weekly basis.
- The family will follow the recommendations of the wraparound team including participating in family therapy and family support groups.
- The family will follow-up on all medication management appointments.
- The family will support the student at home and in the community with regard to school participation including homework, school activities, and so on.

School/Mental Health Staff
- The school staff will involve the family and students in the decision-making process.
- The school staff will follow the recommendation of the wraparound team.
- The school staff will meet with the family to complete all needed documentation for entrance into the program.
- The teacher will oversee the educational program for the student and will develop the individual education plan with support from the wraparound team.
- The teacher will implement behavior management strategies and will oversee the incentive strategies used within the classroom.
- The teacher will work cooperatively with regular education classroom teachers who have SED students within their classroom.
- The case manager will assist the student on a daily basis with improving self-management of the symptoms associated with their diagnosis.

- The case manager will assist the teacher with developing the behavioral plan that will work toward meeting treatment goals developed by the wraparound team.
- The case manager will coordinate services with other service providers and will assist the family in identifying and acquiring community resources.
- The case manager will provide consultation and education to regular education teachers and administration and assessment as necessary in regard to students' mental health.

Stages of Helping

The program consists of five separate stages of helping: The Engagement Phase, The Planning Phase, The Implementation Phase, The Review Phase, and the Termination Phase. The stages are cyclic in nature and will need to be revisited as the child progresses through the program. The following will describe the purpose of each phase, the key activities of each, and the length and activity that marks the end of the stage and the beginning of the next.

The Engagement Phase. The engagement phase is marked by three specific occurrences: referral, assessment, and intake. The engagement phase primarily serves to introduce the family to the program and determine whether the program will meet the needs of that particular child. The engagement phase should be short, from referral to the program to intake lasting no longer than two weeks and most likely much shorter due to the need of an immediate change in placement.

This stage is begun with a referral by the school (teacher, principal, school social worker, school psychologist), a mental health professional (therapist, case manager, psychiatrist), or the parents of the child to the program. This referral would be made if any of the aforementioned individuals have concerns regarding impediments to the educational process due to the behavior of the child. The referral is reviewed in an IEP team meeting. This team reviews the current placement and makes a recommendation to enter the program to the Special Education Director.

Following this, the Special Education Director will schedule a placement meeting with IEP Team and the TLC (therapeutic learning center) Treatment Team. The two teams, along with the parents, will assess the need for services and determine the least restrictive environment. They will then make a recommendation based on this assessment and a change of placement would be indicated on the IEP. It will be at this time that the final step is completed. The parents will be asked to enroll their child in the program through the use of the intake process at the community mental health center. The purpose of this is to allow the child to have access to the array of services available through the program. Upon completion of the intake and acceptance into the program, the engagement phase is completed.

The Planning Phase. This phase begins with the assessment of the child within the classroom. Upon entering the classroom, the teacher and the case manager will have ten days to complete a behavioral assessment and to assess the educational needs of the child. When these ten days have expired, a wraparound meeting will be scheduled by the case manager. All key actors in the child's life will meet to review the IEP (individual education plan) and develop the IEP/POC (individual education plan/plan of care) document that will determine the plan for treatment. The IEP/POC document will need to be completed within the first fourteen days of placement. This phase will end when the IEP/POC document has been produced and the wraparound team has signed off on the plan for treatment.

The Implementation Phase. This phase begins with the implementation of the classroom guidelines and the behavior modification system (the level system, and rewards and consequences). When these have been explained to the child and family, it becomes the duty of the case manager to acquire resources for the family that will help their child to succeed at school. Resource acquisition includes the domains of school, community, and home. School resources will be provided by the TLC instructor and support will be provided for the student at school by both the school and mental health staff. These resources include access to the school social worker, school medical facilities, alternative learning styles (including night school, Saturday school, computer learning, etc.), and any other modifications that need to be made in order to accommodate the unique learning style of each child.

Outside of school, the case manager will work with the child and the family to identify resources that will enable the child to meet the goals and objectives of the treatment plan. These resources include additional mental health resources (individual therapy/counseling, family counseling, medication management, etc.) and community resources including: accessing Social Security benefits, churches, civic organizations, recreational activities, and any other community resources that would facilitate the meeting of treatment goals and objectives. This phase continues until a review is scheduled. The review occurs within three months of the development of the treatment plan.

The Review Phase. The review phase will occur every three months and will allow the wraparound team to assess the effectiveness of the implemented interventions and will allow for changes to IEP/POC to be made as necessary. Upon completion of the wraparound and review of the treatment plan and having every member of the wraparound team sign off on the changes, this phase will be completed. Following this, either the Implementation phase will be revisited or the child has met all goal and objectives of the program and the wraparound team has determined that the child no longer needs the services of the TLC. If this is the case, then the child will enter the termination phase.

The Termination Phase. The termination phase begins with the wraparound team determining that services are no longer needed for the child. At this time, a termination plan will be put into place that transitions the youth with supports as needed to the appropriate placement within the school setting. If the child no longer meets the criteria for community based services through the community mental health center, or if the parents want to terminate, it will then be the responsibility of the case manager to transition the child to other community resources as smoothly as possible. This phase will end with the child exiting the TLC program.

The Ideal Helping Environments

The classroom is set up as to accommodate a maximum of ten students. The walls are painted to encourage learning, preferably in a brighter color such as yellow. The desks are arranged in a manner that allows for each student to have their own cubicle. Due to the nature of the classroom, each student is responsible for his or her individual learning and the ability to be excluded from distraction would be essential. In addition, the classroom is equipped with multimedia including computers at a ratio of one computer to every three students. This allows the students to complete online class work within the classroom. The staff desks are arranged in a manner that provides a clear view, while being seated, of each student.

The classroom has its own entrance and exit to allow students to enter or leave the building. This serves several functions. It allows the students to enter the classroom without the knowledge of the student body thereby reducing stigmatization associated with being in the contained classroom. The classroom would have its own restroom facilities and meeting room/ seclusion room (to be used for behavior modification "time-out," testing, meetings, etc.).

Another environment is access to recreational and art facilities. The facilities should be at an existing school site, allowing for access to both mainstream education classes and the aforementioned facilities. The classroom will be handicapped accessible. The rooms are carpeted and brightly lit, both from natural lighting (windows) and florescent lighting. Modifications will be made to accommodate individual students based on diagnosis.

Transportation during the school year will be provided by the school district. All mental health center staff will dress in a casual business/professional manner and be provided with school identification badges so the student body will be able to identify them. Any activities outside of the school will be conducted in a discrete manner so as to limit any stigmatization the clients may be subject to by participating in mental health services.

The key actors and their behavior required for the child's success are listed in Table 5.2. This includes school and mental health center staff. Ways to elicit each behavior are also identified.

TABLE 5.2. Chart of Key Actors and Their Behavior

Key Actors	Behavior Required	How to Elicit Behavior
TLC School Staff		
1. Special Education Teachers 2. Special Education Para's	1. Oversees the education plan for the child 2. Coordinates with the parents in developing the IEP 3. Implements the behavior management strategies 4. Works cooperatively with the regular education staff 5. Works cooperatively with the mental health staff	1. Educate TLC school staff about their specific role with in the program 2. Provide the school staff with all program guidelines and assessment tools necessary 3. Facilitate contact with school administrators and Pawnee Mental Health Administration 4. Provide the school staff with information regarding the needs of children with SED
TLC Pawnee Staff		
1. School-Based Case Manager 2. School-Based Attendant Care 3. School-Based Therapist	1. Assists child with improving self-management of symptoms associated with their diagnosis 2. Assists the teacher in developing the behavioral plan 3. Works toward goals agreed upon by the family and the treatment team. 4. Coordinates services with other service providers 5. Assists the family with identifying and acquiring community resources 6. Provide consultation, education and ongoing assessment to school staff with regard to students mental health needs	1. Educate TLC Pawnee Staff about their specific role within the program 2. Provide the Pawnee Staff with all program guidelines 3. Facilitate contact with school administrators and Pawnee Mental Health Administration 4. Provide Pawnee staff with continued training with regard to school-based mental health, behavioral management strategies, and school policy / IEP

TABLE 5.2 *(continued)*

Regular Education School Staff

1. School Administrators 2. General Education Teachers 3. School Social Workers 4. School Psychologists	1. Assists the wrap-around process through observation data 2. Assists the TLC staff with transitions into mainstream education classes. 3. Provides additional support outside of TLC program	1. Educate the school staff about the Program 2. Provide the school staff with program guidelines 3. Facilitate communication between school staff and TLC staff 4. Provide the school staff with information regarding the needs of children coping with SED and training with regard to school-based mental health and classroom behavioral management strategies

Non-School Pawnee Staff

1. Parent Support Workers 2. Psychiatrist/ Medical Staff 3. Office-Based Psychotherapists	1. Assists the wrap-around process through professional assessment 2. Provide assistance to the child and family outside of the TLC 3. Provide support to children and families around educational issues	1. Educate the Pawnee staff about the Program 2. Provide Pawnee staff with program guidelines 3. Educate Pawnee staff about Community-Based Services and the wrap-around process

Actual Helping Behaviors: The Quarterly Wraparound

The key component to the success of the program lies in the parent's involvement in the development and monitoring of the child's educational and treatment plans. This involvement is accomplished through regular contact with the parents by the teacher, case manager, and the parent support worker. The formal aspect of this involvement entails the use of the wraparound process. It is the goal of the program to hold a quarterly "wraparound" meeting for each student. This formal gathering of all key actors allows the progress of the child within the educational and treatment plan to be reviewed and modified as necessary on a regular basis. The following will illustrate what occurs at a quarterly wraparound.

Johnny is a fourteen-year-old boy who has been in the Therapeutic Learning Center (TLC) for the past six months. It is now time for his six-month review. The process is initiated by the case manager who contacts each individual listed in the Plan of Care as a key actor in the child's life. In Johnny's case, the case manager invited the Parents, Johnny, the TLC teacher, two regular education teachers, the principal, the therapist, and Johnny's probation officer. When the case manager consulted the parents with regard to the best time, it was decided that before school would work best for them. The case manager scheduled the meeting so as to allow both parents to attend and gave a ten-day notice to the other participants in the group.

On the scheduled day, the Team (parents, Johnny, the TLC teacher, the Case Manager, a science teacher, the therapist, and the probation officer) met in the TLC classroom before school had started. The meeting began by introducing the science teacher who had not been to a wraparound before. The case manager explained the process. "First, we will begin by reviewing the strengths assessment that was completed three months ago. It is at this time that any new strength will be added. Next, we will review the needs we were working on and determine if these needs have been met or it there are additional needs that could be added. Following this, we will review the IEP/POC to determine if the goals and objectives are still appropriate. If they are, then we will continue with the current level of services. If not, then we can look at changing these to better meet Johnny's needs."

After the introductions, the case manager led the group in assessing the strengths. The case manager asked Johnny whether he felt like he had any strength to add since our last meeting. Johnny did not know, but his parents spoke up and said that he had become very involved in the youth group at their church. In addition, since the last meeting, Johnny has added two regular education classes and seems to be doing very well in both. The science teacher stated that, "Johnny does very well in my class, he sits in the front row and asks questions when he does not understand something. Also, I have watched him in the halls and he seems to have a lot of friends." Since Johnny had been working toward developing peer relationships, both the youth group and friends at school were added as strengths. The TLC teacher stated that he had been doing very well in his class also and would soon be adding another class. The probation officer stated, "Johnny has been attending our meeting regularly as scheduled and has been doing very good, it looks like his curfew will be getting moved back to 10 in the next week or so." Both were added to the strengths assessments with the rest of the group agreeing that Johnny had made a lot of improvement.

Following this, needs were reviewed. When the case manager asked Johnny if he felt that there is anything else he needed to be successful, he stated, "I liked my regular education classes but I have a hard time keeping up and I get frustrated when I get behind." This was added to the needs assessment. In addition to this, the probation officer stated that, "Johnny still has not paid his court costs and needs to complete over half of his community service hours."

Following the needs assessment, the case manager passed around a copy of the completed IEP/POC for the team to review. Johnny thought that he had met his goal of making friends so that should be deleted. The team discussed this and agreed that Johnny had been working very hard to meet these goals and objectives so they could be removed from the plan. The case manager wanted Johnny to continue to go to the psychosocial group and Johnny stated that he enjoyed doing this, so a goal of improving social skills was added. Next, the science teacher stated that he would be happy to meet with Johnny after school to help him keep up. The team agreed that this would be a good idea and Johnny said that he would go. The team added an objective to the goal: Johnny will add three regular education classes to his school schedule by the end of the year. The objective stated the following: Johnny will attend two sessions of tutoring after school per week. Finally, Johnny's parents stated that they did not have the money to help Johnny pay for his court expenses. The probation officer stated that he could waive these fees if Johnny would complete twenty hours of community service beyond his required amount, and that this should all be completed before our next meeting. Johnny stated that he could do this, but he could not drive and his parents had to work after school and on the weekends. The case manager stated that he could drive Johnny to his community service on the weekend and after school. Johnny agreed and these were added as objectives to his plan.

After this was complete, the case manager asked whether anyone had any questions or comments. The group seemed satisfied with the work and agreed to meet again in three months. The changes were noted on the plan and the team signed off. Finally, the case manager took Johnny aside and asked him if he felt okay with everything that was decided. Johnny stated that he felt good about it. Following the wraparound, the case manager made copies and distributed them to the team members.

Affective Involvements of Consumers and Staff

The expected emotional responses of consumers and staff to the service transaction are identified in Exhibits 5.2 and 5.3. In each case the most likely emotion is identified in the first column, the appropriate response is listed in the second, and the desired resulting emotion is included in the third.

Exhibit 5.2. Chart of Consumers Expected Affective Involvements

Likely Emotions	Client: Responses	Desired Emotions
1. *Fear:* The child and family will fear a change into a new school placement away from supports and peers.	It will be the workers' responsibility to facilitate the clients' emotional responses from their likely emotions to their desired emotions. This will be accomplished in a variety of manners.	1. *Hope:* The client should feel that success in the program and at school is possible; included in this is a hope for a better life.
2. *Anger:* The clients may be angry with a change in placement. They may feel as if they had no choice in the manner.	To begin, all clients will enter the classroom following strict but consistent guidelines and a level system that rewards positive behavior. As the client becomes accustomed to the structure, they will begin to realize opportunities for self-autonomy. As they rise through the level system, their ability to affect positive change in their lives increases. The staff will facilitate this increase in positive behavior by using active and empathetic listening to students concerns.	2. *Safe:* While in the classroom, the clients should feel that they are in a safe environment. Included in this is the feeling of physical and emotional safety.
3. *Anxiety:* The clients may be anxious about being in a new classroom. Anxiety may also exist as a result of perceived failure at school.		3. *Successful:* As with hope the clients should feel confident about their ability to achieve a successful outcome with regard to school performance.

4. *Confusion:* The clients may feel confused about the reasons behind being "forced" to enter a new classroom. They may be confused by the classroom guidelines and expectations.

5. *Embarrassment:* The clients might be embarrassed by their perceived entrance into a "special education" program.

6. *Powerlessness:* The clients may feel as if they are powerless to control their environment. This can be expressed in a manner that could be construed defiant.

In addition, all successes both behaviorally and educationally will be rewarded. The one-to-one attention given to each student will allow the student to achieve success and failures in a safe and supportive environment. This will lead to increased self-esteem and feelings of safety, success, and encouragement. What begins as negative experience will hopefully turn into a positive experience as the child becomes accustomed to the classroom guidelines and an environment staffed by consistent and caring individuals.

4. *Motivated:* Students should feel motivated to achieve their goals and strive to be successful in both the program and in school.

5. *Encouraged:* Students should be encouraged to try new things. Included in this is an inherit lack of fear of failure and conversely a lack of fear of success.

EXHIBIT 5.3. Chart of Staff Expected Affective Involvement

Likely Emotions:

1. *Frustration:* Staff may become frustrated because of lack of motivation of client. Perceived failure on the part of the staff may lead to this sense of frustration.

2. *Anger:* It is very possible that staff may become angry with the clients. This occurs as a result of frustration, fear, helplessness, and a sense of being overwhelmed.

3. *Fear:* Staff may fear the clients. This happens when clients tend to be emotionally unstable and resort to violence as a coping mechanism. In addition, new staff may fear clients because of a lack of appropriate tools to modify behavior.

Staff Responses:

The ability of the staff to reach their desired emotions will be key to the success of the program. This will be accomplished through several means. The first will be continuing education and training guided toward providing staff with the tools necessary to manage the classroom in a positive and safe manner.

Following this will be consistent communication within the classroom through regular staffing and with other staff including mental health professionals and school administration. In addition, the program will strive to keep a client to staff ratio that facilitates positive interactions between staff and clients. Other responses include setting realistic expectations for clients and reviewing interventions regularly in order to best meet the needs of the individual

Desired Emotions

1. *Hope:* It is the desire of the program that staff have "hope" about the ability to see success in the future of each individual student.

2. *Pride:* The staff should strive to have pride in the accomplishments of both the program and the participants.

3. *Optimism:* This is the ability of the staff to expect the best from each student—the constant belief that each student will succeed.

4. *Overwhelmed*: Staff may feel overwhelmed when they are unable to meet the needs of individual clients because of a lack of support from other staff, regular education staff, and administration.

5. *Sadness*: Staff may feel sadness as they empathize with the client. This is normal and leads to compassionate work.

clients. Other supports would include additional staff to "fill in" when regular staff need to be absent. This would hopefully decrease feelings of burnout. Finally, a set manual of policy and procedures to guide staff in times of crisis and a concrete behavioral plan for each child that has been agreed upon by the parents in order to avoid any miscommunication are needed. Finally, the regular education staff must be educated about special needs children and be willing to work with the TLC staff in order to provide the best learning environment.

4. *Safety*: All staff should be provided with a psychically and emotionally safe environment that is free from physical, verbal, and sexual abuse.

5. *Compassion*: The workers will develop compassion for the students and their struggles in coping with SED. By empathizing with the students, the worker can begin to understand the struggles these children face.

SUMMARY

This is the third and final chapter that presents the elements of the program management framework. As a whole this framework provides a coherent picture of the social problem faced by consumers, the results that they are likely to be achieved by participating in the program, and the means to achieving these results. This picture informs consumers, workers, policymakers, and the larger public. It is as detailed and complex a picture as are the social problems that we seek to ameliorate.

The program framework is also a powerful management tool. By knowing the detailed specifications of the program, the manager can work to establish the conditions that are most likely to result in positive outcomes for consumers. Managers can use this knowledge along with their change skills to influence staff, key actors, policymakers, and others to create and maintain the conditions for success. Managers can also use this framework to guide their actions in acquiring and managing staff, information, and other types of resources.

The Program Mangement Framework—Part 3

Analysis of the social problem
The population: From the general population to the consumer
The theory of helping: Goals, objectives, and expectations
Key people required for consumer success
The helping environment
Emotional responses of consumers and staff
Actual helping behaviors

Chapter 6

Managing Information: Determining Whether the Program Is Operating As Intended

Data that informs on program operations and results are essential to effective management. It is through data that social administrators know whether consumers are achieving desired outcomes. Data of a variety of types let managers know whether workers are feeling rewarded for their efforts and whether necessary resources are being acquired as needed. Although the program framework details how a program is supposed to operate, it is data on program operations that tell whether it is operating as intended with the desired effects.

Information management is an essential tool in the practice of consumer-centered social administration. Along with skills to influence people and to design effective programs, information management allows social administrators to implement the principles of consumer-centered management. Selecting and using measures of consumer outcomes communicates to everyone in the organization that these results are the reason for the program existence and is a concrete step in *creating and maintaining the focus.* Using these data in meetings and memos to communicate the importance of consumers and their achievement is an essential part of *venerating these people.* Social administrators demonstrate *learning for a living* by reading information system reports to learn about consumers and how the program is operating, and to identify ways to improve. Finally, social administrators use reports that show seemingly intractable problems to engage in brainstorming and problem solving with staff as one part of a *healthy disrespect for the impossible.*

Textbook of Social Administration: The Consumer-Centered Approach
© 2007 by The Haworth Press, Inc. All rights reserved.
doi:10.1300/5802_07

Information Management Learning Objectives

- *Recognize the power of measurement.*
- *Learn how to use feedback to influence behavior.*
- *Identify the elements of a learning organization.*
- *Identify the management skills and knowledge required for a learning organization.*
- *Identify the elements of an organizational culture that supports learning.*
- *Identify and apply the skills of designing effective performance reports.*
- *Apply the five principles of performance report design.*
- *Identify at least ten ways to use information to enhance program performance.*
- *Identify the elements of a performance improvement strategy.*
- *Identify and apply at least six ways to search for explanations for inadequate performance.*
- *Identify the characteristics of and set improvement goals.*
- *Create a program improvement strategy.*

Readers experienced with social service organizations and common information system reports may read the introduction of this chapter a bit skeptically. Although management information systems have been developed to meet housekeeping needs (e.g., issuing checks to staff and clients, maintaining client records) and proposed as decision-support aids, not many have focused on managing information as an integral part of a learning organization. Information in this capacity acts as a performance-guidance system whereby performance is monitored, problems and achievements are sensed, and staff are informed. In this context the manager is much like a pilot of a plane who watches the dials and gauges in the cockpit to monitor the plane's performance, to change course when necessary, and to land safely at the desired destination. The various instruments take readings on critical functions; the pilot compares these to various standards and "acts" based on this comparison.

We prepare social administrators to develop and use information systems that make it possible to guide programs to reach intended goals. In this chapter and the next we identify the attitudes, skills, and knowledge necessary to develop, implement, and operate information systems that facilitate organizational learning. This chapter begins by exploring the power of numbers on human behavior and identifies elements of a learning organization; we present principles of report design and demonstrate how managers can pilot the human service enterprise. In Chapter 7, we delve more deeply into the technical skills of selecting outcome measures, measuring critical areas of performance, and exploring innovative report designs.

THE POWER OF MEASUREMENT*

We encounter measurement daily and act upon it. We check the weather forecast to find out the predicted temperature and decide what to wear. We check the clock to see whether it is time to go home or to work or school. What an instructor measures in terms of performance is probably the most powerful determinant of student behavior. Class sessions that cover material needed to complete an assignment are always well attended. Book chapters and articles that are assigned to be read are in fact read if students know that they may be called on to summarize an article and that a grade is assigned to that activity. Inquiries like, "Will this be on the test?" and "How long should this paper be?" are all indicative of a concern, if not preoccupation, with grades over learning. The power of that one measurement!

Think about how you might react if you stepped on a commercial airline, looked left into the cockpit and there were two seats and a large window but no gauges. Would you have confidence in the pilot to get you safely to your destination? Measurement and information is most powerful (i.e., most likely to influence behavior) when the measure is reflective of a goal, a purpose, and an outcome that is important to the person. The measure provides feedback on where we are relative to that purpose or goal. For example, wanting to get out of debt (purpose) may lead you to checking your credit card balance (measurement) before deciding to have dinner at a nice restaurant or at home (decision or action). Other examples of the purpose-measurement-action formula are located in Table 6.1.

To listen to human service managers, one would conclude that the largest obstacle to better performance is not information but some combination of better people and more resources. There is certainly truth to this idea. Since social services are labor intensive, organizational performance is largely dependent on the individual and collective competence of the personnel. Likewise, additional funds to employ more staff and create more programs would help. This is particularly true now, when social workers are being asked to serve more clients with increased effectiveness with static or reduced dol-

*The authors would like to thank Terry Moore for his contributions to this chapter. His "Results oriented management in child welfare" Web site is www.rom.ku.edu.

TABLE 6.1. Examples of the Purpose-Measurement-Action Formula

Measurement	Outcome	Decision/Action
Thermometer	Comfort	What kind of clothing to wear
Speedometer	Safety and avoid traffic ticket	Whether to take your foot off the accelerator of your car
Test scores	Child does well in school	Whether your child should stay home and study tonight
Bathroom scales	Stay healthy, and lose or maintain weight	Whether to forgo dessert today
Checkbook	Sufficient funds to pay a bill	Pay the bill or wait until payday.

Source: From "Results oriented management in child welfare" by T. Moore (2003) www.rom.ku.edu. Reprinted with permission.

lars. More resources and better staff, however, are not necessarily guarantees of better performance nor is better performance dependent on these.

The dilemma, of course, is that these two elements are the most difficult to influence. Administrators already try to hire the best available candidates given the constraints of salary, civil service, geographic location, and the quality of education candidates receive from universities. Some agencies provide staff development programs for their employees, but funds for these have always been and will continue to be rather meager. Similarly, organizations are always chasing dollars through appropriations and grants. The chances of huge increases in social service budgets are slight, and even if budgets were to increase, they would still not satisfactorily serve clients.

Without negating the need for competent staff and more resources, organizational performance can be improved, and improved dramatically in some cases, by exploiting the power of information. As Schoech (2000) states: "Managing information is an organizational process as important to agency success as managing money, personnel, and property. Failure to manage information is wasteful. It causes poor decision making and results in poor goal achievement" (p. 323). Few would quarrel with the premise that information can be influential. However, maybe a few real-life examples of how information has improved organizational performance would help make this proposition come alive.

Case 1

A supported employment program for people with psychiatric disabilities was having a difficulty with job development where employment specialists worked directly with employees to acquire jobs. Employment specialists tended to use passive approaches and were reluctant to directly contact employees. As part of the strategy to increase job development time, the program began monitoring number of employees' contacts each specialist had weekly. Within five months, the employment rate went from 16 to 42 percent (S. Swanson, personal communication, October 21, 2005).

Case 2

A supervisor of case managers working in a Kansas community mental health center received reports that his staff was consistently avoiding goal setting with their clients who were psychiatrically disabled. As a result, much of the work seemed directionless, emphasizing maintenance and crisis intervention over growth and developmental activities. He wanted an increase in the number of goals set and an increase in the amount of goal-directed work. He began posting a summary graph showing the total number of goals that each case manager set with their clients per month. This report was posted on an easily seen bulletin board in the case managers' work area. Within two months, goal setting with clients increased by 25 percent.

Case 3

Rather than allocating resources based on historical trends, contract commitments of future performance, or debates between providers and the state based on anecdotal evidence, New Hampshire designed and implemented a new performance funding system with an empirical methodology based, in part, on performance outcomes. In 1992, the New Hampshire state mental health authority set aside 5 percent of their service budget and allocated it based on contracted agency (community mental health centers) performance in preventing psychiatric hospitalization and increasing competitive employment. From 1992 to 1998, the average number of state hospital bed days across the state decreased from 17.4 to 10.1 days per client per year, the average time in competitive employment per client went from 7.2 percent to 1991 to 17.2 percent in 1999, and the cost per weighted client went from $10,593 to $7,489 per year. It is noteworthy that the percentage of people who were competitively employed went from a statewide average of 11 to 32 percent (Rapp, Huff, & Hansen, 2003).

Case 4

Performance contracting has increased attention to measurement of service elements that have fiscal consequences. When the State of Kansas changed their system of contracting for child welfare services, they specified a penalty for children reentering care within one year of returning home from foster care. The contract included provisions for agencies not to be reimbursed for foster care when children returned to care within one year of returning home. Among other things, contracting agencies carefully counted and reported on when children returned home and the number of months they were there. Kansas is now a state with one of the lowest reentry rates of 3.5 percent compared to the national standard being 8.6 percent (Kansas Department of Social and Rehabilitation Services, 2005).

Exercise

Using an organization that you are familiar with, ask the following questions:

1. *Ask a supervisor to identify one or two things that they measure or pay attention with questions to workers.*
2. *Ask a couple of workers in this unit to list some of the most important elements of their job.*
3. *Identify what the overlap is between what supervisors measure and workers identify as important.*

These short vignettes support what the organization theorist Mason Haire said, "What gets measured gets done" (Quoted in Peters & Waterman, 1982, p. 268). When information is made available, people respond to it. Peters and Waterman (1982) in their study of successful companies observed:

> We are struck by the importance of available information as the basis for peer comparison. Surprisingly, this is the basic control mechanism in the excellent companies. It is not the military model at all. It is not a chain of command wherein nothing happens until the boss tells somebody to do something. General objectives and values are set forward and information is shared so widely that people know quickly whether or not the job is getting done—and who's doing it well or poorly. (p. 266)

They also observed that the data was never used to "browbeat people with numbers" (p. 267). The data alone seemed to motivate people.

THE EFFECTS OF FEEDBACK ON PERFORMANCE

Measurement of something is the first step. Presenting this information in a way that people can act upon it is another. There has been substantial research in organizational settings that have produced important results. Alvero, Bucklin, and Austin (2001) reviewed the research on effectiveness and characteristics of feedback in organizational settings published between 1985 and 1998. Their review followed the methodology and findings of Balcazar, Hopkins, and Suarez (1985), who reviewed this research for an eleven-year period from 1974 through 1984.

Consequently the findings of Alvero, Bucklin, and Austin (2001) cover over twenty years of organizational research. They found that in 58 percent of the 64 recent studies that they reviewed the feedback had consistent positive effects with 41 percent of the studies showing mixed effects and only 1 percent showed no effect. The six conditions of effective feedback in organizations that they identified are presented in the accompanying text and are worth committing to memory and using on a daily basis as an essential management tool. Managers who are committed to increasing performance have at hand a powerful tool. By proactively and systematically collecting and feeding back information, managers can enhance the goal-directed performance of program staff, as well as increase their motivation, professional learning, and sense of reward.

Feedback Was Most Effective When

- *combined with antecedents such as training, task analysis, or supervisory prompts;*
- *provided through graphs combined with written and verbal feedback;*
- *delivered daily, monthly, and the combination of daily and weekly;*
- *provided to the work group;*
- *provided both privately and publicly;*
- *compared group performance with a standard or previous group performance, or individual performance with a standard of individual or previous performance.*

THE LEARNING ORGANIZATION

A learning organization takes periodic readings on its performance and makes adjustments so that performance is improved. If funds are the lifeblood of an organization, then information is its intelligence. A provocative, yet little realized, promise of information systems is that they become a tool for the "learning organization" to improve its performance.

Argyris and Schon (1996, 1978) work on organizational learning started with their 1978 landmark book. They have devoted more than twenty-five years to defining and researching organizational learning with their concept of "double loop" learning. Double-loop learning is how organizations detect errors in performance as well as objectives and values (Argyris, 2004, 1999). He observes that this requires valid information, free and informed choice, and internal commitment to the choice and monitoring of its implementation. This is exactly the information system and organizational climate that we advocate.

For an organization to engage in double-loop learning it must take periodic readings on its performance and *use* these readings to adjust and improve performance. Figure 6.1 depicts the relationship between the elements of the learning organization.

This requires three things:

- There must be an organizational culture that supports learning and that includes contingencies for enhanced learning. Within the organizational culture, performance-enhancing strategies require a supportive environment. This is not to say that if the support environment does not exist, social administrators should throw up their hands and say it is hopeless. The importance of the culture is emphasized to remind administrators that they have an important role in constructing the environment in which management technologies can succeed.
- A manager must have the knowledge and skill in the learning organization to use information to enhance performance. The manager can either sense what is important and bring it to everyone's attention or diffuse attention by focusing on trivial elements.
- There must be an information system, an ongoing system, to measure, store, retrieve, and report performance-enhancing information.

Organizational Culture

The only perfect system is the one you have now to produce what you get. Although a learning organization includes resources, quality of staff, and quality services, it also includes the organizational culture within which people work. Friedman, Lipshitz, and Overmeer (2001) in their explication of the Argyris and Schon model of organizational learning comment that double-loop learning requires a culture that fosters inquiry, openness, and trust.

The elements of organizational culture are more fully developed in Chapter 8. However, one critical element is the norms and values of the social system that drive the way things are done. These define what is impor-

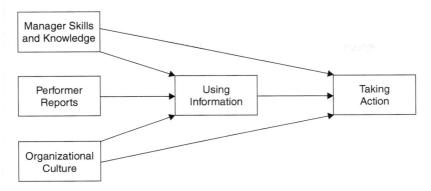

FIGURE 6.1. Elements of the Learning Organization

tant in the organization and the boundaries for behavior. What managers pay attention to is both a primary mechanism for creating norms and a manifestation or symbol of the organizational culture.

Some managers seem to manage by budget, whereby most decisions are made based on the income it can generate or the costs to be saved. Some managers seem to manage by rules and regulations, where as long as these are followed and adhered to, all is well. Often this type of manager's preferred solution to some problem is to create a new policy or rule. Still other managers seem to manage by happy constituents. In this style, good publicity (or at least the absence of bad publicity), contented judges and affiliated agencies, and happy staff are the most important matters. There are managers that seem to manage by problem, whereby their responsibilities are discharged through whatever the latest crisis or problem is, which is brought to them by staff, clients, or external constituencies. The irony is that managing by problems with its lack of proactive behavior and the attention paid to problems by the manager leads to a steady, if not increasing, flow of problems.

Organizational members in a learning organization focus on the continued improvement in client outcome performance and believe people are capable of and have a desire to learn. There is no social program that is so successful that there is nothing left to learn. Yet many organizations block learning by excusing poor performance or blaming others for mistakes. Common excuses include that the caseloads are different and more difficult, lack of resources, and lack of staff or time. Blame often is directed at key players such as families, courts, other agencies, or the clients themselves. Excuses and blame block learning by assuming a protective or defensive stance.

The learning posture assumes that staff are doing their best and that they confront myriad obstacles and constraints. These need to be identified and addressed, not tolerated or assumed to be unchangeable. It also assumes that the organization has much to learn from the higher performers within the agency. The responsibility for these cultural mores is the performance manager, and it is the information system that provides all staff with that valued feedback indicating success, suggesting the possibility for improvement, and directing the staff to the important areas for learning.

Organizational culture not only establishes the desire to learn but it also dictates whether data are interpreted and action taken. For example, a manager of a community program for the people with psychiatric disabilities receives data on the movement of clients into and from independent living situations. Managers will devote time to interpreting the data if they know their superiors are going to question their performance—whether it is inadequate or outstanding. Managers will probably take action if their evaluations are partially based on the movement of clients. In many agencies, the match between the data and the organizational contingencies is discrepant except for financial reports. For example, many personnel evaluation systems still measure such things as punctuality, responsibility, and cooperation, rather than performance.

The point is, when data are reflective of the organizational contingencies, the likelihood of organizational personnel spending time interpreting data and acting upon it is increased. It is the rare organization where

- the desired outcome for clients is clearly stated and regularly communicated;
- client outcomes are a regular and explicit item on staff meeting agenda;
- client outcome data are featured in agency public relations material;
- client outcomes are the subject of agency memos;
- the program's "batting average" on client outcomes is posted; and
- effective staff are featured in board meetings.

Exercise

Use a service unit within an organization with which you are familiar. Identify how many of the following things are done on a regular basis. If the unit does not measure up to your expectations do not use the results to criticize the manager but to identify concrete things that you will do when using information to enhance consumer success.

- *The desired outcome for clients is clearly stated and regularly communicated.*
- *Client outcomes are a regular and explicit item on staff meeting agenda.*
- *Client outcome data are featured in agency public relations material.*
- *Client outcomes are the subject of agency memos.*
- *The program's "batting average" on client outcomes is posted, and effective staff are featured in board meetings.*

Too few social service units follow these practices and this contributes to the slow rise in concern about performance information within organizations or units. Human services rarely get rewarded for effectiveness in terms of client satisfaction, or client outcome. Administrators are rarely reprimanded or even questioned as to how many clients "improved." Staying within the budget, staying out of the press, and continuing to serve an adequate number of clients seems to suffice. Reports for federal and state governments are dominated by concerns for the number of clients served in various categories, dollars spent, and amount of service activity. Rarely do they reflect whether these produced any benefits to clients.

In recent years there has been a definite and potentially powerful trend to developing outcome-oriented human service systems through performance contracting (Martin, 2005). Performance contracting has two major elements: (1) the outcome desired and a performance standard; (2) consequences for achievement and nonachievement. In vocational rehabilitation, Oklahoma has developed a milestone system that reimburses contractors for client movement toward competitive work with the highest reimbursement for the last two steps of job hiring and job maintenance. In Kansas, child welfare services (adoption, foster care, and family preservation) were contracted where the state agency allocated an amount for each child. For example, such children served by the adoption agency received a flat amount of $18,000. The incentives were for the agency to place a child as quickly as possible. In fact, adoptions did increase.

It is likely that client outcome information will be collected and used in agencies operating under such performance-contracting schemes. Regardless, social administrators are responsible for their organization's culture and contingencies. Of the five performance areas, the acquisition of resources and tracking the number of units of service produced are the most frequently attended to and culturally supported areas. The social administrator needs to take responsibility for the organization's culture and goals as they relate to client outcomes. Many of the cultural elements required to support these performance areas are included in other chapters. In the realm of information, the key is to find a variety of ways to have data become important symbols for communicating organizational priorities and accomplishments.

Skills and Knowledge of the Manager

A pilot needs to know how to read the gauges that comprise the cockpit and to interpret the readings, and be skillful in making necessary adjustments. The social administrator is the crucial element in how staff performs, just as the pilot determines the plane's performance. It is largely through the manager's efforts, behaviors, and actions, that an organization transforms its resources into performance. In the learning organization, the manager's attitude is that information and data enhance learning. Along with this, the manager needs to know what performance is and how it can be measured. And finally the manager needs the skills to provide information to staff in ways that will enhance their learning and make them act upon the information to enhance their performance. Friedman, Lipshitz, and Overmeer (2001) further identify the skills as fostering transparency or openness, inquiry by all staff, disconfirmation, and accountability.

A learning stance by organizational members is ignited by a purpose that reflects client outcomes (the principle of creating and maintaining the focus). This purpose must then be reflected in what the organization does and how members behave. It is the performance manager who helps maintain the focus and links managerial behavior, including the use of data, to that purpose. Managers also have to be skilled in reading, interpreting, and using data reports. They have an appreciation for the influence such data can have on staff and performance. As Rapp and Goscha (2006) described:

> There are two levels of purposefulness in case management. The ultimate purpose of our work is to help a person recover, reclaim or transform their lives. The relationship should be goal-directed and growth-oriented; sharing a common agenda that defines the work you do together. This overall vision provides a foundation for the second level, the purpose of each helping encounter.
>
> For many case managers, the work tends to be reactive and passive. The purpose of seeing a client is often described as to "check on," "monitor," "visit" or "see how they are doing." In answer to "how's the clients doing?" the answer is often, "Howard's doing fine." This language is reflective of the perception of the role and purpose of the case manager.
>
> In contrast, a case manager who has adopted the vision of recovery tends to use phases like, "planned next steps in getting a car," "while doing a strengths assessment found the following information helpful

to the person recovery," "reviewed his goal achievement for the last week," "I learned the reasons he doesn't like to take his medications," "we celebrated his first week on the job by going out for coffee together." (p. 74)

Skills in Designing Performance Reports

In human service, managers must know what constitutes performance. It is very difficult to improve performance if you do not know what that performance is. This involves the identification of units and areas of operation that perform adequately, as well as problem areas. The literature and curricula on management are replete with content on problem solving, but relatively little attention has been devoted to problem finding. Yet a number of people have argued that problem-finding skills are a more potent predictor of successful managers than problem-solving skills (Argyris, 2004). Problem-finding information detects errors and disconfirms ideas about how performance is achieved. It is necessary to prevent organizational crises, evaluate staff, and keep the program on course. Data-based management reports focused on performance are in part problem finders. The reports do not tell the manager what to do, only where to do it.

Managers must also know how to measure performance and design meaningful, easy-to-read reports. Measurement frequently conjures up images of program evaluation with the technical expert who comes into an agency and interviews clients, staff, and files. Another inadequate image is the psychometrician who develops measurement instruments for such concepts as self-esteem or locus of control, obsesses about validity and reliability, and is never satisfied with the result.

A manager must be able to judge the relationship between the instrument and what it purports to measure, in this case, performance. A manager may judge that a potential measure does not reflect performance or that the results will not be the best indicator of the desired performance. For example, a report on the level of psychiatric hospitalizations may stimulate a reconsideration of the measure itself. Perhaps length of stay or number of hospital days consumed would be a more accurate reflection of a program's intent. Interpretation is enhanced when the measure says something very directly about the purpose and performance of the agency.

Although measurement is a technical area, there are only a few measurement concepts that managers need and can readily learn. There is a wealth of measurement technologies currently being used from which managers can borrow and learn. Since what gets measured gets attended to, managers must develop the knowledge to measure performance. See Chapter 7 for information on measurement.

Principles of Performance Report Design

Once the social administrator has determined what to measure and how to measure it, the goal is to provide performance information to organizational personnel in such a way as to facilitate its use for improving program performance. Just as the pilot needs to be able to glance at his or her various gauges and judge performance to determine whether action is required, social service staff need to be able to glance at a report and see how the program is performing. Effective feedback is clear and easily understood; it is focused and not overwhelming. How the report is presented, organized, and formatted is critical to how the information will ultimately be used. In this regard, there are five design principles.

Principle #1: Every Report Needs a Standard

Numbers reflecting performance are meaningless if there is nothing to compare them to. If the plane is at an altitude of 25,000 feet, is that where it should be? What does the figure forty-five clients employed in December 2006 mean? Is it adequate performance? Inadequate? Outstanding? From January to December 2006, 523 persons were in day treatment; is this worthy of commendation or castigation? If a standard is not present in the report, the reader must locate the standards on an annual goal sheet or some interdepartmental memo and incorporate the information into the report. This does not facilitate the use of the report to measure or enhance performance. This not only seems to be common sense but is one of the conditions that Alvero, Bucklin, and Austin (2001) found for the effective use of feedback.

When numbers are reported for which no standard has been established it allows people to ignore the report or make up their own standard to make the unit "look good." A report that is discarded is a waste of organizational resources. A report that allows someone to create their own standard creates conflict because one person views the number as reflective of good performance while another would see the same number as poor. In any case, a lack of standards does not help an organization attain its goal.

Establishing performance standards is usually based on historical patterns of the program, of other programs, or practice wisdom. A fourth method of standard setting avoids the use of historical information through the use of ranks.

Past experience: The experience of other program efforts. In an ideal world, standards of performance would come from the experience of those programs that established the intervention as an evidence-based program.

Although no two social programs are exactly the same, the research base includes expectations for the size of the effect of the program that translates into performance standards. The evidence-based practice movement in adult mental health has produced information on levels of client outcomes likely to be produced by implementation of the practice and information on the levels of fidelity that would predict these outcomes levels (Becker, Xie, McHugo, Halliday, & Martinez, 2006; Becker, Smith, Tanzman, Drake, & Tremblay, 2001; Bond & Salyers, 2004).

Either direct communication or a careful reading of the research literature can yield information about the outcome and implementation experience of other programs. It is now reasonably common to find the results of program effort in a wide variety of academic and professional journals. For example, reports of program experience that would be useful in constructing numerical targets can be found regularly in such journals as *Evaluation Quarterly, Policy Studies Review, the Community Mental Health Journal, Social Work, Child Welfare,* and the *Social Service Review,* among others. Authors of these reports are usually quite responsive to requests for further detail if it is needed.

One caution about using performance standards from other programs is in order. Other programs implemented in other places and at other times can be expected to differ. Thus, it pays to take extra care in being clear about similarities and differences of programs. It also pays to implement changes adopted from other programs slowly and audit the results. It may be that the program to which they are being applied is sufficiently different that alternations need to be made or it may be that the standards are appropriate and program performance needs to change. Careful consideration and judgment by the social administrator are required.

Past experience of the program. Most social programs are manifestations of ideas that have a history, and it is from this history that an estimate of a sensible numerical target can be derived. One should be cautious, however, in using prior program history for this purpose. Generalizing from past experience is only safe to the extent that the conditions and the people concerned are the same or at least plausibly similar. For example, prior experience could show that a program reduced commitments of the mentally impaired to state hospitals by fifteen people per month. This program experience can be safely used to project a standard for a new program only if the client population and the level of program effort (staffing, funding, etc.) are similar. Of course, if these differences can be clearly specified, then some creative arithmetic can shade expectations in the appropriate direction.

It may seem reasonable to expect that where programs are replications of past experience, better outcomes can be expected. The principle is that improved program management and outcomes should be expected in repeat performances. A 10 percent improvement over past efforts may be a reasonable expectation, absenting any other basis. Here is where "guesstimates" are appropriate. Note that they are carefully constrained to an estimate of improvement and an "add-on" to the basic expectation derived from concrete experience.

Practice wisdom. Where none of the foregoing sources are available, one often-overlooked source is the practice wisdom of those who have experience with activities and/or clients of concern. A good case can be made for the notion that practice wisdom is seriously underused. Most program designs come from the practical, empirical experience of practitioners who first saw the basic elements of the design operate in a small set of instances. For example, a permanency planning program that intends to free children from what is called "foster care drift" surely originated in the observations of practitioners who saw such things as (1) children in need of care could occasionally be removed permanently from inadequate parents even by the most intransigent and uninterested juvenile judge, (2) even older, or very debilitated, severely multiple handicapped children could sometimes be placed in adoption, and (3) some foster children who were required to be released to what was thought to be inadequate parents turned out all right. Eventually, research was done that more firmly documented these observations, but the point is that some program designs based on these ideas were implemented even before this research was complete. The research later justified the funding for more extensive national programs along the same lines. A fieldworker's practice wisdom is a legitimate source for report standards. For example, many practitioners and administrators had, very early on, fairly clear ideas about how many children were in a condition that was later called "foster care drift," what characteristics they had, and how much and what kind of program effort it would take to impact the problem.

Ranks. Ranking organizational units can serve as a useful method for setting standards. Many people and organizations, in fact, are competitive and motivated toward being "number one" or at least above average. It is important when using ranks as standards to consider the performance area and the measurement involved in assessing this performance. For people to consider their rank as important, they need to consider the performance behaviors themselves to be important. The key is for staff members to be clear about how performance behaviors are explicitly related to the goals for service.

The use of ranks has its weaknesses, however. It is possible that the performance of every unit would be considered inadequate, yet there will always be a number one rank. Similarly, the opposite phenomenon where everyone is performing in outstanding fashion, but someone still had to be ranked last could occur. This in turn could actually reduce motivation and performance.

The selection of a standard (the actual number reflecting desired performance and the type of standard) is based on two factors: achievability (but not too easy) and importance. Achievability involves setting a standard that can be attained for the vast majority (75 to 100 percent) of people or organizational units. This is neither to say that everyone will attain it nor that it will be equally easy for all the parties. An exaggerated example might be to increase the number of psychiatrically disabled individuals in independent living arrangements from 48 percent to 90 percent within three months. There is no way a team could do this without hurting some clients and staff in the process. On the other hand, the standard cannot be too easy to attain. More specifically, if the person or unit needs not to do anything more to achieve the norm, there is little satisfaction in getting it done.

Importance relates to how necessary a given level of performance is. Some outcome indicators may be judged more reflective of organizational mission than others. Perhaps the number of persons being discharged from the hospital within one week may be seen as more central versus the number living at the highest level of independence. The importance of productivity measures often leaves room for discretion. For example, the research indicates that the frequency of worker contact with clients in vivo, ongoing service plan/goal setting, and frequency of contact with clients' significant others/collaterals are all critical to maintaining people in the community. Which is most critical is not known. The manager can make some judgments, however, of which one should receive primary attention during the year. He or she should also reinforce the priority by setting a higher standard on that dimension.

There is as yet no neat formula for setting standards. It requires the knowledge and judgment of the manager. Although much time has been spent discussing the types of standards, the critical element for performance report design is that the standard is present in the report.

Principle #2: Performance Reports Should Be Simple and Contain Few Data Elements

Performance reports are more likely to be used to improve performance if they are simple. That is, they contain only the numbers needed by the manager. London (1997) found in his review of the feedback literature that too much information that is complex may be distorted, ignored, or misunderstood. If a manager has to sort through hundreds of numbers to locate the critical few, they are not likely to spend the time reading it. Several rules of thumb can be proposed:

1. Put one concept, theme, or dimension per page.
2. Data should be distributed only if relevant to the receiver. (If a program manager does not need to know of the performance of other programs, such information should not be routinely provided. The notion is that reports should be tailored to the receiver.)
3. Too much data diffuses efforts by implying a broad range of purposes, goals, and performance indicators. A few key performance indicators can help focus the efforts of semiautonomous staff, units, and agencies.
4. In tables, keep rows and columns to 7, plus or minus 2. A 9 × 9 table contains 81 pieces of information, which is a lot for any normal human mind to read, understand, and analyze.

Principle #3: Aesthetics Are Important
(Pictures Are Worth 1,000 Numbers)

Aesthetics go well beyond the "numbers of numbers" previously mentioned. A performance report should allow the reader to easily read it and evaluate whether the data reflects adequate, inadequate, or outstanding performance. Only when this condition has been met can emphasis be placed on managerial action based on the data.

Alvero, Bucklin, and Austin (2001) found that graphs combined with written or verbal feedback were effect in influencing behavior. Graphs are more likely to be read and understood than data presented in tabular form. Graphic displays are more visual and conclusions are more likely to "leap off the page." Variations are extensive and care must be exercised that the graphic portrait fits the performance information. Variations include many familiar methods, such as bar graphs, pie graphs, line graphs, and the use of maps.

Graphs can illuminate or lie. There are three points to keep in mind when constructing graphs. First, establish the increments for an axis by incorporating the range of the data. Frequently you can simply divide the range by the space available to set the increments. Occasionally there are one or two data points that are very different from the remaining data. In these rare cases, a break can be made in the graph. Second, it is important to keep the increments along the axis uniform. If a space is to represent 100 units, every space needs to represent 100 units. Third, frequently there is a large gap between zero and the first data point. In these cases the axis can be broken. Again it is important to show this on the graph.

Principle #4: Labels Should Be in English

Each table or graph should have a title describing it so that a person not familiar with the agency can understand what is being reported. This is an essential element of having feedback be clear and easily understood (London, 1997). The same principle holds for column and row headings. Abbreviations may have to be used on occasion due to space, but a glossary should be included at the bottom of the page, on the back, or in a cover memo. This principle is particularly important for newly issued reports. When percentages or index numbers are used, a description of how the number was obtained is useful. For a percent, the question, "Percent of what?" should be answered on the table or graph.

Principle #5: The Rule of Aggregation—the Level of Aggregation Used Should Match the Recipients' Place in the Organization

The level of data aggregation included in a report should match the recipient's place in the organization. If serious about providing information to help a person do his or her job better, then the data must say very clearly something about the person's job. For example, statewide data on the allocation of staff time has little import for a team supervisor because it says nothing about his or her domain. Similarly, providing a regional administrator with lists of clients is inappropriate. In general, the direct service worker domain is the client; the program and the agency administrator's domain is the entire agency or the state.

In a small organization with two or three layers it may be possible for audiences at all levels to share the same information. In large multilayered organizations, attending to level of aggregation is more important. For example, frontline workers need data on their cases and data aggregating their caseloads for their supervisor. Similarly, area managers of a statewide organization need data aggregated to report on the performance of their supervisors or program managers and data aggregated for the area.

Principles of Performance Report Design

1. Every report needs a standard. Standards come from the following:
   a. Evidence-based practices
   b. Past performance
   c. Practice wisdom

2. *Performance reports should be simple and contain few data elements.*
   a. *Put one concept, theme, or dimension per page.*
   b. *Data should be distributed only if relevant to the receiver. Reports should be tailored to the receiver.*
   c. *Too much data diffuses efforts by implying a broad range of purposes, goals, and performance indicators.*
   d. *In tables, keep rows and columns to 7, plus or minus 2. A 9 × 9 table contains 81 pieces of information, which is a lot for any normal human mind to read, understand, and analyze.*
3. *Aesthetics are important (pictures are worth 1,000 numbers).*
4. *Labels should be in English.*
5. *The rule of aggregation: The level of aggregation used should match the recipients' place in the organization.*

Skills in Using Information

In human services, managers must have the skills to use information as part of the learning organization's feedback system. Action is unlikely, if not impossible unless the manager can bring meaning to the numbers. Have the results say something about organizational performance. Minimally, this means the manager needs to assign a value to the number. Does the number reflect adequate performance, inadequate performance, or outstanding performance?

Managers should use information to instigate actions, to influence behavior. Datum becomes information only when it can be interpreted and acted upon. Perhaps the most effective information system is that of McDonalds. Upon entering McDonalds, you read or scan the menu, and place your order. The cashier presses a button or two. The information on your order goes directly to the kitchen and includes what you ordered, when it was ordered, and the cost of the meal. McDonalds is the perfect information system in that by pressing a few keys all the symbols necessary for the various employees to do their job is transferred. And there is no waste. Every symbol or piece of data influences the behavior of the staff and is, therefore, information.

In the human services field, data-based performance information can instigate managers to do the following:

- Share information widely
- Reward employees or units for outstanding performance
- Identify factors contributing to high performance
- Identify barriers to adequate performance

- Request a plan of action by which improved performance will be pursued
- Engage in problem solving with subordinates
- Provide training or consultation
- Change policies, procedures, or methods
- Request additional resources or reallocate resources (dollars, effort, etc.)
- Review selected cases
- Enforce current procedures or policies

This list should be merely viewed as a sampler. An information system like McDonalds is nothing more than the mechanism for measuring, collecting the data, storing it, and formatting the data to communicate meaning.

Elements of the Learning Organization

- *Organizational culture that values the following:*
  Openness
  Learning and inquiry
- *Managers' skills and knowledge that includes the following:*
  Knowing the purpose of the unit
  Knowing what performance is
  Skills to measure performance
  Skills to use feedback to effect behavior
- *Performance reports that contain the following features:*
  Include critical performance areas
  Are easy to read
  Instigate action

THE HUMAN SERVICE COCKPIT

Kaplan and Norton (1992, 1993, 1996) developed the idea of "The Balanced Scorecard" following the airplane pilot analogy. They viewed the balanced scorecard as the performance-guidance system for business executives.

Think of the balance scorecard as the dials and indicators in an airplane cockpit. For the complex task of navigating and flying an airplane, pilots need detailed information about many aspects of the flight. They need information on fuel, air speed, altitude, bearing, destination, and other predicted environment. Reliance on one instrument can be fatal. Similarly, the complexity of managing an organization today requires that managers be able to view performance in several areas simultaneously. (Kaplan and Norton, 1992, p. 72)

The experience of developing and using the Balanced Scorecard in business includes the following:

1. Bringing disparate elements of an enterprise together into a single management report that reinforces the organization mission, purposes, and vision
2. Analyzing the possible relationship between organizational elements reflected in the scorecard

Creating a cockpit involves engineers, scientists, computer specialists, and designers. Using the cockpit is the principal responsibility of the pilot (Figure 6.2). This goes on in the context of a culture (from the general citizens to the Federal Aviation Administration) that places a primacy on safety. In the human services, a manager is part engineer, part designer, part pilot, and part shaper of the culture. The manager receives assistance from

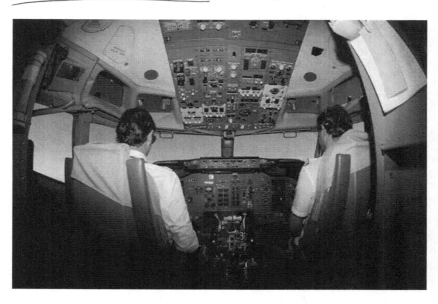

FIGURE 6.2. Airline Cockpit.

computer specialists, other managers, funders, consumers, and university experts but if the cockpit is really going to work, the consumer-centered manager needs to take a leadership role. Like a pilot, the social administrators' job is to steer the organizational unit to achieve its performance goals by making mid-course corrections and adjustments.

The information system for the consumer-centered performance manager within a learning organization produces key performance indicators (KPI) and the ability for managers to "drill down" to better understand performance. Drilling down refers to the information system's ability to configure reports tailored to the manager to answer questions through increasing level of detail. For example, a manager who oversees four teams of case managers notes (from a KPI report) that last month's client employment rate was 25 percent, which was 5 percent below the agency goal. The first question may be what is the contributing performance on this outcome for each of the four teams? Drilling down means that the manager can immediately get such a breakdown on the computer by "pressing a few keys." We will return to drilling down later in the chapter.

The gauges in an airplane cockpit assess essential elements of the plane's performance. Similarly, key performance indicators are the core of the social service performance-guidance system and report on program performance. Performance includes client outcomes and key service events and can include measures of resource acquisition, efficiency, and staff morale.* Depending on one's level within the organization, each of these could vary in importance. For example, the manager of a statewide social service agency would necessarily focus on resource acquisition, as well as client outcomes and key service events and other measures of productivity. In contrast, a frontline supervisor would need information on client outcome, productivity, and staff morale, with less concern with resource acquisition.

The goal is to produce performance information to organizational personnel in such a way as to facilitate its use for improving program performance. This means that the reports must

1. contain the right information for each person's location and responsibilities in the organization;
2. provide data that is accurate, trustworthy and timely; and
3. be formatted to be easy to read and use.

---

*This chapter focuses on client outcomes and key service events, which we believe to be the indispensable core of managing information for performance. The measurement of resource acquisition, efficiency, staff morale, and summary measures of productivity are addressed in the Chapter 7.

The Cockpit: Key Performance Indicators

An example of key performance indicators for an employment program for people with psychiatric disabilities is presented in Figure 6.3. The left column of dials measure client outcome performance in two areas: competitive employment and enrollment in post-secondary education. The right column captures the three service events that are key to producing the outcomes: number of contacts with employers, number of hours in the community, and number of clients where first employer contact was more than one month from referral (desired performance is within one month). The area to the left of the dials reflects below standard performance. The agency requires employment specialist to enter the data for these five dials by 9 a.m. the day following a change. This allows each worker and the employment program supervisor to have always current information, which enhances the power of the feedback and allows the supervisor to intervene, if necessary, in a timely manner. The data need not be formatted as a series of dials. It could be bar graphs or other depictions. The KPI system for this agency was designed so that every time a manager turns his or her computer on the KPI page is on the screen.

PILOTING THE HUMAN SERVICE PROGRAM: ESTABLISHING AND USING A PERFORMANCE-IMPROVEMENT STRATEGY

If the KPIs have been designed correctly, in terms of measurement and formatting, then the likelihood of managers using the data to steer the enterprise is more likely but far from assured. Factors such as the manager's comfort or discomfort with reading and interpreting data and his or her skill in using information will influence its use. There are two obstacles that most profoundly lead to nonuse.

First, the degree to which managers apply an outcome focus and are leaders of their domain in their quest for client outcomes will be a determinant. There is evidence that managers who are reactive, having a laissez-faire leadership style, contribute to lower rates of consumer outcomes and consumer satisfaction (Corrigan, Lickey, Campion, and Rashid, 2000), greater burnout, and less cohesion of staff (Corrigan, Giffort, Rashid, Leary, & Okeke, 1999). Managers who spend their day responding to problems and crises brought to them by staff or attending a lot of administrative meetings not related to client outcomes will have little interest in reading,

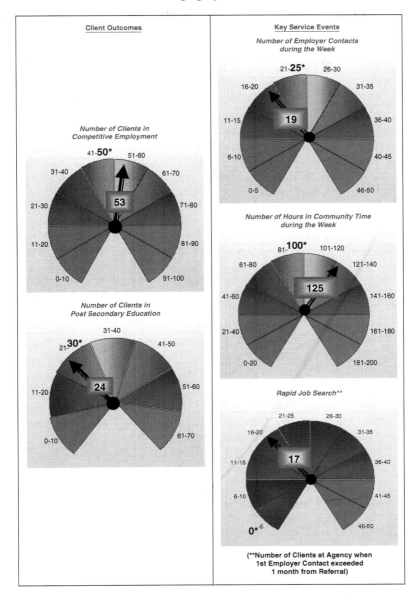

FIGURE 6.3. Cockpit for Employment Service Supervision. *Denotes Agency Standard

interpreting, and using the KPIs contained in the cockpit. In fact, it is an oxymoron that a manager can be reactive or laissez-faire and lead.

Second, the data itself must not only be reasonably accurate but must also be timely. Receiving a performance report six months after the period of performance is of minimal use to the client-centered manager. It would be like a pilot receiving data on the plane's altitude based on its position an hour ago. Feedback is most influential when it is timely, if not immediate. Some computer systems in the human services only produce reports at pre-set periods and often at considerable delay. Timeliness is also affected by delays in staff entering data. In business, a salesperson enters sales immediately upon an order. When checking into a hotel, it is automatically entered. The UPS worker immediately records the status of a package. Therefore, the customer and anyone in the organization can have a current status report. In human services, it is more frequent to expect weekly or monthly entering of data. Beside "fear" of employees, there is little reason that workers should not be expected to be current on a daily basis (except in the case of a crisis of some sort).

Prerequisites to Implementing a Performance-Improvement Strategy

1. Social administrators apply an outcome focus and are leaders of their domain in their quest for client outcomes.
2. The data must not only be reasonably accurate but must be timely.

Here is a social service example. Sitka is the team leader for the supported employment team serving people with psychiatric disabilities within a community support program. At 8:30 a.m., she turns on her computer and reviews "the people employed" KPI. She also reads the "number of job development contacts" KPI (a powerful predictor of employment outcomes) and sees that there were only six contacts yesterday for her staff of five. She then calls upon the computer to provide the breakdown of contacts by staff member. She finds that one worker had three contacts, one had two, and another had one. As she sees her staff that day, she is in a position to ask about how the job development contacts went and reinforce the link between these contacts and employment outcomes. She can also review with the three staff having one or no contacts their use of time yesterday or barriers they may have confronted, and then reinforce the expectation of two employer contacts a day, and ask them about today's schedule. This mode of managing/leading, is so much more powerful than getting a report a month later and reviewing it with the staff (although this would be better than not doing it at all).

The Search for Explanation

Similar to the pilot who sees a discrepancy between what a gauge should be showing and what it indicates and chooses an action, a performance-improvement strategy in a learning organization begins with the information system detecting an error or inadequacy in performance. Explaining or understanding inadequate performance is focused on locating factors contributing to it. These factors often become the target of performance-improvement efforts. There are almost always multiple factors that come together to impact performance on any given outcome indicator. The manager has a better chance of developing a lasting solution to the performance problem when one considers these multiple factors. Each of them can provide important clues about what to do. It usually starts with questions such as the following:

1. Does each worker (team) contribute equally to the performance? Are some workers doing exceptional and others inadequately?
2. Are the key service events sufficiently frequent to produce the desired performances?
3. Is there a subset of cases that are negatively affecting the performance?

Exhibit 6.1 contains a beginning list of dimensions and factors (variables) that often impinge on performance. To answer these types of questions, a manager can use a combination of computer-based tools, the manager's own knowledge, and that of the staff.

Drilling Down

Information systems can have the capacity for a manager to query the data base for answers to questions such as the ones mentioned earlier. The current information technology (IT) term is "drilling down." Examples of current systems with this capacity include the Results Oriented Management system (www.rom.ku.edu). The term "drilling down" is used to convey that the user can obtain more detailed information about cases comprising the performance numbers that can be sorted, analyzed, and verified. This helps with interpreting the results and ultimately informs managers on where to target program improvement efforts.

> Let's say that Mike the manager sees that children are re-entering placement at a rate higher than the performance standard. A manager can pull up a list of those children re-entering and sort it by length of time from reunification to re-entry, age, county or management unit, judicial distinct, whether it was an abuse/neglect or non-abuse/ neglect case, or whatever information is provided. If any of these factors seem to stand out as having some relationship with the outcome, the manager can target the action they take to improve performance. (Moore, 2003)

Using drop-down menus, the manager can get data organized in a myriad of ways. For example, a manager notices that the rate of psychiatric hospitalization was above standard (poor performance) for the last three months. She wants to answer the question about staff's possible contribution to the situation. On the drop-down menu, she selects the indicator (hospitalization), the time period (most recent quarter), and by worker. On her screen is the incidence of hospitalization for the last quarter for each worker. She could also ask the computer for a listing of clients who were hospitalized in order of the amount of service hours they received. The clients on the bottom would be clients who had few service hours, which could have been a contributing factor to the hospitalization. Further, she could query the data to break down service hours into the type of service.

Without this computer capacity, the quest for answers to these questions is more cumbersome involving requests for special reports from the IT staff, case record reviews, discussions with staff, and so on.

The Best Guess Approach

One approach starts with your best guesses (hypothesis) about what is contributing to this performance (Moore, 2003). A guess by someone familiar with the field (educated guess) frequently turns out to be very close to what is really happening. Hunches or practice wisdom are great places to start.

> In our example, Mike the manager, hypothesized that the kids who came into placement due to behavior (non-abuse/neglect) was the population that re-entered at greater rates. He later analyzed re-entry rates for both abuse/neglect and non-abuse/neglect populations in order to test his hypotheses. This analysis supported his guess (hypothesis). (Moore, 2003)

The Observation Approach

Another approach suggested by Moore (2003) is to observe patterns from looking at groups of consumers where performance was either met or not. It is easy for practitioners to suggest reasons for consumers succeeding or failing. These suggestions can then be treated as hypotheses to be tested through data.

> In our example, Mike had his field staff look at a list of cases where children re-entered out of home placement, to look for patterns and commonalities. The staff noticed that these cases did not stay in out-of-home care long, moved frequently, and came back quickly. Then they analyzed their data that confirmed these associations. They also noticed that most of these cases were ones where judges did not follow agency recommendations. Except for one judge, this checked out to not be true. (Moore, 2003)

Intensive Case Review

Case review may be the oldest approach in social work. In some agencies supervisors are expected to review each and every case file every time a worker has an encounter with a consumer. Some agencies practice something known as "grand rounds." This is a practice borrowed from medicine where a particularly troublesome case is presented to a group of agency staff. This is followed by discussion of the consumers' situation or condition and different approaches available to staff. Quality improvement systems usually include taking a random sample of the case and filling out a questionnaire regarding consumers' situation and worker action to determine whether workers are employing "best practices." As Moore suggests (2003) not only do common themes emerge that can be useful in taking action but staff also learn a tremendous amount from the process.

Field Supervision

At times, the root of a performance deficiency is not what is being done (e.g., frequency of job development contacts with employers) but how it is being done (e.g., various engagement and interviewing skills of the workers). The *only* way to truly assess worker skills is to accompany them as they conduct their work. It also provides great opportunities to provide feedback and model specific methods. Any deficits uncovered could be addressed by training, role-playing, or, most powerfully, by additional in-field supervision.

A combination of methods is often used to analyze and explain a given performance deficit. The result is usually one or more salient factors that will be targeted for correction. (See Exhibit 6.1.)

EXHIBIT 6.1. Checklist of Factors to Consider in Analysis

- Client Factors: Are any client characteristics correlated with the outcome you seek to explain? The following is a starter list to consider:
  — Demographics (e.g., age, sex, race)
  — County of residence
  — Disability types
  — Family/parent characteristics
  — Case plan goal
  — Special needs or strengths of children of family (e.g., poverty, supportive extended family, drug/alcohol usage, mental illness, parenting skills, school performance)
  — Referral reason (e.g., abuse or neglect types)

- Services factors: Can the quantity of quality of services or the type of services provided help to explain the outcome being achieved?
  — Services provided (e.g., mental health services, respite care, parent training, substance abuse treatment, or any specialized programs or treatment)
  — Placement type (e.g., residential, family foster care, kinship, independent living)
  — Duration of services
  — Conformity with policies and procedures (e.g., case plan reviews within time requirements, court recommendations approved by the supervisor)
  — Quantity of service units (e.g., contacts with parents or child, parent-child visitation)
  — Quality of services (e.g., engagement of family, placement proximity, licensing)

- Organizational factors: Does anything the organization (agency) is doing or not doing impact on the achievement of this outcome?
  — Management units (area, county, unit)
  — Policies and procedures
  — Staffing (e.g., caseload size, vacancies, conflicts between and among staff, staff morale)
  — Available resources (e.g., placement, treatment, funding)

— Program design—the array of services provided to whom under what conditions [e.g., aftercare (reunification) services provided, concurrent case planning, separation or integration of permanency and adoption staff.)]
— Values and culture—he attitudes, beliefs, and behaviors reinforced by the organization

- Community factors
  — County of venue (judges or county/district attorneys)
  — Availability and cooperation of community resources (e.g., education, housing, employment, child care, mental health, dental)
  — Child and parent attorneys

From "Results oriented management in child welfare" by T. Moore (2003), www.rom.ku.edu. Reprinted with permission.

Setting Improvement Goals

Before generating strategies to address the inadequate performance, the manager needs to begin setting a relevant improvement goal. As Lawler (1996) states:

Considerable research in psychology on goal setting shows that the highest performance comes when individuals are committed to reaching such goals. It also shows that individuals are more likely to be committed to those goals when there are rewards that are attached to achieving them and when individuals believe that the goals agree with their value systems and contribute to objectives they share. (p. 66)

Goals are also cognitive representations of a future and, as such, influence motivation (Lawler, 1996; Locke & Latham, 1990).

Goals should be challenging yet achievable. Of particular interest is which goals do you think are most effective, easy, or difficult goals? Surprising, more difficult goals lead to a higher level of performance than do easy goals, if the task is voluntary and the person has the ability to achieve the goal (Lawler, 1996; Locke & Latham, 1990). People tend to expend more effort to attain a goal they perceive as difficult. However, the goal must not be so difficult that it seems to be unachievable because most people will avoid a task they perceive as impossible. One way of setting challenging goals is to decompose a six-month goal into monthly goals.

The goal is often derived from the problem or factor. The goal restates the problem as a statement reflecting a positive view of the future. This is not just semantics. People simply react more positively to statements of a desired future than to problems. They begin to see a goal rather than a problem. They then begin to imagine how to achieve this goal or desired state. With problems it is common for people to react with defensiveness, helplessness, and negativity. In defining your desired future you have changed from a focus on problems to a focus on possibilities.

Goals can be of several levels. One level should be reflective of the relevant client outcome or result area (KPI):

- Decrease the number of incidence of hospitalization by four during the next quarter.
- Increase the number of adoptions by 10 percent next month.
- Increase the supported employment fidelity score from sixty to sixty-five by January.

A second level is frequently reflective of the previous analysis where specific factors have been identified. In the example of Manager Mike, one goal, given the analysis, could have been:

By March, 95 percent of non-abuse/neglect cases in foster care will have an aftercare plan that has been reviewed by the supervisor for quality.

Social administrators might find a monthly form useful for setting improvement goals. Figure 6.4 is an example that can assist managers to use data reports to celebrate success and/or set goals. It has all of the ingredients of a tool that promotes action.

Improvement Goals

- *Should motivate staff and represent a shared future*
- *Should be challenging but achievable*
- *Should reflect the desired consumer outcome*
- *Should reflect specific identified factors that are thought to contribute inadequate performance*

Are you satisfied with your team's performance for this reporting period?

YES- What data from the report reflects exceptional performance?

How will you Celebrate and Acknowledge your team's SUCCESS?

NO- Our team CAN do better!
What numbers from the report data reflects performance you would like to improve?

What resources or information are necessary to improve performance?

GOAL (1)	GOAL (2)
Right now, our report data says we are here:	Right now, our report data says we are here:
_____	_____
By the end of the next report period, our report data will improve to:	By the end of the next report period, our report data will improve to:
	_____

 What FIRST STEPS will the team take to accomplish each GOAL?

GOAL (1) Step 1	GOAL (2) Step 1
GOAL (1) Step 2	GOAL (2) Step 2

FIGURE 6.4. Form for Celebrating Success and Setting Goals.

Creating a Performance-Improvement Strategy

This step of the performance-improvement process answers the question: How will we achieve our goal? This entails developing a general strategy, defining specific tasks, assigning responsibility for those tasks, and dates for meeting the responsibilities. Management actions taken to optimize outcomes can take many different forms. Here are a few:

- Taking action on individual cases or group of cases
- Making refinements or changes in program design, policy, or procedures
- Securing needed resources
- Developing skills and knowledge of your staff
- Influencing stakeholders either internal and external to your agency
- Enforcing existing expectations

Since each situation is unique, Moore (2003) suggests guidelines for developing performance-improvement strategies that are useful across situations. The following are his guidelines.

Breaking Down into Manageable Pieces

The saying widely attributed to Chinese philosopher Lao-Tzu is appropriate here: "A journey of a thousand miles begins with a single step." Helping a consumer manage an addiction, a worker manage a caseload, or an agency implement a new strategy to improve outcomes requires breaking the seemingly overwhelming task into small first steps. The work days of managers and staff are already filled. However, even within a busy day, a phone call can be made, a case record can be reviewed, a letter can be written, or even a meeting can be held. Breaking large performance-improvement efforts into discrete tasks lets the work become manageable and avoids feelings of being overwhelmed.

Documenting Your Plan in Writing Is a Good Idea

Most of us are familiar with the telephone game. Form a circle and whisper something to the person next to you. That person passes the message on to the next and so on until the message is back to the originator. The message is seldom the same. The best designed plans formed in your mind or by a group fall into this same trap. People forget or misunderstand or do not hear it quite the same way. To keep everyone on the same page there needs to be a page. According to Moore (2003) among the elements to be recorded are the following:

1. The outcome goal (and any intermediate goals)
2. General strategies

3. Measurable objectives
4. Tasks, establish responsibilities, and determine timelines

Determine General Strategy

The general strategy follows almost naturally from previous analysis. The improvement plan started the outcome goal. The search for an explanation of a discrepancy between expected performance and what data are showing generated ideas or hypotheses that are useful for forming a general strategy. The general strategy may be as simple as selecting those hypotheses that are best supported by the data and are most feasible to implement.

In our example of children reentering foster care, the hypothesis that most of these children had entered care due to behavior problems turned out to be the case. This suggested that although the child successfully adjusted to living in a foster home and was judged ready to return home, the home was not ready for the child. Therefore, the general strategy that the team agreed with included the following:

- Prior to reunification, provide parents with behavior management strategies and techniques specific to the difficult behaviors they have identified, those that led the child to being placed in foster care and those identified by the foster parents.
- Immediately upon reunification, have a worker visit the home on a daily basis and review with the parents the child's behavior and the use of behavior management techniques. The worker should be prepared to practice the techniques with the parent and bring in a behavioral specialist as needed. As the child's behavior becomes manageable, the frequency of the visits decreases.
- Have a behavioral specialist available to the parent and caseworker on a 24/7 basis until the behavior stabilizes.

Involving Others or Not

Deciding who needs to be involved in creating a performance-improvement strategy is an important management task. The old adage that too many cooks can spoil the soup is appropriate. At the same time, too few ingredients makes a thin unsatisfying soup or, in this case, an unsuccessful attempt to improve performance. Moore (2003) suggests the following advantages for involving others.

1. Enriched understanding of the problem due to the input from multiple perspectives
2. More ideas for how to improve performance
3. Increased focus on outcomes you are striving to achieve
4. Greater ownership and cooperation for carrying out the action plan

In general, who these others are depends on (1) who has the knowledge to be helpful and (2) who is needed to implement the strategy.

Clearly consumers and workers provide the perspective of the day-to-day successes or failures of current practices. Content experts such as the behavior specialist in the previous example can help fit effective interventions to real-world situations. Policy or contract staff can help determine where the resources can come from to implement the strategy. Judges, police, or other "key actors" identified in the program specifications (Chapter 5) need to know their role and be willing to perform it for consumers to be successful.

An example of how consumer involvement can be helpful comes from Sedgwick County, Kansas (Wichita).

Community Support Program staff became aware that only 12 of out 874 clients were enrolled in postsecondary education. They knew that a sizable increase could not be accomplished by the program alone. The staff invited representatives from affiliate mental health agencies, the Kansas Alliance for the Mentally Ill, consumers from the program's advisory board, consumer drop-in center, representatives from universities and junior colleges, and a few employers.

At the meeting, the CSP Director, Kevin Bomhoff, distributed the data and expressed his dismay. He went on to say, "We need to do something about this and the people in this group are the ones who could make it happen. The purpose of this meeting is to figure out how."

One result was the hiring of a person whose only responsibility was supported education. A liaison with each postsecondary institution was designated, and responsibility for collecting information on scholarships, financial aid, and various courses of study was delegated. Methods for educating consumers, parents, and case managers were formulated. Within six months, there was a 58 percent increase in the number of clients enrolled in college.

Brainstorming

In the process of refining the details of a performance-improvement strategy, those involved in the process frequently identify obstacles or roadblocks to the success of the plan. Stopping the process and brainstorming with those you choose to involve in the process is a useful technique to generate creative ideas to overcome these problems. Moore (2003) reminds us of rules for successful brainstorming.

1. Collect as many ideas as possible
2. Be creative (all ideas welcomed)
3. Build on other's ideas
4. Record ideas for all to see
5. Set a time limit
6. Do not judge or evaluate ideas
7. Do not discuss ideas in depth

Assign Responsibilities and Timeline

Unassigned tasks rarely get done. The written plan contains tasks, responsibilities, and timelines. Each task needs to be linked to a person responsible for its accomplishment by the time specified.

Careful consideration of who is responsible for each task is also important. A task assigned to someone without the expertise of interest in it is unlikely to be successfully accomplished. Although asking for volunteers has the potential advantage of the person volunteering being motivated, this should be balanced with their ability to successfully accomplish the task. Frequently a mix of assigning tasks to some people, asking specific people if they would be willing to take on a task, and seeking general volunteers is what occurs.

Establishing and Using a Performance-Improvement Strategy

- *The search for explanation*
- *Setting improvement goals*
- *Creating a performance-improvement strategy*
    Break it into manageable pieces
    Write the plan
    Determine a general strategy
    Involving others?
    Brainstorming
    Assigning responsibilities and timelines

Chapter 7

Selection and Measurement of Performance Indicators

Chapter 6 focused on the tasks of the consumer-centered manager converting data to outcomes for consumers. The social administrator guides the social service program like a pilot guides the plane by creating a learning organization, nurturing a culture of inquiry, and using the power of data to provide feedback in a helpful manner. The selection of measures that ultimately emerge as cockpit gauges requires a different set of technical and conceptual skills.

Learning Objectives for Selection and Measurement of Performance Indicators

- *Understand the criteria for individual performance measures.*
- *Understand the criteria for a set of program performance measures.*
- *Select consumer outcome measures that match the type of desired outcome.*
- *Determine measures for program performance in the areas of service events, acquisition of resources, efficiency, and staff morale.*
- *Become familiar with the innovative report designs of movement tables and event history graphs.*

SELECTING OUTCOME MEASURES

The airline cockpit has a set of gauges that report measures that aeronautical experts agree are essential for safely piloting the plane to a destination. The social administrator has the challenge of not only piloting the program

Textbook of Social Administration: The Consumer-Centered Approach
© 2007 by The Haworth Press, Inc. All rights reserved.
doi:10.1300/5802_08

but also determining the measures that will guide it. This challenge has two parts. First, administrators must choose individual measures that are accurate. Second, administrators must place these measures in a context where they collectively are a valid reflection of program performance.

Selecting Individual Measures

Readers will remember the standard measurement criteria of validity and reliability. In the context of a social program we add a few additional considerations. To guide a social program, measures also need to be understandable, susceptible to change, and efficient.

Measures Need to Be Understandable

A measure needs to use words that everyone understands. A learning organization has a culture of shared norms and values and communicates these through a common language. If different individuals or units have different understandings of a measure, the single focus on that result is lost. From a measurement perspective, development of a valid and reliable measure starts with an unambiguous definition of the concept.

Outcome measures should also pass the commonsense test for users of the data. Reporting to key stakeholders is a critical aspect of the balanced scorecard of Kaplan and Norton (2001). Social services exist because the public invests valuable resources in working with victims of social problems. Consequently, the public is a key stakeholder with which we have an obligation to communicate. A public that does not understand what we are talking about is unlikely to support our efforts.

For example, "family-centered services" has become a popular phrase. This is widely used in child welfare agencies and seems to resonate with social work values. However, it is difficult to find a consistent behavioral definition. The National Resource Center for Family-Centered Practice and Permanency Planning at Hunter College provides a definition that identifies the following four essential components of family-centered services:

1. The family unit is the focus of attention.
2. Strengthening the capacity of families to function effectively is emphasized.
3. Families are engaged in designing all aspects of the policies, services, and program evaluation.
4. Families are linked with more comprehensive, diverse, and community-based networks of supports and services. (Mallon, 2005)

This definition captures important ideas about how families might be engaged in services. However, it is difficult to envision how several people working in the same agency would implement these concepts in the same way. For example, different workers would very likely have various ideas about the meaning of effective family functioning. One can imagine the protracted discussions that are necessary to develop a common understanding of this term. A measure of family functioning without a consensually understood definition is not likely to be useful. This is not to criticize the important work of this center but to point out the difficulty of concretely defining many of the words we use. In mental health, empowerment, social support, and recovery are commonly used terms that, to date, have defied consensual and precise definition.

Measure Should Be Valid

The concept of validity is reflected in the common question: Does the instrument measure what it intends to? This criterion is related to the first, since a concept that is not clearly understood is not likely to be measured in a valid manner. Measures that are not defined in a concrete observable manner cannot be validly measured.

An agency interested in measuring family functioning must first arrive at an unambiguous definition. Considering the complexity of families with multiple members and tasks, this is a daunting undertaking. Although it is possible to identify the many contexts that families operate in and eventually arrive at observable instances of effective functioning in those settings, it may be beyond the resources of a particular program to do so.

Given the complexity of so many of the situations that social workers intervene in, there is a temptation to skip the step of clearly defining a concept and to just adopt a measure developed by someone else. It is costly and time consuming to develop a valid instrument and not to be undertaken without sufficient expertise and resources. At the same time, when a measure is selected the user is also adopting the definition of those that developed it. The step of clearly defining what it is that you want to measure cannot be ignored.

Once a concept is defined and a measure is selected, validity can be discussed. Although it is a difficult task to determine whether everyone in the unit has a shared meaning for a concept, it is even more difficult to determine the validity of a measure. There is a tendency for those who want to be critical of a measure to question its validity by saying; "This instrument is not valid." Although this may be true, the statement also implies a misunderstanding of the concept of validity. Measurement validity is not a yes or no concept. Instruments are more or less valid with different types of evidence for validity. The question is: "What is the validity evidence for this instrument?"

Experts in measurement have a variety of ways to gather evidence for validity including construct, concurrent, and predictive. These technical aspects of validity will not be undertaken here. Social administrators are familiar with the basic types of validity from introductory research courses and should consult with measurement experts when examining a particular instrument.

Measures Should Be Reliable

The basic idea of reliability is consistency. If the concept being measured does not change, the measure should not change. In an agency context, this also means the results should not vary simply because a different worker completes the measure.

For example, placement stability is an important child welfare outcome. Most people would agree that when children are removed from their homes due to abuse or neglect they should be in stable placements. But what does this mean? Most people think about stability in terms of placement changes. When a child is removed from his or her foster home, this change of placement represents a disruption in stability. However, some argue that a child being removed from a foster home for psychiatric treatment in a hospital is not an indication of instability but rather an indication of responding to the needs of the child. Some argue that if a foster child runs away but returns to that same home, this is not an indication of instability. Others disagree with one or the other of these situations. One can easily see how several workers or agencies would count placement changes differently and consequently arrive at different stability results for the same performance.

Again, a carefully thought-out operational definition is a prerequisite to having a reliable measure. Everyone who uses the measure also needs to agree to use this same definition. This is the reason that repeated training in the use of a measure is a standard method for maintaining or improving the reliability of a measure.

Although validity was discussed first, reliability is a prerequisite. If a measure shows different results when the underlying phenomenon does not change, it is impossible to know what it is measuring. Consequently, discussing validity is meaningless. A measure must hit a target consistently before it is possible to determine whether it is the right target.

Measures Should Be Susceptible to Change

Social administration is about helping consumers achieve desired changes. The measures that administrators use to pilot the program must detect these changes. At first reading this may seem to contradict the idea of reliability, but keep in mind that reliability is consistency of the measure, assuming the underlying concept has not changed. When change has occurred it needs to be detected.

An important part of this criterion in the context of social programs is the time frame involved. When selecting performance measures, managers need to think about what changes they expect to see in what time. Measures and reporting periods can then be matched to expected changes. The measure needs to be able to detect real changes that occur in the desired time frame.

A program that helps people with disabilities enroll and progress through postsecondary education would not see many changes if the report was generated monthly. Enrollment and course completion usually occurs only three times a year. For most months, progress measured by enrollments and courses completed would be zero. Likewise, a monthly report on the number of interagency agreements signed is unlikely to make sense since these tend to happen infrequently.

On the other hand, some events, although rare, may be so important that frequent reporting is desired. Fortunately, abuse of a child in foster care is rare. However, given the importance of such an event, a manager may want a daily report on any child in the caseload experiencing abuse.

Measures Should Be Efficient

The costs and benefits of data collection are an important consideration. Information system costs are substantial and are often not recognized because much of the cost is staff time. Yet everyone in an organization is aware, at some level, of the cost of collecting data. Substantial resources are devoted to data collection, storage, and retrieval, from the caseworker filling out forms to the supervisor receiving data entry error reports, to the number of staff positions in the data processing department.

For example, SACWIS is a government supported program to help states improve their child welfare information systems. A government accounting office report includes estimates from the states that a sum of more than $2.4 billion dollars has been invested in the design and implementation of SACWIS information systems (United States General Accounting Office, 2003). This is an enormous amount of money that did not go to services for children and families. These opportunity costs deserve consideration. In addition to the developmental costs, workers filling out forms in their office are missing the opportunity to spend time working directly with or on behalf of families.

The considerable costs of data collection may be a useful argument for not implementing a new measure. On the other hand, data collection costs may lead managers to accept measures based on existing, but inferior, data. Osborne and Plastrik (2000) warn managers against taking these types of "measurement shortcuts." These authors observe that much of the existing data in organizations is probably not relevant and the best response is to stop gathering data that is not useful so that resources are available to collect data that is.

The challenge of constructing measures at the least cost takes considerable effort and thought. Measurement starts with a definition that identifies aspects of the concept. It is these aspects that are then measured. This is followed with the design of a data collection instrument that includes each of the aspects and is implemented at the expense of a worker taking time away from consumers to fill out another form. The first stage of identifying key elements of the concept is critical to developing a consensual definition of the term. However, rather than trying to capture each and every aspect of the concept being measured, finding a single indicator that captures the heart of the idea is a worthwhile activity.

The child outcome area of well-being provides an example. Measures of child well-being are expensive to implement. For example, education as a well-being category for foster children is often discussed in terms of different aspects of education. This frequently includes grades, grade level, presence of an individual educational plan (IEP), absences or attendance, graduation, suspensions, expulsions, and so on. Asking workers to report on each of these features places a large burden on them and would probably result in missing and inaccurate data.

At the same time Sharon Freagon (2001) of the Center for Child Welfare and Education at Northern Illinois University identifies age in grade as one of the best predictors of educational success or failure. The idea is that if a child is in the grade that is usual for his or her age, then it is likely that the child is making adequate educational progress. On the other hand if he or she is older than others in the grade, this is an indicator of falling behind in educational achievement. Although this may not be the best educational outcome measure, it raises the possibility of selecting a single indicator to assess a critical aspect of child well-being.

This example also indicates the usefulness of consulting with content experts in the selection of measures and indicators, a suggestion that is echoed by Osborne and Plastrik (2000). With child welfare including every aspect of a child's life, it is impossible for a manager to be an expert in every area. Experts in health, education, and other areas can help identify indicators that they regard as good outcome measures.

Individual Performance Measures Need to Be

- *Understandable*
- *Valid*
- *Reliable*
- *Susceptible to change*
- *Efficient*

Criteria for Sets of Performance Measures*

Picking individual performance measures that help managers pilot social programs takes a lot of effort. Creating the set of measures that constitute the gauges in the cockpit is another challenge. The cockpit represents a set of measures that allows the pilot to safely guide the plane to its destination. The challenge to the social administrator is to select the set of outcome measure that will assist in guiding the program to achieving results for consumers. The question is: What criteria does a set of outcome measures need to satisfy to provide a valid picture of the outcome performance of the system. The following criteria are proposed:

1. The set of measures should include as few as possible.
2. All outcomes that occur as consumers move through the system should be captured.
3. Perverse incentives should be avoided.
4. Real changes are captured while avoiding manipulation.
5. The set includes counterbalancing measures.

The Set Should Contain As Few Measures As Possible

A program manager's need for information is great, yet his or her ability to focus is limited (Osborne & Plastrik, 2000; Kaplan & Norton, 2001). Lawler (1996), among others, suggests that organizations get the kinds of behaviors that they measure and reward. Yet too much data diffuses this

---

*Much of this section is based upon *Managing for child welfare outcome: The selection of outcome measures* by J. Poertner, T. Moore, & T. P. McDonald. Reprinted with permission.

attention and energy, allowing people to select those measures that reflect positively on their performance and ignore the rest, or simply ignore all of the data because it is too voluminous (Rapp & Poertner, 1992). Yet when developing a set of performance measures, Osborne and Plastrik (2000) observe that there is a tendency for "measurement creep" to occur. This is an almost natural drive for more and "better" information, leading to complex systems that no one can understand and use. They admonish managers; "Don't measure what you won't use, and stop measuring what you don't need" (p. 261). This advice fits into that large category of "easier said that done." Judgments about what is needed and used require constant examination of successes, failures, and the link between data and decision making.

Kaplan and Norton (2001) have found in their work with many organizations that sixteen to twenty-five measures for an organizational scorecard are usually adequate. The measures in the organizational scorecard would include consumer outcomes, service events, resources acquired, staff morale, and efficiency, and could also include measures of innovation, stakeholder opinion, and so on. A focused scorecard serves to establish common organization purpose and effort in complex organizations with multiple units. Kaplan and Norton (2001) have found that organizational performance is enhanced when there is a scorecard that is small enough for everyone to be able to understand and attend to.

These authors also indicate that within a complex organization with several units there may be additional scorecards. For example, in a large child welfare agency, there is likely to be a need for one scorecard for protective services and another for permanency units, in addition to one overall scorecard. In addition, major outcome measures can be disaggregated (drilling down) for different populations (e.g., recurrence for neglect or maintaining relative placements). This is particularly useful when a program unit is striving to improve performance in a specific area.

Limiting the number of measures is a difficult task and there are few guidelines on how it is done. Osborne and Plastrik's (2000) admonition not to measure what will not be used and stop measuring what is not needed is difficult to achieve. However, actual use of a measure is a reasonable test for outcomes measures in any system. Has this report ever been used to make a decision or is it simply interesting? If no decision is made based upon a measure, it ought to be eliminated. The "interesting" test leads to large and cumbersome data sets.

Another way to limit the number of outcome indicators is to make certain that they truly identify outcomes. This is obvious but it is not uncommon to find process measures in many sets of outcome indicators. Placement stability is frequently identified as an outcome. Stability is important to children.

However, it may be more of a service response than an outcome or result for children. One can imagine that stability may be associated with child well-being and if this is the case this may be an important process measure. Alternatively, it may be a highly held value that is important to key stakeholders and, therefore, measured, and reported in that critical performance area.

The Kansas Consumer Status Reporting System (CSR) provides a good example. There are many outcomes for adults with severe psychiatric disabilities that are of interest. The list could include social supports, quality of life, feelings of confidence, hope and empowerment, social involvements, control of symptoms, daily living skills, pre-vocational skills, social functioning, family burden, and so forth. Further complicating the issue is that each consumer brings specific and unique goals to the service program. The CSR system was established in 1988 and refined over the years. Four consumer outcomes are measured and tracked for every consumer receiving community mental health services:

- Reduce psychiatric hospital usage
- Increase independent living status
- Increase competitive employment
- Increase postsecondary education involvement

Each of these outcomes reflects the desires of most people with psychiatric disabilities. They are also valued by critical stakeholders: families, mental health professionals, and legislators. These measures are also reflective of the overall ethos of mental health services that places a premium on community integration, normalization, and recovery. There are services and methods that affect these outcomes and, therefore, the outcomes are susceptible to change.

Although there are not many rules for helping managers limit the number of consumer outcome indicators, having a target such as four to six is useful. As a set of indicators grows in size, a manager should seek to drop a measure in response to the need for adding one. A useful question might be: "If you could only have one indicator of _____, what do you think is most important?" The answer to this question might be a matter of expert judgment, practice wisdom, or managerial judgment. In all cases it can and should be empirically tested. Selecting an indicator, using it, and checking whether it is accurately reflecting real changes for consumers is a necessary part of every information system.

Osborne and Plastirk (2000) also suggest asking for a cost estimate when a new measure is proposed. If careful attention is paid to all of the measurement costs including data collection, storage, and retrieval, the real cost of the measure will be identified. This may produce a powerful rationale for not implementing a new measure.

The Set of Indicators Should Count All Outcomes
That Occur As Consumers Move Through the System

It is important that the outcome status of all consumers is on the radar screen. A set of outcome measures should not exclude any consumer. Once an agency has accepted responsibility to work with a consumer, the status of that person is in the managers' hands.

In child welfare, for some children the placement experience is completed in a very short period of time and for others it continues for years. The Adoption and Safe Families Act (ASFA) provision regarding a child spending fifteen of twenty-two months in care draws our attention to the initial months of care, as do measures that concern themselves with exiting care in twelve months. However, public accountability as well as management responsibility does not end after a child has been in care for twelve or twenty-two months. A safety measure that counts maltreatment for all children once they have come into contact with the child welfare system is an example of a measure that includes all of the outcome events for which the system is responsible.

Perverse Incentives Should Be Avoided

Closely related to the criteria of counting all outcome events during consumers' experience with a social program is avoiding perverse incentives. A perverse incentive is one that unintentionally causes an agency to avoid a positive outcome.

In child welfare, counting children in care during some time periods and not others is one way that perverse incentives are created. This may cause managers to attend to desired outcomes during the time periods of interest but not after that time period (e.g., two years) has ended. For example, attention to children adopted within a specific time period establishes an incentive to place major attention on those children during that time. Once a child has been in care beyond that time period, there is less incentive to consider adoption for this child.

People with disabilities who want to work in integrated, "normal" setting should be helped to do so. Over 60 percent of people with psychiatric disabilities want to work in competitive employment. But what is "competitive"? Clarity and completeness of definitions is important. Some mental health and vocational rehabilitation systems define competitive employment as a job that is in an integrated setting (not a separate sheltered facility) and pays at least minimum wage. This definition created an incentive to place consumers in janitorial jobs within mental health centers and others placed in transitional employment positions that are supervised by mental health staff. In both situations, the jobs are "set aside" for consumers. These job arrangements hardly match most people's (including consumers) ideas of competitive employment and constrict the choices available to consumers. Some mental health programs achieve seemingly high levels of employment but the majority of jobs are as described earlier. Tightening the definition of competitive employment, by excluding mental health center work and transitional jobs which are a form of "sheltered" employment and often not open to nondisabled applicants, encourages the agency to find "real" jobs in the community for consumers.

There is no magic formula for avoiding establishment of perverse incentives. Making certain that all outcome events are counted is one way to avoid some negative incentives. Careful thought about what an indicator will draw focus and energy to, as well as what it ignores, is also important to consider. Perverse incentives are unintended. Unintended consequences are not seen before they occur. This suggests carefully monitoring all outcomes after a set of indicators is implemented to determine whether the way an outcome measure is defined is causing poor performance in other areas.

A Set of Measures Needs to Be Able to Capture Real Changes and Avoid Being Susceptible to Administrative Manipulation (Gaming the System)

For a set of measures to be a useful management tool it must have the ability to capture changes in policy and practice. Although perverse incentives are unintentional, some sets of measures encourage some managers to manipulate the agency procedures and definitions to "look good." Although it is arguably possible to "game" every set of outcome indicators, establishing incentives for positive results for all consumers and capturing real changes in policy and practice is the goal.

It is likely that some measures are more easily manipulated than others. A measure that is based upon a vague definition is an example of one that is more easily manipulated. Comparing national child welfare data with the complexity of more than fifty child welfare systems and key terms determined by state statute, there are likely to be many examples of concepts that are difficult to define.

To avoid administrative manipulation, it is instructive to consider what a manager can do to make apparent changes in outcome indicators that do not accurately reflect results for consumers. To administratively manipulate results, a manager can influence which consumers enter the system or choose a subgroup already in the system in order to achieve some desired outcome, at the expense of others. For example, consider a reunification measure that focuses on the first twelve months that a child is in care. To perform well on this measure, a manager might encourage an intake policy that places children in out of home care who are at low or no risk of abuse and who may be easier to reunify quickly. Most states' child abuse and neglect statutes are sufficiently vague to make this possible. In Kansas, for example, over 40 percent of the children who entered foster care in the 2005 fiscal year were not identified as victims of abuse or neglect (Social and Rehabilitation Services, 2005). Conversely, a manager might find ways to discourage taking children into care who are thought to be difficult to reunify. Children with severe disabilities are an example. A manager might argue that these children are not victims of abuse or neglect and are more properly the responsibility of the developmental disabilities system. Either of these strategies has the promise of demonstrating improved short-term reunification results.

Another way to discourage administrative manipulation is to develop a culture that rewards openness and positive performance. A punitive culture that emphasizes sanctions generates defensiveness and administrative manipulation. Friedman, Kipshitz, and Overmeer (2001) observe that organizational learning takes place in a climate that fosters inquiry, openness, and trust. This requires a context that includes a tolerance for admitting errors, judgments based upon substance, egalitarianism, and a commitment to learning. Sets of outcome indicators used in this context will encourage learning and not manipulation.

The Set Should Include Indicators That Counterbalance Each Other

In any set of outcome indicators there is a concern about interactions between them. These interactions suggest the need for measures that account for or counterbalance these interactions. A social administrator does not want to produce a negative outcome for a consumer while working to achieve a related positive result.

Child welfare, for example, has always had difficulty balancing outcomes such as safety and permanency. Placing too much emphasis on family preservation and reunification may place some children at risk of abuse. Similarly, placing too much emphasis on child safety may result in more children entering foster care and staying longer. Consequently, measures of both safety and permanence are required. The proper balance between safety and permanency is unknown but must be a management concern.

Criteria for Sets of Performance Measures

1. The set should contain as few measures as possible.

2. The set of indicators should count all outcomes that occur as consumers move through the system.

3. Perverse incentives should be avoided.

4. A set of measures needs to be able to capture real changes and avoid being susceptible to administrative manipulation (gaming the system).

5. The set should include indicators that counterbalance each other.

MEASURING CONSUMER OUTCOMES

One element of our model of social administration is that managers must produce performance in five management areas: consumer outcomes, service events, resource acquisition, efficiency, and staff morale. For a social program (or manager) to succeed, they must produce benefits for consumers through the social program and the efforts of staff. This can only occur if resources are acquired and used efficiently, events that result in benefits to consumers happen, and staff morale is maintained. Each of these performance areas requires systematic monitoring, but it is the measurement of consumer outcomes that is the centerpiece of the consumer-centered manager.

The goals and objectives established during the program design phase drive consumer-outcome measurement. This statement, however, camouflages the myriad of critical decisions that the human service manager is required to make. The most central decision concerns how to measure the outcomes. We urge managers not to develop their own consumer outcome measures. A manager should use instruments that have already been developed whenever possible. The development of a measure that meets all of the criteria listed at the start of this chapter is costly and technical and is best done by a person with specialized measurement knowledge.

The selection of the "best" instrument should be based, in part, on the basic measurement concepts described earlier (e.g., validity, susceptible to change, efficient). One would also like instruments that have been tested and used with the same or a similar population to the one that the program is serving. There are excellent sources for such instruments, including the work of Corcoran and Fisher (2000a,b) *Measures for Clinical Practice: A Sourcebook Vol. 1: Couples, Families and Children* (Third Edition) and *Measures for Clinical Practice: A Sourcebook* Vol. 2: Adults (Third Edition). Many well-tested instruments have been copyrighted and require permission for the author to use the instrument. This frequently requires a small fee and it is well worth the small cost per consumer to use a well-tested instrument that matches a program's goal.

In addition to the basic concepts of validity and reliability, it is useful for managers to be knowledgeable about the most common measurement approaches. This will allow managers to make better decisions when selecting consumer outcome measures. Social work interventions are most often designed to work with consumers to produce outcomes in one or more of these categories: changes in psychological states, knowledge acquisition, behavior change, status change, and environmental changes. This section will review existing measurement approaches for these types of changes.

Changes in Psychological Status (Affective Change)

Changes in feelings and perceptions are a frequent target of human service programs. Efforts are made to help improve consumers' self-esteem, empowerment, and satisfaction with life, or decrease such feelings as sense of hopefulness, anxiety, or loneliness. Other programs seek to change beliefs about racism, homophobia, and other forms of discrimination.

Researchers have devised many ways to assess or measure attitudes. Typically, attitude measurement is accomplished with a set of questions derived from the definition of the concept and the person completing the scale indicates their response on a scale. There is a wide variety of response scales. Perhaps the most frequent are agree/disagree, true/false, or frequently/never. The number of choices also varies and frequently ranges from five to eleven or more. The responses to the individual items are added to produce a score.

The Hope Scales of Snyder (2000) provide useful examples. Snyder first defined hope from scholarly writing about the topic. He arrived at a definition with three central concepts. People tend to exhibit hopefulness when they have goals, plans to achieve a goal, and some level of goal-directed energy. The scale includes items to assess each of these three dimensions. For example, an item that assesses plans to meet a goal is; "I can think of many ways to get out of a jam." Goal-directed energy is assessed by items such as; "I energetically pursue my goals." Respondents are asked to select a response to each item that "best describes YOU." There are eight choices that people can make on a true/false continuum, ranging from definitely false to definitely true.

Selecting a scale to use as a consumer outcome attitude measure involves locating one that is based upon a definition of the concept that is consistent with that of the program. It is also important to try to select a scale that has evidence of reliability and validity. For example, the Hope Scale usually achieves a reliability rating ranging from .7 to .8 and is judged to have excellent construct validity (Lopez, Ciarlelli, Coffman, Stone, & Wyatt, 2000). Finally a judgment needs to be made as to its fit between the language of the items and the culture and educational background of consumers. This might best be done by using a consumer advisory group to examine the scale and to judge its appropriateness.

The Acquisition of Knowledge

Many human service programs have a knowledge acquisition purpose or component: parent education, self-help groups, health promotion programs, crime prevention programs. Even many psychotherapeutic or counseling approaches are focused on learning "insight" or "self-awareness." Readers are familiar with assessing knowledge acquisition, since that is what educational testing seeks to achieve.

If you have decided that a main component of your program is educational, then you will want to measure this outcome. As with all measurement you must first define what it is that consumers are to learn. Suppose you want to find out whether consumers have increased their knowledge of self-protective behaviors. Through the program specifications you have already decided what you would like them to learn.

One of the best-known knowledge outcome assessment technologies is the pretest/posttest technique. Although it not a research method that can establish a causal relationship, it may be reasonable to attribute improvements in posttest scores to the educational intervention. Pre- and posttests can be developed using true/false, multiple-choice, or open-ended questions. The type of questions used is determined by several factors, such as the verbal skills of the consumer and the level of learning to be assessed.

True/False Questions

This type of assessment is designed to measure simple recognition or recall of the material. If the questions are written carefully, this formant generally does not require a high level of verbal skills. Consequently, this format may work well with children or with adults having a lower-than-average reading level.

Multiple Choice Questions

Multiple choice questions can be written to evaluate higher levels of learning, such as application (problem solving or applying ideas in new situations) or comprehension (restating or reorganizing material to show understanding). Multiple choice items are most useful when the person being assessed possesses adequate reading skills.

Multiple choice item tests require consumers to select the correct answer from an array of possible answers. Typically, the multiple choice question presents the problem in one of two formats: the complete question (e.g., "What should you do first if you suspected a child has been abused?") or the incomplete statement (e.g., "The first thing you should do if you suspect a child is being abused is to . . ."). With these two formats, the respondent selects either the correct answer or the best answer from the list of options provided.

> In the correct answer form, the answer is correct beyond question or doubt while the others are definitely incorrect. In the best answer version, more than one option may be appropriate in varying degrees; however, it is essential that the best response be the one that competent experts agree upon. (Clegg & Cashin, 1986, p. 2)

The multiple choice format is simple; it is constructing a meaningful and worthwhile item that is so difficult and time-consuming. An item that a test developer thinks will identify those who have learned a concept may fail miserably when actually used. A useful multiple choice test requires writing many questions, using them with the intended audience, and careful evaluation of each item. Fortunately, multiple choice tests are a popular method of conducting educational evaluation, so a social administrator should be able to obtain expert consultation from educational assessment experts at a nearby college or university.

Open-Ended Questions

Open-ended questions can be written in much the same way as multiple choice questions, only the consumer must supply the answer(s). An open-ended item requires that a consumer know material well enough to either solve a problem or recall the material, instead of merely recognizing an answer provided in a correct-answer form question. Although it is often appealing to use open-ended questions, they should be written and used with great care. If consumers are not highly articulate, it is unfair to expect them to respond to open-ended questions.

Every social administrator can recall writing volumes in response to essay questions in college, with the hope that the correct response is included. The best open-ended question is the one for which the correct answer can be identified succinctly, clearly, and unambiguously. For example, "Identify the three rules of anti-victimization presented in the film."

Writing test questions or items is no easy task. They need to be written and refined over time. Only in actually using the items can you determine whether they are measuring the knowledge you intend for consumers to learn. The instruments that you use need not be limited to only one type. For instance, you may want to use both multiple choice and true/false items on the tests in order to get at varying levels of cognitive changes.

After you have decided on what items to use to measure knowledge acquisition, the instrument is ready to administer. The pretest should be given to consumers before the intervention begins. This will allow you to see how much knowledge consumers have about the subject before they become involved in the learning of the material you are going to present. The time interval at which the posttest is administered will vary depending on the service. For example, the posttest can be given at the end of the last session of a parent education program, or it can be given weeks or months after the last session to assess retention of knowledge. Once the assessment is complete, tests are scored. A comparison of the pre- and posttest scores is evidence of knowledge gained.

Behavior Change

Measures of behavior change fall into two categories: skills and performance. Skills refer to a person's ability to exhibit a behavior and the program's ability to help people learn these behaviors. The test for this is usually whether consumers have the behavior in their repertoire. In other words, if I gave this person a million dollars (or some other equally grand reward) would she or he be able to do the requested behavior. This is of a different order than the cognitive mastery of a subject. For example, an individual with a development disability enrolled in a prevocational program may be able to list the specific tasks needed to find a job, but may not be able to do the actual tasks of finding a job (e.g., search want ads or engage a prospective employer). Another example is the parent who can describe three techniques for nonphysical discipline, but when asked to demonstrate the techniques, cannot do it. Skill training is a major element of a wide variety of social programs, including vocational programs, day treatment and partial hospitalization programs, programs for people with developmental disabilities, and so on.

This distinction between skills and performance is recognition that there is an interaction between behavior and the environment. What a person can do in one environment may not be attainable in another. Measuring skills always requires observation of the consumer either through role-playing or in the natural environment. Behavioral checklists guide the observer. To test discrimination and generalization, observations in a variety of settings is necessary.

We are most often interested in behavior change that results in performance in the consumer's natural environment. Performance asks the question: Do consumers use the knowledge and/or skill in their lives? Does the mother use time-out or privilege restrictions instead of paddling a child? Does the person who knows how to ride the bus system do so? How often? Behavior change measures seeking to capture behavioral performance can be designed for consumer self-reports and professional or significant other evaluations.

There are several ways to measure behavior change. Ollendick, Alvarez, and Greene (2004) identify behavioral interviews, rating and checklists, self-reports, self-monitoring, and behavioral observation as current methods for measuring behavior. An essential element of all of these methods is an attention to unambiguously identifying the behavior. This is not easy and may not always be practical.

For example, a highly regarded and widely used behavioral measure for children is Achenbach's Child Behavior Checklist (CBCL) (Achenbach, 2001). The core of this instrument is a list of over 100 behaviors that the observer rates as 0 = not true, 1 = somewhat or sometimes true, or 2 = very true or often true. The list includes unambiguous items such as the following:

- Bites fingernails
- Vomiting, throwing up
- Refuses to talk

Although it is ideal to have behavioral checklists contain unambiguously stated behaviors, this is not always possible. There are many challenges facing children that are difficult to identify in a behavioral statement and if specified through identification of the individual behaviors, the behavioral list becomes meaningless. For example, Achenbach's CBCL also includes items such as the following:

- Easily jealous
- Feels he or she has to be perfect
- Not liked by other kids

One can easily see that rating of these child behaviors will vary by environment (e.g., school, home, boys, and girls club) and by the observer (e.g., parent, teacher, foster parent). What appears to be jealous behavior to one observer is not perceived that way by another. It may be important to have more than one key actor complete the behavioral assessment. Many programs that use the CBCL have both teachers and parents complete the assessment form and compare the perspectives. Recall that differences may be due to the point of view of the rater, or they may be due to environmental factors.

Status Changes

Movement of people between statuses is a characteristic of many social systems. The central idea is that the goal of the service system is to move a person to a more desirable status or to maintain the person in a "most desirable" status. The permanency planning movement in child welfare, recidivism in corrections, and in-home care of the elderly are inherently concerned with status change or status maintenance.

The development of status measures must meet the following four criteria.

1. The list of possible statuses needs to be exhaustive.
2. The statuses need to be mutually exclusive. A person should not be able to be in two statuses at the same time.
3. It should be possible for the statuses to be hierarchically ordered from least desirable to most desirable. It is important that there be a reasonable degree of consensus on this ordering among people familiar with the program.
4. The measures need to be sensitive to change.

Being sensitive to change generally means carefully considering the time interval for observation of consumers. If the interval between reporting periods is too short, little change would be seen, and the paperwork burden would increase. If the interval is too long, there may be multiple transitions and camouflaging patterns of movement. In addition, long intervals between reporting do not allow a reasonable degree of immediate feedback and prevent timely corrective actions. Two examples of status hierarchies for people with psychiatric disabilities in two life domains are shown in Table 7.1. One measure assesses the consumer's living arrangement and the other vocational status. It is easy to see how this instrument can be used to assess status change. A worker or consumer simply identifies the applicable status at some point in time, such as during the intake phase, and again at some later time point. The difference between these ratings is the status change over the time period.

The use of statuses has a number of appealing qualities. First, it has the ability to unify the agendas and performance expectations of the agency's multiple constituencies. Frequently status maintenance or change is the avowed goal of public policy (e.g., maintaining children in a safe and permanent home). Consequently, existing administrative data systems frequently contain the information needed to report status changes. In addition, statuses in any social service program are finite. In contrast, models of behavior change and goal attainment are often formulated through the interaction between the consumer and the worker, and can be highly idiosyncratic. The finite property of status change can enhance organizational control and the process of supervision, and allow for increased focus at multiple organizational levels.

TABLE 7.1. Example Status Change Measures

Living Arrangement Status	Vocational Status
1. Psychiatric hospital ward	1. No vocational activity
2. General hospital psychiatric ward	2. Prevocational classes
3. Nursing home	3. Screening and evaluation of vocational interests and abilities
4. Emergency shelter	4. Active job search
5. Adult foster care	5. Participating in work program at MHC
6. Lives with relatives and largely dependent	6. Employed at sheltered employment
7. Group home	7. Participating in ongoing volunteer
8. Half-way house	8. Any job or set of jobs requiring less than thirty hours per week
9. Boarding house	9. Any job or set of jobs requiring more than thirty hours per week
10. Lives with relatives, but is largely independent	10. Other (specify)
11. Supervised apartment program of MHC	11. Retired
12. Shares apartment and capable of self-care	
13. Lives alone or with spouse and is capable of self-care	
14. Other (specify):	

A major drawback of status change is the possibility of it being subject to administrative manipulation, rather than being based on consumers' progress. For example, it is possible that children could be "dumped" out of foster care due to budget constraints, not due to improved families. Such administrative actions tend to be rare, however, and when they occur they are usually accompanied by a public outcry. When focus on change is subject to organizational, programmatic, and managerial efforts, then such measures are realistic and helpful. Status change also poses fewer dangers to validity and reliability, and the data are often already available in case files or data bases.

Environmental Changes

Measurement of environments is a developing area. Although social workers recognize the importance of the environment to understanding human behavior, little attention has been given to its measurement. This is an important area for social work research.

Assessing an environment, as any measurement, starts by clearly identifying what is meant. A definition of an environment identifies aspects that are considered essential to some consumer outcome. For example, the Family Day Care Rating Scale by Thelma Harms and Richard M. Clifford (2000) is designed to assess day care environments that promote child development. This scale defines a quality day care setting with six categories: space and furnishings for care and learning, basic care, language and reasoning, learning activities, social development, and adult needs. Through research on child development, the researchers have determined that these categories are important to child development. Notice that the concept of environment goes beyond the physical environment and includes such features as child care, learning, and relationships between people in that environment.

The next step is to identify items that characterize each of the identified categories. These are like subscales that operationally define the category. For example, the Family Day Care Rating Scale dimension of language and reasoning includes communication and has four items that operationalized this as informal use of language, helping children understand language, helping children use language, and helping children reason. The entire rating scale includes thirty-two items, operationalizing the six categories.

Finally, each item in each category must be rated. Each item of The Family Day Care Rating Scale can be rated as follows: inadequate (does not even meet custodial care needs), minimal (meets custodial needs and, to some degree, basic developmental needs); good (meets developmental needs), and excellent (high-quality personalized care). The total number of good or excellent ratings can serve as a measure of this environment. Similarly the inadequate or minimal ratings can identify areas for correction.

This example demonstrates the complexity of developing and using a measure of environmental change. Considerable research is required to identify environmental features that are important to the desirable outcome. Great care and extensive research is required to operationalize the critical features. Then the scale must be tested for the usual characteristics of measurement, such as reliability and validity.

The reader might have questioned the ability of a rater to make distinctions required by the Family Day Care Rating Scale. Someone with little or no training in child development would have difficulty in reliably identifying examples of activities that helped children understand language. This underscores the importance of adequately training those who will use the instrument and conducting periodic retraining so that measurement results are reliable. This also underscores the importance of continued development of reliable and valid environmental assessment instruments.

MEASURING PERFORMANCE
THAT SUPPORTS CONSUMER OUTCOMES

Piloting a social program requires monitoring performance in those areas that make it possible for an agency to achieve consumer outcomes. The performance model presented in this text identifies these areas as the service events that produce the outcome, the acquisition of resources, efficiency, and staff morale. A cockpit that takes readings in each of these areas along with the intended consumer outcomes is an information system that is likely to assist everyone associated with the program keep the program on course and achieve desired results.

Measuring Service Events

Social work interventions include two types of elements that are considered in this performance category—structural and clinical. Structural elements include such dimensions as caseload size, composition of teams, nature of supervision, and location of work (e.g., outreach). Clinical elements reflect the intervention done with and on behalf of consumers. Service events are the occurrence of these elements of the intervention.

Evidence-based practices are the first source for identifying critical service events. The program theory similarly identifies key service events that in an ideal world are identical to those of evidence-based practices. Practice wisdom is also a useful source for identifying these events. Staff who have been successful in working directly with the program's consumers to achieve mutually defined goals generally know what it is they do that produces results. From these three sources, the social administrator creates a list of key service events that, if increased in frequency or quality, would increase the rate of successful consumer outcomes and, therefore, improve attainment of the organization's purpose. There are three ways of measuring service events: discrete events, service episodes, and elapsed time.

Measuring *discrete events* requires the counting of specific actions on the part of the worker. These actions are derived from the program design and could include such events as a group session, an interview, a home visit, a class session, a home-delivered meal, a physical examination, a case review, or a telephone call. The primary strength of this unit of measurement is its ability to represent the implementation of the program design. A major disadvantage is that counting worker actions tends to camouflage the dramatic differences between such events. Some events are more crucial to producing consumer outcomes than others, and some events require more time or intensity than others. It follows then that a measure that counts all events equally can be very misleading.

Second, service events can be measured by counting *episodes*. A service episode is the complete period in which a service is provided. One service episode could include recognition of the problem, the effort to find help, a period of working with one or more professional helpers, and termination. A service episode encompasses more than one discrete event. Counting service episodes is particularly well suited for short-term or emergency services, such as crisis hotlines or emergency room service. These services are quick and rather uniform, and the possibility of contact with consumers more than once is high. The chief disadvantage is that service episodes are not applicable to services that are long term or could vary considerably from consumer to consumer.

Elapsed time is another method for measuring service events. In this case, the units are time oriented, such as days of nursing home care, hours of counseling, or hours spent delivering home health services to the elderly. The great advantage of elapsed time as a measure is its precision with respect to the use of resources. It is possible to show the hours of worker's time and, therefore, resources allocated to different types of cases and to one particular consumer, or to the caseload as a whole. The measure also has a special utility when making budget presentations, since there is a direct correspondence between elapsed time of the worker and cost of the program. The great disadvantage of elapsed time is that it focuses on the expenditure of time by the worker without any attention to the number of consumers served, their characteristics, the amount of help received, or even the service activity performed in the program. However, if the activity of the worker over time is in some sense constant then this unit might be useful.

As an example of selecting which service events should be part of an information system, a manager of a program for adults with psychiatric disabilities knows that Assertive Community Treatment (ACT) has been identified as an evidence-based practice. A recent literature review identifies the standard for frequency of contact in such programs as "At least four contacts per week per consumer; at least four contacts per month with consumer's family or support system" (Lewin Group, 2000, p. 26). Treatment is also identified as occurring in the community 75 to 80 percent of the time. This means that the program manager will include in the information system measures of contacts between workers and consumers that occur in the community as well as contacts with family or support systems. The manager also knows that Illness Management and Recovery is an evidence-based practice and that the fidelity instrument for such programs specifies that consumers receive at least three months of weekly or six months of bi-weekly sessions (SAMSHA, 2005). Consequently the manager includes measures of consumers attending weekly sessions for three months in the information system.

In the child welfare area, a program was concerned about the number of youth who were exhibiting behavior that was difficult to manage. An examination of the files of these children found that many were victims of sexual abuse and may be exhibiting symptoms of posttraumatic stress. A review of the literature identified several programs that had been evaluated using randomized clinical trials. Two of these programs appeared to be particularly promising since they demonstrated large or medium positive effects on the desired outcome variables.

Both of these programs used a variation of cognitive-behavioral therapy. The program reported by Cohen and Mannarion (1997) and Cohen, Mannarion, and Knudsen (2005) involved children and their caretakers in twelve sessions of forty-five minutes duration each. King and colleagues (2000) reported research that involved comparing working with the children only in twenty weekly fifty-minute sessions and a program that involved children in this same format and their non-offending parent in twenty weekly sessions.

The child welfare program manager wanting to implement one of these programs must select the relevant service events to be part of the information system based upon the program as it was evaluated through randomized clinical trials. In either case, it appears that the information system will count sessions attended by children and those attended by parents or care-givers and that they will involve either a twelve-week or twenty-week format.

Acquisition of Resources

All social administrators must spend time acquiring resources. The systematic measurement of these resources may or may not be needed depending on the nature of the resource and size of the organization.

Funds

All human service organizations need funds. For example, a large mental health center may receive funds from Medicaid, state grants, private insurance carriers, endowment funds, corporate and private gifts, contracts with schools and industries, local tax levies, and consumer fees for service. The manager usually knows how much money is needed for agency services to be maintained or for expansion of services to occur. Based on the estimate of need, the manager would want to systematically monitor how much money is being received from what source. The danger in not doing so is that the "books" will not balance at the end of the fiscal year. In contrast, a small community-based volunteer program, which receives its modest funding from only one source like the United Way, may not need a formal system of monitoring the acquisition of funds.

Personnel

A large complex organization may want to systematically measure the particular qualifications and talents of its staff. These same organizations may want to measure the number of women and minorities at various organizational levels to help insure their presence in higher-level positions. A small agency may not need to. Some organizations benefit greatly from the use of volunteers and others. These agencies would want to measure the number of volunteers, the number of hours of service, and the length of tenure that the volunteers have with the agency.

Consumers

All agencies need to acquire consumers whose characteristics are consonant with the agency's target population. It is also true that the capacity of virtually all programs is less than the number of people who could benefit from the service. In many cases, people can meet the target population criteria but still not be the "most in need." For example, a program designed to provide education to families with psychiatrically disabled members would typically include content on medications, the etiology of mental illness, coping strategies, and community resources. These psycho-educational approaches have demonstrated consistently good results in terms of decreasing patient symptoms and hospital admissions, increasing knowledge gained, and satisfying family participants. What is also clear is that these increasingly prevalent programs tend to reach middle- and upper-class families. Poorer families with fewer resources tend not to participate and have resisted becoming involved. In such a situation, the manager would want to carefully monitor consumer characteristics even within the target population.

Acquiring consumers that match the program often requires multiple referral sources. Depending on the program, referral sources could include the police and courts, family and friends, other agencies, self-referrals, schools and corporations, and in large agencies, staff from other programs or divisions. In many cases, the manager needs to monitor the number of consumers being referred from various sources. In some cases, monitoring the number of people referred who meet the target population criteria from each source is important. No manager wants to devote resources to consumers who will not benefit from the program nor contribute to the discomfort of people who get "turned down" because they do not meet the criteria.

Technology

The human service manager also needs to acquire the technology that will produce the consumer benefit. This includes equipment (computers, cars) and supplies (paper, desks, forms), as well as the intervention knowledge identified in the program specifications, training experiences, agency libraries, and so on. Although the need for systematic measurement will vary by agency, it is nonetheless important that the manager attend to these resources. In particular, the number of hours of training in which content areas and for which personnel applies to most agencies.

Public Support

Public support and influence is critical to all agencies. This is the most amorphous of resources, the measurement of which could include surveys of the general public or key informants, awards and other forms of recognition (e.g., complementary letters), scrapbooks of newspaper articles, and number of requests to take part in professional, community, or state planning or work groups. A more powerful measure of public support and influence would be based on the behavior of the key actors identified in the program specifications. Under this approach, the manager would systematically measure the degree to which each key actor behaved as desired by the program. For example, the permanency planning supervisor may want to keep score on the frequency with which a judge has verified that "reasonable" efforts had been made by frontline staff to prevent placement of children. An influential agency would be the one where key actors achieve high levels of consistent compliance. It could be in terms of such actions as making funding decisions, setting policy, or making referrals and getting them accepted. This approach has the added benefit of being focused on the primary reason for public support: the improvement of consumer outcomes.

Efficiency

Efficiency is a ratio between program inputs and outputs. Since the consumer-centered manager is always trying to deliver the most effective service to as many consumers as possible, measures of efficiency are one means of monitoring how well the agency is doing. The most common measure of efficiency is the cost per unit of service: the cost of an hour of counseling or a day of nursing home care. The computation is merely total program funds divided by the total units of service. Contracting agencies often use such calculations to compare the performance of similar programs. Efficiency, however, is seldom considered beyond these examples.

There are several measures of efficiency that are particularly useful to the consumer-centered manager. One measure is the percentage of available direct service time that is spent in direct consumer (or collateral) contact. Total direct service time (per week) is the number of direct service workers (full-time equivalents) times thirty-six hours (forty hours minus 10 percent for vacation time, sick leave, personal days, holiday). This figure is divided into the number of hours spent in contact with consumers. This will provide an approximation of the amount of time consumed by paperwork, meetings, travel, and so on. Since consumers get helped primarily through contact with staff, managers want a high level of worker time spent with consumers.

Another potentially powerful efficiency measure is the percentage of direct service time devoted to key events. For example, an outreach community-based mode of service delivery is a critical factor in producing consumer benefits for case management with the people with psychiatric disabilities. The manager of such a program would want to monitor the percentage of contact with consumers that occur in the community.

The selection of the most useful efficiency measures is a difficult task, which in large part is derived from the program design and the consumer-centered management principles contained in this book. Table 7.2 contains a sample of efficiency measures, the consumer-centered principle it relates to, and qualifications on its use. For example, the principle of serving as many people in the target population as possible needs to be weighed against possible harmful effects to effectiveness and staff morale.

Staff Morale

Staff morale as a performance area refers to the attitude or feelings of staff about their work environment and the degree to which this environment satisfies their needs. Chapter 8 on personnel management contains a more detailed discussion of job satisfaction, its meaning, and common elements. In this section, we will briefly review current technologies for measuring job satisfaction.

TABLE 7.2. Efficiency Measures

Computation No. of Consumers Served	Indicator	Consumer-Centered Management Principles
No. of people in target population	Percentage of target population	Program should serve as many of the target population as possible. (Possible trade-offs: effectiveness, morale)
$\dfrac{\text{\$s expended in direct service}}{\text{total program \$s}}$	Percentage of dollars going to direct service	As many dollars as possible should be used in the trenches. Corollary—keep administrative costs low as possible.
$\dfrac{\text{\$s in direct service}}{\text{\$s in administration}}$	Amount of dollars for direct service per \$1 of administration	As many dollars as possible should be used in the trenches. Corollary—keep administrative costs low as possible
$\dfrac{\text{No. of hours of key events}}{\text{No. of direct service time, available}}$ or $\dfrac{\text{No. of hours of key events}}{\text{No. of direct service hours provided}}$	Percentage of available direct service time devoted to key events Percentage of actual direct service time devote to key events	As much direct service time should be devoted to key events (possible trade-off: morale).

Informal Approach

For the social administrator with a small staff and with frequent contact, there really is no better way to assess staff morale than on a one-to-one basis and through small group conversations. A personal relationship that includes mutual respect and openness will elicit useful and honest responses to questions about job satisfaction. Noticing the interaction of people in the work unit and their apparent pleasures and frustrations derived from the work is a genuine way to assess staff morale.

Although this personal and informal approach to measuring job satisfaction may be ideal, there are several problems that threaten its reliability and validity. The first and most obvious hindrance to this approach is the possibility of inflated or inaccurate feedback because of the perception that the manager controls rewards and resources. Many people within organizations have difficulty openly showing success or frustration with a person who is "their boss."

Second, the informal approach can easily get pushed off the manager's agenda. The demands of the agency or the program's multiple constituents requiring immediate attention frequently results in a delay of attending to staff needs.

Third, it is difficult for an administrator to remember the job values and needs of several workers. Buckingham and Coffman (1999) have identified a dozen job values important to most people. Individuals value these dimensions differently and may have additional values not shared by others in the workplace. For a manager to keep in mind the top six job values of seven different staff members is difficult.

More Structured Approaches

Given these drawbacks, we suggest that every social administrator use some more formal method to structure assessment of job satisfaction while attempting to retain the personal relationship with each staff person.

The first, and perhaps the easiest, way to keep staff morale on the agenda within a small work group is to develop one to five open-ended questions to which staff respond in writing or within a staff meeting. At specified intervals staff can be asked to respond to questions such as the following:

- What are some of the ways I can help you do a better job?
- What are some of the things around here that I can help change to make this a better place to work?
- What are some things I could do to help you feel better about your work?

These questions are only examples; managers need to develop questions that fit their style and that will tell them how their staff value their jobs. The preceding questions do have two features that we have found useful. First, they ask what the manager can do, rather than how the staff person feels. Second, the questions reflect important, commonly held job values: the work itself, working conditions, and rewards and feedback. As is true with all measurements, there is great value in just keeping staff morale on the agency agenda. Use of the questions and acting on staff responses will communicate to staff that these are important questions to which they can respond openly and honestly.

A second method of measuring staff morale is really just a variation on the use of open-ended questions. Each staff person receives six note cards. Staff are requested to use three cards to list "What on the job has gone well in the last month?" One incident or item is written on each card. The other three cards are used to list "What would you like to see done differently?" The administrator can collect all of the cards in two piles and even shuffle the cards in each pile to preserve anonymity if necessary. The cards that list what has gone well are a rich source of data on the critical incidents contributing to staff morale. Managers can use these to reward themselves for their efforts and construct situations so staff can continue to have the same types of experiences. The cards that identify what staff would like to see done differently can be used to improve the working environment.

The work of Buckingham and Coffman (1999) yielded a "measuring stick" that makes a formal staff morale measurement instrument. The twelve questions are answered with a yes or no. This provides a quick and easy way for people to respond. Similarly administrators can easily tabulate the results, construct a report, and discuss the results in a unit meeting.

INNOVATIVE AND POWERFUL REPORT DESIGNS

The ideal cockpit for the consumer-centered manager is accurate, timely, and simple to respond to. The system upon which the cockpit is designed needs to contain varying levels of information. It starts with key performance indicators. It should also allow the manager to "drill-down" to different levels of aggregation (e.g., program, team, individual worker), different types of consumers, and link the two. In short, the system should be interactive, allowing the manager to answer questions that can more finely direct their actions.

Within this interactive capacity or within a preset data report package, a variety of displays can be produced. Basic tables, such as bar graphs and line graphs, are the most common. A report that is designed according to the "Principles of Performance Report Design" influences the conclusions that the reader will draw with the use of the data. This section introduces two innovative types of analyses and displays that are particularly relevant to many human service managers: (1) movement tables; (2) event history graphs.

Movement Tables

Movement tables are a useful way to show changes in consumer status. Deinstitutionalization in mental health and child welfare, recidivism in corrections, and in-home care for the elderly are all focused on the movement of consumers through the service system. Movement tables provide more information than the traditional end-of-the-time-period (weekly, monthly, etc.) report on consumer status.

The traditional method used to report consumer status change and program performance is to compare, for example, vocational/educational situations by month (Table 7.3). Although the distribution and totals are similar, this data tells the manager very little about how consumers have moved from one status to another. For instance, is the "17" showing "No Vocational Activity" in month 2 comprised entirely of new people in the program, or did consumers who were employed drop to this status in month 2? If the latter is true, it means that very different management action needs to occur from what would be needed if the former is true.

The first step in constructing a movement table is to group the list of discrete statuses into a meaningful set of categories. The number of categories is important and is usually no more than five. Movement tables with more than five categories are difficult to read and interpret. The list that follows

TABLE 7.3. Example Consumer Vocational Status Change Report

Vocational Status	Month 1	Month 2
No activity	14	17
Moderate activity	10	14
Substantial activity	27	31
Competitive activity	12	12
Total	63	64

provides an example of grouping eleven vocational/educational statuses relevant to people with psychiatric disabilities into five categories or levels.

1. *Consumers with no vocational activity*
   No vocational activity
2. *Prevocational activity*
   Prevocational activity
   Screening and evaluation of vocational interests and abilities
3. *Substantial vocational activity*
   Active job search
   Participating in work program at MHC
   Employed in sheltered employment
   Participating in ongoing volunteer activity
4. *Competitive vocational activity*
   Any job or set of jobs requiring less than thirty hours per week
   Any job or set of jobs requiring more than thirty hours/week
5. *Other respected social status*
   Any person who remains home to take care of children or others
   Retired

Once the categories have been established, a movement table can be constructed. Table 7.4 is an example of a movement table for vocational/educational statuses. The columns represent the number of consumers who moved *to* a given level and the rows represent the number who moved *from* a given level. For example, the second row that is labeled "Prevocational Activity" includes the numbers 9, 20, 6, 1.

   9 represents the number of clients who moved from prevocational activities to no vocational activity
  20 represents the number of clients who moved from prevocational activity to prevocational activity, in other words, remained at the same level
   6 represents the number of clients who moved from prevocational activity to substantial activity
   1 represents the number of clients who moved from prevocational activity to competitive activity

Movement tables, if designed properly, provide much information in an economical fashion. The levels of statuses are in hierarchical order in terms of desirability. For example, moving people with psychiatric disabilities from no vocational activity to moderate activity is viewed as progress.

TABLE 7.4. Vocational Movement Table To Fiscal Year: 2005 Quarter: 4

From: Fiscal Year: 2005 Quarter: 3	None	Prevocational	Substantial	Competitive
None	350	20	5	11
Prevocational	9	20	6	1
Substantial	9	5	31	9
Competitive	4	1	5	55
Total	372	46	47	76

Note: Movement Score: 1.5758 Cases with vocational status in both quarters: 541.

Movement tables are also a way of capturing consumer outcomes in a more sensitive manner and thereby allowing the program to receive credit for small but significant progress. For example, due to the severity of the illness and stage of recovery, not all consumers with disabilities can or desire to hold a full-time competitive job. For others, this goal may take several years of rehabilitation. The movement tables capture increments of progress. The consumer who has not worked for fifteen years but is now volunteering in a meals program for the elderly has made a significant improvement, for which the program and the consumer should receive credit.

A second use of movement tables for measuring vocational outcomes is that an index of movement can be compared to a standard. Using the data in Table 7.4, the index is computed by ignoring the numbers on the diagonal (top left cell to bottom right cell—12, 350, 20, 31, 55) and then dividing the number of persons who moved "up" in vocational status ($N = 52$) by the number who moved "down" ($N = 33$).

Index = (Movement number of Consumers with Improved Vocational Status: Above Diagonal) / (Number of Consumers with Declining Vocational Status: Below Diagonal)

The number of persons moving toward improved vocational status can be found adding the numbers above the diagonal. The number of persons declining in vocational status can be computed by adding the numbers below the diagonal. If the index is above 1.0, performance is in the desired direction, with more people moving "up" than "down." In contrast, performance below 1.0 indicates a program that is not moving consumers toward improved vocational status. At 1.0, program performance is unchanged. In Table 7.4 the index is:

$$\frac{20+5+11+6+1+9}{9+9+5+4+1+5}=\frac{52}{33}=1.57$$

This table indicates that the ratio of consumers progressing to regressing is almost 2 to 1, which is certainly solid performance for that month.

A second way of summarizing a movement table into a single performance measure is to assign weights to each "cell." The weights are illustrated in Table 7.5. Each "cell" of the table is weighted to reflect positive, neutral, or negative values for consumer movement. The number of people in each cell is multiplied by the weight assigned to that cell and then summed. To standardize the resulting table across programs of varying caseload sizes, the sum is divided by the total number of cases. To illustrate this measure, the numbers in Table 7.4 and the weighting in Table 7.5 are multiplied to produce Table 7.6. This figure (31) is then divided by caseload size (134) resulting in the number .23, which can then be used to compare the performance of teams or programs.

The strength of this method over the movement index is threefold. First, this method includes more consumer data in its computation by giving assigned values to the upper-left and lower-right cells. Second, this measure distinguishes consumer movement involving two or more levels from consumers who move only one level. Third, this measure clearly explicates the

TABLE 7.5. Weighting System Approach to Vocational Movement Table

	None	Prevocational Activity	Substantial Activity	Competitive Activity
None	−1	+1	+2	+3
Prevocational Activity	−1	0	+1	+2
Substantial Vocational Activity	−2	−1	0	+1
Competitive Vocational Activity	−3	−2	−1	+1

TABLE 7.6. Weights Applied to Table 7.4

−12	+9	+8	+15	+4
−6	0	+5	+6	+6
−2	−2	0	+7	+12
−12	−10	−3	0	+9
0	−9	0	−4	+10
−32+	−12+	+10+	+24+	+ 41 = 31

differential value placed on certain statuses. The main drawbacks are that the summary figure only has meaning when compared to similarly derived figures (in itself, this measure has no intuitive meaning, and the calculations are complex).

Event History Graphs

A common characteristic of social services is the desired outcome being an event where timing is important. In our recurrent mental health example, people enter a community support program and important milestone events include completing an illness management and recovery component or moving to substantial vocational activity. In child welfare, exiting foster care is important for children who enter care, and that includes returning home, becoming adopted, or having someone other than the state becoming the child's guardian. In school social work, important events for children at risk of school failure can include suspensions or movement to a mainstream classroom.

Similar to the movement table, event history graphs account for more than just the status of a group of consumers at a point in time. The usual information system report which counts events at a particular point in time frequently produces biased results. This bias results from not counting some events and overrepresenting those consumers who have been in the system the longest. For example, a child entering foster care and leaving before the end of the time period of the report is not counted since he or she is not an open case at the time the report is run. Similarly, a child in foster care for four years will be counted in each report over that time period, but a child in care for only one year will be counted many fewer times.

The most unbiased information derives from keeping track of all of the events of interest for a group of consumers entering a program during a specified time period. This is called an entry cohort. The period of time could be a week, month, quarter, year, or longer. The choice of the time period is based upon service volume and frequency of the event of interest. For example, a large child welfare program may want to keep track of monthly entry cohorts, while a small program may want to keep track of quarterly or yearly entry cohorts. Event history analysis reports on the events of interest at specified time periods until everyone in the entry cohort has experienced the event(s) of interest.

Event history analysis is an efficient way to display a set of movement tables for a group of consumers that entered the program during the same time period. A movement table is then generated for each succeeding month until all of the consumers exited the program. For example, a group of children enters foster care in one month, and a movement table of foster care exits is generated for this group of youth each month. Each new movement table is displayed next to the one from last month and so on, until all of the children in the group have exited. Each month, there is an added movement table for each existing cohort and another for the cohort entering care. One can see how quickly this becomes complex, difficult to understand, and unmanageable.

Event history data is typically displayed graphically to simplify the presentation of all of this information in a user friendly format. Recall that when feedback is presented graphically, it tends to be more effective; this is an added benefit of event history analysis (Alvero, Bucklin, & Austin, 2001). Event history permanency graphs of entry cohorts provide a powerful picture of how the program is doing for the consumers. All consumers and all events are counted. Further, time lapsed until the event of interest is a central focus of these graphs. Although time is important to consumers, it is not always easy for a manager to maintain a sense of urgency for producing outcomes. Event history graphs, by their very nature, aid this effort.

The reader has probably noted that since event history graphs are produced for entry cohorts, a separate function or curve is required for each entry cohort and this adds to the complexity of such a report. This is correct. The advantage of this approach that offsets added complexity is that these curves allow instant comparison of outcomes for consumers who entered in different time periods.

For example, if the entry cohorts are children entering foster care during the state fiscal year, then the reporting system includes functions or curves showing achievement of permanency for each entry cohort until all of the children have exited. If some children remain in care for ten years, there will be a curve for that tenth year as well as for all of the other years. One advantage of this is a continued focus on permanency for children who have been in care for a number of years. For example, a manager confronted with an event history graph for a cohort of children who entered care six years ago can use the "drill down" feature of the information system to determine who these children are, and use the creativity of the team to find new ways to help these children achieve permanency.

Another advantage of these multiple curves is the ability to compare outcomes for different cohorts of consumers following changes in programs or policies. Comparing outcomes of consumers who entered the program prior to program changes to those who entered in the next time period provides important evidence on the effectiveness of the program changes.

A simple child welfare event history graph is presented in Figure 7.1. This is an example report for a cohort of children entering foster care in

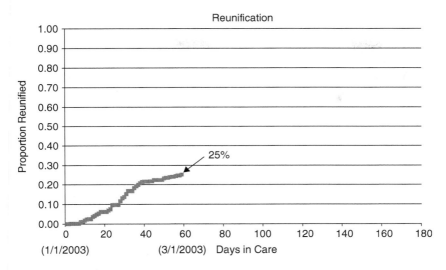

FIGURE 7.1. Example Event History Graph

2003. This report was generated on the first of March to report on the first two months of the outcome of reunification. The horizontal or X axis counts the days in care and the vertical or Y axis shows the proportion of children in this entry cohort returned home. This graph shows that after sixty days in care, or by March 1, about .25 or 25 percent of the children were reunified. This is a positive outcome. At the same time without making it explicit, the graph reminds the staff that 75 percent of these children are still in care. The horizontal axis of the graph only extends to 180 days so that the curve showing the proportion of reunifications would not be so small that it would appear inconsequential. At the same time it communicates that time for these children is "marching on." As the year(s) progresses, the horizontal axis will be extended. This report does not include a standard and, there-fore, does not meet this important criterion. However, a standard could be easily added based upon the goal of the program. For example, if the pro-gram goal is that 50 percent of the children are reunified within one year, the line at .5 could be made a different color and labeled as the twelve-month goal to show the destination of the program. The standard could also be an event history curve that represents the ideal pattern of exits.

An even better way to present the data is to display the outcome over time for different entry cohorts. A good example is the work by T. P. Mc-Donald, A. Press, P. Billings, & T. Moore (2003) titled "Outcomes Research Report #4: Predictors of timely adoption—A cohort analysis." Since the graph (p. 12) requires color to tell the story, it is not included here. It is available at http://www.socwel.ku.edu/occ/bac/rr4.pdf.

This particular set of data focuses on finalized adoption as the outcome of interest. The graphs show this outcome for children in five different entry cohorts. The horizontal or X axis shows the total number of days from an adoptive placement to finalization. The vertical or Y axis shows the proportion of children reaching finalized adoption. Each of the individual graphs reaches the top of the chart where the proportion reaching finalization is "1" and shows that the outcome of interest was achieved for all children in the cohort. The X axis was extended to nearly three years so that the individual graphs were able to reach the goal of all children in each cohort achieving finalized adoption. This permits a visual comparison of the results for each of these cohorts.

The fact that the individual graphs are different suggests that children had different experiences based upon the year that they were placed for adoption. The line for the 1997 entry cohort runs nearly diagonally across the chart with the other lines much more vertical. This shows that children who were placed for adoption in the later years achieved adoption finalization much more quickly. For example, drawing a vertical line through the 360-day point on the X axis shows that for the 1997 cohort about .40 or 40 percent achieved adoption finalization while approximately 80 percent of the 1999 cohort achieved the same result. Clearly whatever program changes occurred between 1997 and 1999 had an important effect on the time it took for children to achieve adoption finalization.

These two examples demonstrate the potential of event history graphs. They can report on outcomes for an entry cohort of consumers. They can compare outcomes of different entry cohorts. They can also be used to represent consumers' experiences with a part of a program or to track one important outcome. There are many possibilities.

Chapter 8

Personnel Management

What is more important than the people who work directly with consumers to achieve mutually desired outcomes? Consumer-centered social administration comprises managing for consumer outcomes and these results depend on regular interactions with social workers. People with serious mental illness obtain and maintain jobs through the efforts of social workers dedicated to this outcome. Families learn how to manage the difficult behavior of their children through the work of social workers. Older vulnerable citizens remain in households longer through the efforts of social workers.

In each of these examples the social worker is not the only person responsible for the outcome. The social worker interacts with a variety of people and operates within a variety of contexts to achieve the desired result. The social administrator operates within these same contexts with the recognition that creating the conditions and interactions in which staff are successful will result in consumers' success.

PRINCIPLES OF CONSUMER-CENTERED SOCIAL ADMINISTRATION AND PERSONNEL MANAGEMENT

Perhaps the best way for social administrators to *venerate consumers* is to create the conditions that help staff achieve results with consumers of services. One of these conditions is *maintaining the focus* on outcomes. Direct service workers are confronted with a myriad of demands that take their time and attention from consumers. Paperwork, staff meetings, or meetings with other professionals may have an indirect benefit but certainly not as powerfully as when workers have the tools and time to spend with consumers. An organization led by someone who helps workers spend time with and on behalf of consumers is maintaining a consumer-centered focus.

Textbook of Social Administration: The Consumer-Centered Approach
© 2007 by The Haworth Press, Inc. All rights reserved.
doi:10.1300/5802_09

Managers operating with a *healthy disrespect for the impossible* are responding to consumers who are confronted with immense problems that bring them to interact with social workers. Struggling with a major mental illness, being a part of the community as the effects of age sap independence, or being excluded from school because of an inappropriate behavior are difficult conditions to confront as a consumer. Workers sometimes struggle with these problems and are often frustrated by barriers to success. The social administrator's disrespect for the impossible engages workers in mutual problem solving to identify creative possibilities for consumers. This may require flexibility in applying what appear to be rigid policies and in blending community and consumer agendas.

Every challenge confronted by workers and consumers is an opportunity for social administrators to demonstrate *learning for a living*. Although interactions between consumers and workers are guided by evidence-based practices, their use requires great skill in individualizing the intervention to the consumer. This is not always a trouble-free exercise. In a dynamic society, new challenges continually arise, creating new problems for consumers. Learning from these challenges and passing this learning on to others in the agency and community is an essential part of creating and maintaining a learning organization.

Consumer-centered social administration relies on managers and others engaging in persistent interactions over time. No one is more deserving of this interaction than those people who are working directly with consumers. Learning, creating new possibilities, maintaining an outcome focus, and venerating consumers takes place in personal interactions with direct service staff. Organizational change follows repeated interactions with staff using the change skills identified in Chapter 2.

Social administrators are operating according to the principles of client-centered management when they create the conditions for direct service workers to work with consumers to achieve desired results.

THE TASKS OF MANAGING PEOPLE*

A core concept of this chapter is that a job is a set of tasks and that the more clearly the tasks are identified, the more likely it is that people will un-

---

*Other chapters include a list of learning objectives. The personnel management tasks are the learning objectives for this chapter.

derstand what is expected of them. To model this, we present the social administrator's personnel management job as a set of tasks. Strictly speaking, the following list does not meet all of our criteria for task statements. We present them here in general terms with the required detail following:

The consumer-centered supervisor

1. uses a variety of mechanisms to create and maintain an organizational culture that implements the principles of consumer-centered social administration:
   a. Venerating the people called clients/consumers.
   b. Maintaining the focus on results for consumers.
   c. A healthy disrespect for the impossible.
   d. Learning for a living.
2. uses program specifications and evidence-based practices to identify the tasks required to achieve desired consumer outcomes and to designs jobs so that workers achieve their job values and consumers are successful.
3. uses formal and informal channels of communication for recruitment and equitable procedures for selection that match people to jobs and maximize the fit between consumer and consumer cultures.
4. uses a variety of information collection strategies including those identified in previous chapters to establish and maintain a system of performance appraisal, feedback, and rewards that informs and energizes staff.
5. assists workers to develop skills and enhance their careers through the mechanisms of supervision and training.
6. uses standard procedures specific to a field of practice to maintain policies, procedures, and training that focus on worker and consumer safety.

THE SPECIAL CASE OF VOLUNTEERS

Volunteers are truly special people who give of themselves by working alongside other staff without pay. They should not be an afterthought. The discussion of volunteers occurs here because it is our belief that they should be given the same consideration as any other member of the organization. In an ideal world, there would be no need to have a special section on volunteers. Unfortunately, this is not always the case. Consequently, we use this section to emphasize that each of the six sets of tasks identified in this chapter applies as much to volunteers as it does to those that are on the payroll.

Volunteer responsibilities require the same carefully designed jobs of anyone else. Too often volunteers are recruited to complete unclear tasks with less than specific direction. Volunteers need to know what they are to do as well as how to do it so they can have a satisfying role and continue to work in the agency. They deserve and should have the benefit of the same training and assistance to do their job as any other member of the agency.

Recruitment and selection of volunteers needs to be done as carefully as other staff. Fortunately, many communities have volunteer centers that assist with recruitment and match volunteer skills to agency needs. Many local newspapers include periodic lists of volunteer opportunities that can aid recruitment. However, these channels of communication may not produce the results you desire. It may be necessary to augment these efforts with others that target particular populations in the community to enhance the mix of people in the agency.

Although performance appraisal does not have the exact same meaning when working with volunteers, it is a necessary component. Recall that the reward-based environment is an essential component of the appraisal system. Volunteers work in your agency for the reward of being a part of everyone's efforts to assist consumers. Volunteers who are part of a richly rewarding environment are more likely to continue their efforts.

At the same time, it is necessary to recognize that some matches of volunteers and agency assignments do not work. It is necessary to conduct some type of performance appraisal to assure that the volunteer experience is beneficial to both the person and the agency. Some people think that they would love to take on a particular responsibility, only to find that they do not have the skills or motivation to be successful. Working with these people to find other opportunities or to help them leave with dignity and recognition for their good intentions is important not only to them but also to consumers, the agency, and the community. A volunteer with a positive experience with an agency, even though it might have been short-lived, is a public relations asset.

THE ENVIRONMENTS OF PERSONNEL MANAGEMENT

The tasks of personnel management that are developed in this chapter occur within a large number of environments or contexts that influence the behavior of everyone concerned, including consumers, frontline social workers, and administrators. When addressing a specific personnel management task such as writing job descriptions, it is easy to forget the multiple contexts that influence the work. It is beyond the scope of this chapter to specify all of the ways that these contexts influence supervisors and the ways that they have reciprocal influence. However, it is useful to recognize that the social administrator's personnel management job includes but goes beyond direct interaction with staff.

Example Environments That Influence Personnel Management

- *Consumers or clients together with their families and friends*
- *Neighborhoods and communities*
- *Agency operations*
- *Policy: agency, local, state, national*
- *Legal*

Mental Exercise

Using your experience of working in organizations, think of one example of how each of the aforementioned environments effects personnel management.

Social services are provided at the behest of the larger public. Traditionally, a social problem is identified and community awareness and concern for the problem is raised. This results in the garnering of resources to mount a response that is sanctioned by the community. Since the community is multifaceted, so is the response.

For example, our current response to child abuse and neglect had such an evolution—advocacy on behalf of abused children resulted in abuse-and-neglect reporting laws, judicial intervention required to remove a child from his or her family, and placement in foster care as the dominant response, in order to protect children. Child welfare workers investigate and visit families in their homes and in neighborhood schools. These workers interact with a variety of attorneys and judges to provide information that will protect the child. Although a worker might determine that a child could be safe in his or her home if someone was available to visit on a daily basis, this may not be possible due to the way that funding mechanisms support foster care over other services.

The consumer, neighborhood, community, agency, and policy contexts are all evident in this example. The selection, training, and supervision of direct service workers in this context are affected by the need to have them visit with families in their own homes. They must have the skills to empathically respond to families and at the same time collect evidence and testify in court. They must be creative in identifying family and community resources that may be available to protect children because the agency services are dominated by a narrow range of formal placement services.

Although multifaceted, other less visible environments or contexts such as antidiscrimination laws, employee organizations such as unions and large agency personnel policies are also important. It is not possible within this chapter to adequately cover all of the ways these contexts affect the personnel management tasks. However, examples will be provided to demonstrate how some of these contexts influence the social administrator's job and some of the ways that she or he can influence these contexts.

Agency size is worthy of special note. Large organizations normally have specialized units dedicated to aspects of personnel management, or human resource management, as they like to call it. In the labor law environment of today, these units play a vital role in assuring that agency personal policies are fairly and equitably applied. These units are necessarily bureaucracies that can also make it difficult to make changes in response to changing needs. For example, new evidence-based practices may require a change in tasks that everyone agrees upon but the procedure to change job descriptions may be slow and burdensome.

Alternatively, it may seem like personnel management in the small agency is easier since change can occur through the leadership of one person or through consensus of a group of like-minded people. Although this may be true, it may also be an environment where personnel policies may be taken too informally and result in a lack of clear expectations, outdated job descriptions, and inequitable practices. The social administrator's personnel management tasks are the same in both environments but how these tasks are accomplished are very different. Throughout this chapter the differences in the tasks due to agency size are discussed.

OVERVIEW OF RELATED RESEARCH

There are no clinical trials of social administration practices that inform the personnel management job. However, there is an emerging body of research linking administrative behaviors to results for consumers. This research was reviewed in detail in Chapter 1. Since the majority of this research is focused on supervisory behavior, it is useful to briefly review that group of studies here.

First, it is important to know that supervisory behavior makes a difference to consumers. Some administrators choose a supervisory position after being a direct service worker for some time. Occasionally, these administrators say that they miss direct service work because they miss having a direct effect on consumers. The study by Corrigan, Lickey, Campion, and Rashid (2000) provides some important guidance for supervisors. Being an active manager by providing inspiration to workers, being considerate, and using rewards linked to important behaviors which produce desired outcomes benefits consumers.

Supervisors Have a Powerful Effect on Consumers

Corrigan, Lickey, Campion, and Rashid (2000) found that consumer satisfaction was higher when served by workers whose leaders

- *rated themselves high in inspiration;*
- *more frequently used contingent rewards; and*
- *rated themselves low in passive management by exception and laissez-faire management.*

Consumers with higher quality of life were served by teams whose workers rated their supervisors as

- *charismatic and inspiring; and*
- *considerate of the interests of individual staff members.*

The research of Sosin (1986), Harkness and Hensley (1991), and Harkness (1997) all provide additional examples of how active managers make a difference. In Sosin's study, supervisors simply reminded child welfare workers that it was time to review cases. In the studies by Harkness, supervisors asked questions about client outcomes and the selection of interventions that might produce the desired outcome. In another study by Harkness (1995), supervisory helpfulness and problem solving were associated with better consumer outcomes.

In this same study, Harkness found that the relationship between the supervisor and worker, including the supervisor being empathic, was associated with better outcomes. Ahearn (1999) found that workers who rated their supervisors more highly on interpersonal skills and client centeredness had caseloads with higher rates of permanency. The specific items used to assess interpersonal skills make this dimension more concrete:

- I find it easy to envision myself in the position of others.
- I am able to make most people feel comfortable and at ease around me.
- It is easy for me to develop good rapport with most people.

- I understand people well.
- I am good at getting others to respond positively to me.
- I usually try to find common ground with others.

In summary, the research on the relationship between supervisory behavior and consumer outcomes, although meager, indicates that consumer outcomes are better when served by workers who are led by people who

- are inspiring;
- direct workers by aiding in problem solving and asking consumer-oriented questions; and
- with whom they have a relationship characterized by empathy, mutual understanding, and rapport.

TASK 1:
CREATING AND REINFORCING
A CONSUMER-CENTERED UNIT CULTURE

In our job description for the consumer-centered social administrator, the first task is to create and maintain a cultural context that supports consumer-centered values and principles. Although controversial, we believe that the idea of healthy or toxic organizational cultures is important. Glisson (2000) defines organizational culture as a property of a social system, such as the work unit, whether it is a team or a large multifaceted organization, that comprises the norms and values of that social system that drive the way things are done in the organization. Glisson goes on to distinguish the concepts of organizational climate from culture. Climate differs from culture in that climate is the psychological impact of the work environment on the individual. This includes concepts such as job satisfaction, discussed later in this chapter.

Organizational Culture

Culture is defined as a property of the collective social system. It comprises the norms and values of that social system that drive the way things are done in the organization. (Glisson, 2000, p. 198)

In recognition of the interactive nature of people and social systems, social administrators both influence and are influenced by the norms and values of the work unit. When a person is new to a work unit, they frequently have questions about why some things are done as they are. The answer may be that the practice is driven by policy or is evidence-based, or it may be a powerful norm or value that is influencing people to behave in a specific way.

Mental Exercise

Think about a work unit that you have been a part of and identify a behavior that you would attribute to a norm or value. Identify the norm or value.

Although social administrators are being influenced by the organization's norms and values, they also have an important role in influencing or changing them. Changing organizational norms and values is not easy. It requires conscious efforts to identify the desired values and use the change strategies of Chapter 2 along with important elements of social systems to arrive at the desired result.

To change a unit culture requires having a list of norms and values that the manager would like to have in place. Some supervisors have conducted staff meetings with the explicit goal of identifying existing norms and values and discussing what the team would like to reinforce, add, or eliminate. Others have a list that they articulate to the team. Some important norms and values are embedded in the consumer centered administrative principles listed in Chapter 1. Although we believe that this list is a necessary part of the organizational culture, it is not likely to be sufficient. Specific practice contexts would have additional norms and values and might reword some to fit the consumer served. For example, there may be explicit mention of the use of evidence-based practices as a norm, the use of certain language that venerates consumers, or a principle respecting cultural differences within the work environment. In any case, taking time to explicitly list the values and norms of the work unit is a necessary first step. The following example of consumer and unit values from a program for people with psychiatric disabilities demonstrates the idea (see Exhibit 8.1).

Reminder: Consumer-Centered Social Administration Norms and Values

- *Venerating the people called clients/consumers*
- *Creating and maintaining the focus*
- *A healthy disrespect for the impossible*
- *Learning for a living*

EXHIBIT 8.1. Example Set of Unit Values

Consumer Values

1. People with psychiatric disabilities can recover and can be helped to do so.
2. People with psychiatric disabilities have the right to self-determination in the goals they set and the help they receive.
3. People with psychiatric disabilities have the right and the ability to live, love, learn, work, and play in the same fashion and in the same locations as others.
4. People with psychiatric disabilities possess considerable talents, strengths, and abilities. They are not the disability but rather the disability is one small part of them.
5. Our community contains opportunities, people, and resources that are sufficient to support our clients' journey of recovery.

Agency Values: What We Stand For

1. *"Walking the Walk"*—All our work will reflect a predominant concern for people with psychiatric disabilities and their welfare. We seek the means to amplify their voice. Our behavior perfectly reflects this preoccupation.
2. *Results-Oriented*—The test of our work will always be whether clients are identifiably better off. We recognize that knowledge gained and professional satisfaction with our efforts, the establishment of a new program, or a change in policy are intermediate measures. The real crucible is to what degree these redound to clients in life-improving ways. This also means that critical reflection and introspection are constantly needed by all members.
3. *Innovative*—We seek to always be on the leading edge. We are creative and flexible in our efforts to help people work smarter. We push the boundaries; break mind barriers, instigate innovation in others. "Just Try Another Way" is the motto. We are maniacs about continuously adding value to our work. We possess a healthy disrespect for the impossible.
4. *Competent*—We are knowledgeable, current about the most recent thinking and practices in the field. We know how to convert the state-of-the-art to practical advice and guidance in arriving at solutions.
5. *"Take it to the Bank"*
    We are dependable—we do what we say by when we say we are going to do it.
    We are responsive to people's requests in terms of understanding, effort, timeliness, relevancy, and practicality. We create partnerships.
6. *Passion*—We are contagious, infectious. We build hope because without it there is no possibility. We seek to motivate and excite people towards our vision; to bring meaning to their work.
7. *Fun*—People smile and laugh; they feel good. We remind people that this is "good" work and it should be a source of personal satisfaction. We bring fun to our work.

Once a social administrator has a list of norms and values by which she or he is going to lead the work unit, the task is to establish these within the unit so that they "belong" to the unit and not the manager. The work of Deal and Peterson (1999) and Deal and Kennedy (1982) identified characteristics of organizational cultures that are useful for changing and/or reinforcing work unit values and norms.

Rites, Rituals, and Ceremonies

These are the day-to-day repetitive interactions that occur within a social system that demonstrate a norm or value. As people within a social system interact on a daily basis, there are a large number of rituals and ceremonies that are established. The simple act of cheerfully saying good morning when coming to work is a ritual that demonstrates that people in the work unit respect each other as individuals. Informal celebrations of achievements of consumers are behavioral demonstrations of the value of venerating consumers. Similar celebrations of the achievements of the worker demonstrate the importance of workers in achieving desired results. Celebrations of holidays that are important to cultures within the community and work group demonstrate the value of respecting cultural differences.

The social administrator can use these as tools to establish or maintain desired norms and values. Observation of existing rituals will identify which ones reinforce desired values and which ones should be eliminated. Starting new rituals and ceremonies that reinforce desired values is an essential administrative task.

Signs and Symbols

The cartoons pinned to the cubical wall and the reports circulated within the unit are just two examples of the signs and symbols that communicate the norms and values within a work unit. Many people enjoy the workplace cartoon Dilbert. Although wickedly funny, it frequently communicates negative workplace norms and values, such as disrespecting your colleagues and customers. On the other hand, a butterfly motif in a child welfare family preservation unit was used to explicitly communicate that some families were going through difficult changes that, like the pupa, were not attractive. The message was that families, like caterpillars, could emerge as beautiful butterflies. Similarly, a chart that keeps current the number of consumers employed helps reinforce the focus on this important outcome.

Social administrators can use signs and symbols to shape organizational culture by taking a fresh look at those that exist within the work unit to identify the norms and values that they communicate. Conscious selection of signs and symbols that reinforce desired norms and values is a powerful tool. Questioning the norms and values communicated through existing signs and symbols that do not reinforce what is desired can lead to their replacement.

Exercise

Take a cultural tour through a work unit that you are familiar with:

- *Notice the ritualistic interactions between people.*
- *Look at what is displayed on bulletin boards and office walls.*
- *Take note of the language used to describe the work.*
- *Ask people for examples of stories that are frequently told within the unit.*

List the norms and values that you think are demonstrated by these cultural elements.

History and Stories

Within every work unit, people tell stories that communicate norms and values. Some of these stories are about consumers, others are about workers, and still others are about people in the community with whom workers interact. These stories communicate norms and values. Examples include upbeat stories about what a consumer has achieved despite seemingly insurmountable obstacles, or an "impossible" teacher who contributes to a vulnerable child's learning difficulties.

These stories exist and can be an instrument of consumer-centered administration by reinforcing desired norms and values, or they can undermine them. Social administrators need an ever-changing group of stories to use as a powerful cultural element to reinforce norms and values. Fortunately, daily successes of consumers, workers, and key individuals necessary to accomplishing desired outcomes are the natural material for creating and refreshing these stories.

Heroes

The stories just discussed include people. They are the heroes of the work unit. When a story is told about a consumer with a psychiatrist disability who has completed a month working at a job, this person is a hero. The story communicates what is possible and the hero serves as a role model. Like any story, a detailed description of how this was accomplished communicates a great deal. The way that the employer responded to problematic symptoms of the mental illness, and the way that the worker prepared the employer and consumer for success are just two "details" that communicate more than a training event.

The consumer-centered social administrator is cognizant of the heroes identified by the work unit. Not all of the stories describe a positive hero. Yet the people identified in the story are heroes in the sense of communicating norms and values. Social administrators recognize and create positive heroes that reinforce the types of role models necessary for success of consumers. These administrators also ignore, question, or extinguish the stories that create negative heroes.

Cultural Networks

The communication network that shares signs, symbols, stories, and heroes is another mechanism for maintaining a consumer-centered organizational culture. So far this section has identified what is communicated. The communication network is equally important. The manager seeking to establish or reinforce consumer-centered norms and values identifies the channels of cultural communication. She or he uses these same channels to share the rituals, symbols, and stories that communicate desired values.

Language

The words we use both reflect and shape the organizational culture. Some organizations allow the use of labels when referring to consumers: "that person is schizophrenic"; "she is an abuser"; "he is a drunk." Labeling language often depersonalizes the individuals we serve and conveys that the person can be known by their label. Other organizations require respectful language where the schizophrenic becomes "the person with schizophrenia" or "the person with a psychiatric disability" or maybe just "Mabel." Language that is dominated by pathology, problems, and weaknesses tends to disempower, whereas the language of strengths, achievement, and resiliency seems to empower. The latter conveys an expectation of growth and possibility.

Creating and Maintaining Consumer-Centered Organizational Norms and Values

- *Write a list of desired organizational norms and values.*
- *Establish or reinforce these norms and values through*
  —rites, rituals, and ceremonies;
  —symbols;

—*history and stories;*
—*heroes;*
—*cultural networks;*
—*language.*
• *Elicit desired behavior through the change model described in Chapter 2.*

Eliciting the Desired Behavior

The mechanisms that create or maintain desired organizational norms and values require behavior. People talk to others in the cultural network, tell stories among themselves, tape cartoons or newspaper clippings on the wall, and participate in rituals and ceremonies. These are all behaviors. In those cases where the elements of organizational culture are communicating and reinforcing desired norms and values, the manager simply needs to reinforce these behaviors and update ceremonies, symbols, and stories. Where rituals, symbols, and stories are reinforcing undesirable norms and values, the manager undertakes the difficult task of changing these elements of culture.

The theory of behavioral intention (Chapter 2, Figure 2.1), which is the model for change in this text, provides the manager with tools for influencing the organizational culture. Behavior that has existed within the work unit that the social administrator would like to eliminate or change has probably existed for some time and has been, at some level, rewarding to workers. Recall that *perceived behavioral control* is one element of the model of change. The existing behavior is easy and natural, and elimination of a behavior or replacement with a new behavior is likely to be perceived to be difficult. A second element of the change model is the person's *attitude concerning the behavior* and the strength of this belief. An existing behavior is likely to be accompanied by a strong belief that it is normal and appropriate. A third element of the change model is *social norms,* which is an element of organizational culture. The change model predicts that these three elements lead to an *intention to act* and consequently the *behavior.*

Thinking about existing behavior using this model demonstrates how difficult it is to change organizational norms and values. Existing behavior is easy and expected by the work group. Replacement behavior is perceived to be difficult, not desirable, and not what is expected in the workplace. It will take considerable effort on the part of the manager to change workers' beliefs about the new behavior and their intention to participate in it. We recommend the full range of change strategies identified in Chapter 2 as tools to bring about desired cultural change.

Using your experience in a work unit,

1. *identify a norm or value that you would have liked to change;*
2. *identify one or two elements of organizational culture that you think maintained the norm or value; and*
3. *pick a change strategy from Chapter 2 and describe how you would use it as the manager of the unit.*

Large and Small Organizations

It is likely to be easier to change the culture of a small organization than that of a large one, although a long-lasting culture within a small organization presents significant challenges. Most social administrators within a large organization manage a particular work unit. The change strategies used within the small unit may present a challenge because they run counter to the norms and values of the larger organization, not based on the skill of the manager. Stories abound of unit managers who were "punished" by co-workers who considered changes to be in conflict with existing norms and values. Despite the difficulties, the supervisor of the team has the most contact and influence with team members and can often elicit the necessary changes.

Reminder: Summary of Change Strategies

Strategies to enhance perceived behavioral control are as follows:

1. *Obstacle removal*
   a. *Task groups*
   b. *Forms and paperwork*
   c. *Education and training*
2. *Modeling*
3. *Behavioral rehearsal*
4. *Provide verbal encouragement*
5. *Provide information*

Strategies to change an attitude toward a behavior:

1. *Add a new reason to think positively about the behavior*
2. *Increase or decrease the importance of an existing belief about the behavior*
   a. *Emphasize advantages and rewards*
   b. *Cite proven results/weight of the evidence*
   c. *Specify the consequences of a stance*
3. *Try it–"foot in the door technique"*

Strategies to affect the normative component are as follows:

1. Link message to a new important person
2. Increase the importance of an existing key actor
3. Change the belief attributed to a current key actor—either positive or negative.

Strategies to enhance the link between intention and behavior are as follows:

1. Enhance perceived relevance of behavior
2. Encourage anticipation of feelings
3. Induce feelings of hypocrisy

The task of changing a culture within a larger organization having conflicting norms and values is extremely difficult. The change strategies available to the manager are the same. The target of change is a different level of the organization. We do not claim that the use of these strategies will yield positive results quickly. It can be a long and difficult task to influence other administrators to engage in changing norms and values. There is also a feeling of being overwhelmed with the task of managing a unit and changing others. This text suggests that social administrators think in terms of the conscious and persistent use of day-to-day interactions with others to exercise influence and bring about organizational change.

A Note About Other Cultures

Social work units with their cultures are not only embedded within larger organizations; they are also part of and embedded in other cultures such as that of a neighborhood or community. These cultures also have norms, values, heroes, stories, rituals, and ceremonies that are important to that group and to the social administrator. These cultures influence the work unit. Consumers also bring their cultural traits to their interactions with workers. Workers, who we contend should be representative of the cultures of consumers, bring their cultural traits to work.

Keeping in mind that a culture is defined by its norms, values, heroes, stories, and rituals, we all have grown and developed in a dizzying array of cultures. Some of these cultures include our family of origin, the neighborhood and community in which we grew up, the schools we attended (elementary, high school, college, and university), and the communities and organizations where we have worked. The cultural characteristics that we adopt from any of these cultures are uniquely ours and cannot be reliably predicted by simply identifying a culture by a label. An awareness of the influences of these cultures can assist us in asking individuals how various cultures influence their current beliefs and behaviors. The relevant section of the NASW Code of Ethics is reproduced here to remind us of the importance of culture to practice.

Cultural Exercise

1. *Using one of the cultural groups that you have been a part of, identify an important norm or value. This may be difficult because it is difficult to think about our own culture.*
2. *Identify one or two examples of signs, symbols, rituals, ceremonies, stories, or heroes that maintain this norm or value.*
3. *Identify one way that this influences your behavior at work.*

Reminder—NASW Code of Ethics

1.05 Cultural Competence and Social Diversity

(a) Social workers should understand culture and its function in human behavior and society, recognizing the strengths that exist in all cultures.

(b) Social workers should have a knowledge base of their clients' cultures and be able to demonstrate competence in the provision of services that are sensitive to clients' cultures and to differences among people and cultural groups.

(c) Social workers should obtain education about and seek to understand the nature of social diversity and oppression with respect to race, ethnicity, national origin, color, sex, sexual orientation, age, marital status, political belief, religion, and mental or physical disability.

Reprinted with permission of NASW Press.

TASK 2: DESIGNING JOBS SO THAT CONSUMERS AND WORKERS ACHIEVE DESIRED RESULTS

This simple statement is more than a single task and obscures the multitude of social administration behaviors, methods, knowledge, and skills required. In this section we develop this set of tasks through the following topics:

- Consumer outcomes and worker behaviors—what produces results?
- Tasks—clarifying expectations—behavior, methods, results
- Characteristics of helpful job descriptions; getting the work done in large and small organizations

Consumer Outcomes and Worker Behaviors

It is a premise of this text that consumers of social services achieve desired results primarily through interactions with direct service workers and other "key actors." These interactions are more successful when they are carefully structured and occur consistently over time. For example, school social workers help children at risk of school failure through regular interactions with the children, their teachers, parents, and possibly other professionals. Social workers working with individuals with psychiatric disabilities help them maintain an apartment by regular interactions with the consumer, landlord, and other professionals that need to be involved.

The social administrator has the responsibility of assuring that these interactions between workers, consumers, and others are structured so that they produce the desired results. Workers exhibit behaviors in these interactions that reflect methods that are shown to produce desired results and rely on the skills and knowledge that they acquired through education, training, and supervision. One critical supervision skill is to consistently communicate and clarify expectations for worker behaviors that produce results. The program specifications developed in Chapters 3, 4, and 5 include worker expectations or behaviors necessary for consumer success. These expectations come from the following:

- Evidence-based practices
- Policy and procedure
- Organizational norms

In the ideal organization, there is a wonderful consistency between worker expectations and those that derive from these three sources. However, the world changes too fast for this to occur often. Evidence-based practices emerge from the research literature and it takes time for them to be incorporated into practice. A finding from health care research makes this point well. In a report by the Agency for Healthcare Research and Quality (AHRQ), they report as follows.

> Recent studies indicate an average of 17 years is needed before new knowledge generated through research, such as randomized clinical trials, is incorporated into widespread clinical practice—and even then the application of the knowledge is very uneven. (AHRQ, 2004)

Agency policy documents tend to be products that are written and changed over time. In larger organizations, there is usually a process for changing policy that takes multiple approvals. This takes time, and frequently means that many of these documents are out of date. Gray (2001) devotes considerable attention to ways of creating the evidence-based organization and suggests that an evidence center is useful to help bridge the gap between knowledge, policy, and practice. An evidence center is a collection of staff (or a part-time staff member) with the skills and resources to evaluate evidence and influence agency operations to achieve timely consistency between research evidence and agency practice. In the framework of this text, it is the evidence center that continually examines program specifications in light of new research. Unfortunately, it is still the rare social service organization that has such an evidence center.

Organizational norms or expectations also direct workers in their jobs. These norms are frequently the result of the work unit doing the job in certain ways that have "worked" for them over time. Since the definition of "worked" has only recently been defined as producing desired results for consumers, it is possible that there are discontinuities between agency norms for worker behavior with consumers and desired results. It is from this context of emerging research, agency policy, and organizational norms that social administrators identify worker tasks.

Evidence-based interventions are arguably the best place for a supervisor to identify worker behaviors that are linked to consumer results. This was a primary idea guiding the writing of program specifications throughout Chapters 4, 5, and 6. Fidelity instruments were discussed and are an important source of worker expectations. In their ideal world, researchers who tested the intervention identified worker behavior shown through randomized controlled experiments to yield desired outcomes for consumers. The importance of such lists of behaviors is exemplified by a study conducted by the Washington State Institute for Public Policy, which was an evaluation of programs for juvenile offenders (Washington State Institute for Public Policy, 2004). In this study, the researchers made a judgment about the degree to which the intervention was implemented as intended and called this "competent" or "not competent." Among their findings was that when a program called Functional Family Therapy was competently implemented, it resulted in a 38 percent *decrease* in juvenile offender recidivism but when it was not competently implemented the result was a 16 percent *increase* in recidivism. This is just one example of how worker behavior makes a difference.

Clarifying Expectations Through Task Statements

Job descriptions are one way that worker expectations are communicated. Developing a useful job description requires identification of the behavior required of workers to produce the desired results, writing these behaviors as task statement, and grouping them together to define a job or position. In the previous section we discussed identifying the desired behavior. In this section we show you how to turn these behaviors into task statement.

Sidney Fine's work on job analysis and writing task statements goes back to the early 1970s and continues to be important (Fine & Cronshaw, 1999). Exhibit 8.2 is a slightly modified form of the Fine and Cronshaw task statement structure. As the example shows, the resulting task statement may not exactly adhere to the structure but it does contain the five essential elements.

There will be other deviations for the "ideal" form as well. A set of statements that all describe a worker's tasks may omit repeating the "who" in every statement. One might also question the inclusion of "To whom?" in every statement if the consumer is always the focus of the statement. However, recall that consumers achieve results through interactions with workers and also through their efforts with other key individuals. Do not forget these "key actors" who are critical to consumer success. It is important in clarifying expectations to include the methods to be used. At the same time, writing out in detail all of the methods to be used would be very tedious and would result in a statement of such length that most people would not read it all of the way through. Evidence-based manuals are an important source for specifying the methods to be used. This also enhances the transfer of training by reminding workers that they are expected to implement the intervention in the form that demonstrated positive results.

To clearly communicate expectations, it is important to think about the words used in writing task statements. This is particularly important for the

---

EXHIBIT 8.2. Task Statement Structure

Who?	Performs what action?	With whom?	Using what methods?	To produce what consumer benefit?

Example

The child welfare workers talks with the parent in their home about how they have rewarded their child for positive behavior using the methods described in the "Assisting Parent" handbook so that the parents can respond more positively to their child's behavior.

"action" words. This needs to be a behavior that everyone in the unit understands in the same way. One of the difficulties in writing behavioral statements is our professional language. Frequently we use words that are abstract. For example, some child welfare supervisors say that "workers should contact each family once a week." Although the supervisor may have a specific definition in mind when they use the word contact, it may not be the same as what a new worker is thinking. However, if this supervisor listed every action that they had in mind, the conversation might be long and people might stop listening. Words like contact act as a kind of shorthand. In settings where everyone shares the same definition, the use of these words makes communication more efficient. Unfortunately, in many cases these types of terms are used and people do not share a common definition.

Exercise

Think of two or three commonly used words in an organization in which you have worked that have had multiple meanings and write out the different definitions. Which definition do you think would be most beneficial to consumers?

Careful selection of the words used in task statements is important but can become tedious and unhelpful if carried to extremes. One way to think through this problem is to decide which definition is most important and use that term. For example, although families may be contacted in a variety of ways including telephone, e-mail, and in person, it may be the evidence-based practice or the experience of the supervisor that indicates that meeting the family in their home is most effective. In this case, the word contact would be replaced by meeting the family in their home. Another idea is to establish a glossary of the most important terms and keep that readily accessible to workers. This might be a useful appendix in a manual that describes the evidence-based practice that is in use.

We have been discussing task statements that identify worker behavior essential to producing consumer outcomes. Although these are arguably the most important task statements, there are other expectations of workers that must be communicated clearly. The framework used in this book includes consideration of additional performance areas. Different positions within an agency have different levels of responsibilities for producing results in each of these areas. The same task statement format is used to write these.

Reminder: Performance Areas

Social program performance includes the following:

- *Results for consumers*
- *Service events*
- *Resource acquisition and management*
- *Efficiency*
- *Staff morale.*

There is considerable interaction between the performance areas. For example, direct service workers' responsibilities for producing service events may be related to results for consumers and resource acquisition. It is the service event that yields the benefit to consumers and may be the primary funding mechanism for the program, such as the fee for service arrangement under Medicaid. Consequently, it is doubly important to clearly communicate to workers their responsibility for producing a given number of service events in a specific time frame.

Another resource acquisition example is staff morale, which is discussed in more depth later in this chapter. Direct service workers are the most important members of the organization in helping consumers achieve results. Workers who are exhausted, feel badgered, and are cynical are unlikely to be helpful to consumers. The research of Glisson and Hemmelgarn (1998) showed that human relations' dimensions of fairness, role clarity, role overload, role conflict, cooperation, growth and advancement, job satisfaction, emotional exhaustion, personal accomplishment, and depersonalization had the expected effect on results for consumers. Although administrators have the primary responsibility for these dimensions, co-workers play an important role in maintaining a positive work environment. We contend that task statements regarding staff morale should be included in expectations of workers.

Although we have not yet discussed what constitutes staff morale, we now provide one example. Buckingham and Coffman (1999) found that an important indicator of staff morale was a person saying that they have received recognition or praise for doing good work in the last seven days. It is not difficult to envision a task statement such as the following: mental health counselors will tell a co-worker when they have done a good job with a consumer when an outcome is achieved.

Characteristics of Helpful Job Descriptions:
Getting the Work Done in Large and Small Organizations

The set of tasks that clarify work expectations are most often communicated to workers and throughout the organization in the form of job descriptions. In small organizations, administrators have a great deal of discretion in compiling tasks into job descriptions. In large organizations, there is likely to be a standard format that may or may not be helpful in supervision. There is also likely to be a specialized human resources unit whose responsibilities include approving job description according to a set of standards and classifying jobs for purposes of pay. Working with human resource units to establish positions and job descriptions can be helpful in assuring compliance with labor laws, affirmative action goals, and to assure equity across the organization. It can also be frustrating.

Klingner and Nalbandian (2003), writing from a public administration point of view, identify five different perspectives that sometimes conflict but explain various forms of job descriptions. The specific perspectives are not repeated here because they are less important than the conclusion that, as a consequence, traditional job descriptions do not help supervisors manage the work, and they do not help employees manage their careers. They have found that the most useful job descriptions include the following elements:

1. Tasks—What work duties are important to the job?
2. Conditions—What things make the job easy or hard?
3. Standards—What objective performance levels can reasonably be set for each task?
4. Competencies—What knowledge, skills, and abilities are required to perform each at the minimum standard?
5. Qualifications—What education, experience, and other qualifications are needed to ensure that employees have the necessary competencies? (p. 120)

The work of these authors comes from public administration. In social administration there is a sixth requirement.

6. Job descriptions should include a statement of the desired consumer outcome.

Regardless of what type of organization a social administrator is working within, it is useful to think of job description in these terms. In a small organization, the administrator may have the latitude to include all six features. In a large organization, the administrator may not. In this case we urge managers to use their organizational change skills to try to influence the human resource unit to develop useful job descriptions. Since this is likely to be a long and difficult task, we also urge managers to have informal job descriptions that contain these six elements for their workers while recognizing the legitimacy of the formal ones. It is extremely unlikely that this will produce any conflict with the formal personnel management system.

TASK 3: RECRUITMENT AND SELECTION TO MATCH PEOPLE TO JOBS

Now that you have done the hard work of writing task statements and have identified the conditions, standards, competencies, and qualifications that make up the job, you are prepared to recruit staff. This is also an important time to consider the role of consumers in matching people to jobs. Consumers who have been involved with the program for some time have insights into the job and the organization and can make important contributions to the recruitment and selection of staff.

Recruitment

The importance of recruitment cannot be overemphasized. The work of the social service organization is primarily carried out through people. It is the interaction between the direct service worker and the consumer that achieves results. The social administrator's best interest is served by recruiting and selecting the most skilled people. Recruitment efforts are driven by the need to obtain the largest possible pool of skilled people matching the culture and needs of consumers. We firmly believe that recruitment involves actively reaching out to a diverse group of audiences to achieve a workforce which adequately represents the diversity of consumers and the community within which the organization functions.

Although this is a highly held value, there are also laws and policies that support this perspective. Equal employment opportunity (EEO) is a commonly used term to cover a variety of mechanisms to eliminate discrimination by assuring fairness in employment decisions. Affirmative action (AA) is designed to help insure diversity in recruitment and selection of staff. There are a variety of federal and state laws that support these ideas. They include the Civil Rights Act of 1964, the Age Discrimination in Employment Act of 1967, and the Vocational Rehabilitation Act of 1973. Although the values of social administrators are consistent with the ideal and intent of this type of legislation, we recommend consulting an expert in this type of labor law to assure that recruitment and selection processes are legally compliant. In a small organization, this may involve hiring an outside expert, usually a local lawyer who specializes in this type of law. In the large organization, the human resources department normally includes this type of expertise.

Recruitment involves getting the word out in ways that assure equal access to job information. Affirmative action goals also help us identify diversity needs for our organizations. An important part of the recruitment process is to reexamine the diversity of current staff and identify types of individuals that we would like to have as part of the workplace. This can then help direct recruitment efforts to reach out to the desired groups to find qualified job candidates. It is worth the time and effort to identify channels of communications to specific groups to increase the likelihood of identifying qualified people and bringing them into the organization.

Although recruitment is critical, it is difficult for people in organizations to focus on recruitment for many good reasons, including the press of day-to-day business—the thought that someone else is taking care of it, the job is posted on our Web site, and the advertisement is in the paper. We encourage administrators at all levels of the organization to counter this natural tendency and actively engage in recruitment. The task is easy; completing it is difficult. Since you have identified the tasks, competences, and qualifications, identify the places where you are most likely to find people who match these requirements and reach out to them.

Recruitment Exercise

For each of the following groups, identify channels of communication to use for recruitment.

- *Women*
- *African Americans*
- *Native Americans*
- *Hispanic Americans*
- *Gays and lesbians*
- *People with disabilities*
- *Consumers*

Selection

Selecting staff from a rich and diverse pool of qualified candidates is the next challenge. Although this sounds like a one-way street, where the employer picks the person to be hired, it is actually a mutual process of identifying whether there is a match between the person and the organization. The candidate for the job is also judging the organization, its culture, the job, and supervisor as well as the work, pay, and benefits.

In its most simple form, the "right" person for the job is the person who has performed the desired tasks with a high level of competence and shares the organization's values and goals. It is unlikely that this person is in the employment pool and highly unlikely that they would want the job. People like to grow and develop and a job that one has mastered is unlikely to be a challenge. The next choice is to select the person who has mastered many of the tasks and wants to develop the remaining skills while sharing the unit's values and goals.

Identification of the ideal person from the pool of candidates is a process of information sharing. The employer shares as much information about the job and the organization as possible and seeks as much information about the candidates' work skills and desires as possible. There are essentially the following four primary mechanisms for the sharing of job information:

- Application
- Job previews
- References
- Interview

The Application

The selection process typically begins with the job application. This may be an application form that the organization has designed or it may be a letter expressing interest in the job along with a resumé. It is important to remember that the job application, like all aspects of the selection process, must seek information related to the job. Extraneous information may insert bias into the process and, if requested by the potential employer, is probably illegal. If you are designing an application for your organization, it is important to have it examined by a personnel expert.

As a document intended to share job information, the focus for both parties is on identifying that the applicant has the qualifications, the competencies, and has demonstrated the skills that make up the job. Most of the other information, including the type font size and paper used, is a distraction.

Relevant information includes prior education that meets the qualifications, employment, or volunteer experiences of the same type as the job. References of people who have observed the person doing the work are useful.

The Realistic Job Preview

Sims (2002) discusses realistic job previews (RJP) as an emerging personnel recruitment mechanism. The RJP is an attempt to bridge the gap between what an organization might say about itself and the job in an effort to recruit staff and the reality of the job. We believe that the RJP would make an even better mechanism for sharing information about the job and the organization. A RJP is nothing more than allowing the job candidate to observe the work as it is being done. This can be done by having them observe workers currently doing the job or having a video of workers doing the job. This not only allows the job candidate to see the necessary skills being used, but it also allows them to observe the organizational culture and make a judgment about the fit between personal values and those of the organization.

Checking References

Many people believe that checking with references in today's legal environment does not provide useful information because so many references are not candid about the candidate's prior job performance. Although there is some truth to this, checking references is an essential step in the process. Checking references is usually done for only the few candidates who are finalists for the job and usually by phone.

The most important references are those people who have actually observed the candidate doing tasks of the desired type. Prior supervisors are probably the best source of this information. Keep the reference interview focused on the candidates' qualifications, competencies, and demonstration of tasks. Specifics about when and where the person has observed the candidate demonstrate the required tasks are far more important than vague personality characteristics.

The Job Interview

The job interview is a particularly valuable mechanism for sharing information about the qualifications and competencies required by the job and possessed by the candidate. The interview is usually a face-to-face meeting or set of meetings between the top job candidates and key organizational staff and consumers. It is an opportunity to see the candidate in action. It is also an opportunity to make critical mistakes. The best interview is the one that shares job information between the candidate and the organization in a valid and reliable manner.

There has been extensive research on the reliability and validity of the employment interview. This research is difficult to synthesize and sometimes appears to yield contradictory results. Two different and useful reviews of this vast array of research were published by Posthuma, Morgeson, and Campion (2002) and Judge, Higgins, and Cable (2000). There is agreement in these reviews regarding the potential for the employment interview to be a reliable and valid method for selecting staff. Both reviews agree that the interview can introduce bias based upon the applicant's appearance and nonverbal cues such as eye contact. Relatively more weight is given to negative rather than positive information, decisions can be based upon similarities between interviewer and interviewee, and decisions are frequently made within the first few minutes, with the remainder of the interview used to justify the decision.

Given these results, it is important to work to minimize biases. The aforementioned reviews also agree that this body of research finds that structured interviews tend to be more valid and reliable than those that are unstructured. Consequently, it is important to carefully consider the structure prior to interviewing any of the candidates. In the large organization, there is likely to be a standard interview format to assure equal treatment of all candidates. In the small organization, the person doing the hiring may be the one who designs the interview. In any case, the focus is on obtaining valid and reliable information that demonstrates that the candidate has accomplished the job tasks and the quality of this work.

Most interviews consist of questions about the candidates' past experiences that relate to the job. However, demonstration of selected job tasks is worth considering as part of the interview. This could be demonstrated through a role-play with a staff member. This could also be conducted with a consumer who is involved in the hiring process.

Once again it is critical not to be influenced by factors that are not relevant to the job. Symphony orchestras only started hiring women when they conducted the interview by having candidates play their instrument behind a curtain so that the gender of the person was unknown to the selection committee. Other research has shown that people involved in the job interview make a quick decision to hire or eliminate a candidate from consideration and then use the rest of the interview to justify their decision. Carefully structuring the interview to be fair and equitable will yield positive results in selecting the person for the job.

TASK 4: MAINTAINING A SYSTEM
OF PERFORMANCE APPRAISAL, FEEDBACK,
AND REWARDS THAT INFORMS AND ENERGIZES STAFF

Performance appraisal, feedback, and rewards are three related topics that include a great deal of complexity. Just as this chapter began with the topic of organizational culture, this section begins with creating a rewards-based environment. We believe that creating a rewards-based environment is a necessary precursor to meaningful feedback and performance-appraisal systems.

The Reward-Based Environment

This environment is one in which all staff continually celebrate the accomplishments of consumers and the staff that participated in these successes. It is easy to see that this is consistent with the consumer-centered norms and values that are essential elements in the organizational culture. When everyone is focused on consumers and what they achieve, it is an easy next step for everyone in the unit to celebrate each others' successes.

Although these values are a necessary part of this reward-based environment, they are not sufficient. There are specific consumer successes that are most important to the unit and they are identified in the program specifications. Recall that these specifications include objectives identifing consumer outcomes necessary to achieve the ultimate program goal. Although every success of the consumer should be celebrated, those identified in the program goal and objectives are the most important.

The reward-based environment also includes the explicit expectation that everyone, not just the administrator, is responsible for the others' job satisfaction. People choose a career and a particular job in an organization because they have reason to believe that their job values will be satisfied within this context. This is the reason that some people choose social work, while others would much rather become medical doctors or mechanics. Job satisfaction is the degree to which a person's job values are satisfied. A person who is very unhappy with his or her job has job values that are not being met.

Although everyone has a unique set of job values, there are also values that are common to subgroups of people in a particular profession and another group that is common to most people. The values related to being a social worker with a particular consumer group are likely to be shared by those working with that group. For example, social workers who work with vulnerable elderly people tend to share some of the same values. It is only the broadest set of job values that are common to people that are measured by job satisfaction surveys.

Since there are so many possible job values, it is not surprising that there is no consensus on what is the best satisfaction survey. However, one of the more interesting attempts to identify these values was done by the Gallup Organization and was complied in a book entitled *First, Break All The Rules* (Buckingham & Coffman, 1999). Their research involved thousands of work units that resulted in identifying twelve questions that they say "measure the core elements needed to attract, focus and keep the most talented employees."

The Measuring Stick

1. *Do I know what is expected of me at work?*
2. *Do I have the materials and equipment I need to do my work right?*
3. *At work, do I have the opportunity to do what I do best every day?*
4. *In the last seven days, have I received recognition or praise for doing good work?*
5. *Does my supervisor, or someone at work, seem to care about me as a person?*
6. *Is there someone at work who encourages my development?*
7. *At work, do my opinions seem to count?*
8. *Does the mission/purpose of my company make me feel my job is important?*
9. *Are my co-workers committed to doing quality work?*
10. *Do I have a best friend at work?*
11. *In the last six months, has someone at work talked to me about my progress?*
12. *This last year, have I had opportunities at work to learn and grow? (Buckingham & Coffman, 1999, p. 28)*

Most readers of this set of questions are not surprised by the implied values. This is because they identify some of the reader's job values. However, you may also be surprised by some of the questions. This is because they identify a value that is less important to you. This underscores an important point about job values. That is, each person has a unique set of values that are important to her or him.

Notice that none of these questions identify the supervisor as the person solely responsible for fulfilling these job values. Nearly all of the questions focus on a characteristic of the work or an event that has occurred. In other words, people place more importance on these considerations than on who is responsible. However, consistent with this point of view is the position that it is the social administrator who is responsible for establishing the expectations and environmental conditions so that people have rewarding jobs.

Exercise

1. Write a list of your job values.

2. Interview someone who works in a job that is very different from what you would like to do.

3. Compare and contrast the values identified in the two lists.

Notice that few of the questions focus on concrete rewards. Only one question mentions praise or recognition. In other words, the rewards-based environment is much more than the concrete rewards, although they are important. In most social work contexts the most powerful and available awards are verbal recognition. There are also a variety of ways that verbal recognition can be carried out. Consideration of the various audiences and channels of communication greatly increases the ways that verbal rewards can be expressed. For example, going to a person's workplace and telling them that they did a good job helping Ms. Jones monitor her medications is just one way of delivering the reward. Saying the same thing in the presence of other workers has another effect, as does including the consumer. Cards, notes, and e-mail are just a few additional ways of delivering the message.

Exercise

Brainstorm as many ways as possible of delivering praise or recognition for a worker's role in a consumer accomplishment. Consider both the various people who could be involved as well as different ways that the message could be delivered.

The Reward-Based Environment

- *Establish the organizational norm that everyone is responsible for celebrating consumer's and worker's successes that are identified in the program specifications.*
- *Identify the job values shared by most people in the unit and establish the expectation that everyone helps each other satisfy these values.*
- *Identify the job values unique to each person that you supervise and talk with them about how to best satisfy these values.*

Feedback

The reward-based environment is rich in feedback. At the same time, it is important to consider ways of giving feedback and its potential effect on staff. Recall that one of the twelve working conditions that Buckingham and Coffman (1999) found important to workers was that of someone talking with them about their progress in the last twelve months.

Feedback, in this context, is information given to a person about job performance. This information can have various effects on people depending on a number of variables. Readers are likely to know of examples where performance feedback had a negative effect because of the way that it was provided. It is important for workers to receive feedback and for managers to provide it in ways that help people grow and develop.

For many supervisors in social services, giving critical feedback is uncomfortable. Not only can it be uncomfortable, but some supervisors avoid giving critical feedback. When feedback is avoided, the undesired behaviors continue until the situation worsens and some kind of formal action must be taken, such as a formal reprimand or steps toward termination. Having a framework for giving feedback successfully can increase the supervisors' comfort level and can improve their ability to use feedback to get positive results.

Alvero, Bucklin, and Austin (2001) conducted an extensive review of research on performance feedback in organizational settings and identified the conditions that produced the most consistent positive results. The results of their review along with the work of Buckingham and Coffman (1999) are useful to managers in designing a feedback system so that they have positive effects.

Clear Expectations

The first item on Buckingham and Coffman's "measuring stick" is clear expectations. Similarly, Alvero, Bucklin, and Austin (2001) found the most consistent positive effects from feedback when it was used along with training, task analysis, weekly task objectives, and supervisory prompts. These are simply mechanisms for making expectations clear. Clear expectations are a precursor to providing feedback.

These expectations include behaviors, attitudes, and process methods in the work. The more precise and measurable the standards and expectations, the more effective they will be in guiding the feedback. Being clear about what is wanted or needed for successful performance in the workplace assists the supervisor in guiding staff toward improved performance and allows for consistency in expectations. It is important to know what you want with regard to performance rather than relying on what you do not want.

A Learning Environment

One element of the organizational culture discussed early in this chapter is a value on learning and growth. The finding of Buckingham and Coffman (1999) that workers value an opportunity to learn and grow shows that they prefer to work in such a culture. This learning environment includes the expectation that critical performance feedback is part of learning and growth for all staff members. This can aid the supervisor in the delivery of feedback. If critical (in the sense of analytic) performance feedback is inundated within the culture, there is less defensiveness and more acceptance of feedback. An agency that uses feedback as a learning, growth-producing, tool rather than primarily when someone is "in trouble" is more effective.

In order to create this learning environment, feedback, both critical and rewarding, must occur constantly and consistently for all staff members, including the supervisor. The supervisor modeling receipt of feedback can also be helpful in creating this learning environment. This includes the supervisor asking for feedback on a regular basis as well as receiving feedback in a healthy and positive manner. The supervisor also clarifies to make sure he or she understands the feedback, asking for feedback that is specific and behavioral, and then changing behavior based on feedback. In a culture where performance feedback is critical for the purpose of learning and improving as a part of agency culture, feedback is shared throughout the agency; direct service staff give feedback to each other and to their supervisors, as well as supervisors giving feedback to their staff.

Timely Feedback

Systems of structured feedback tend to specify timing of the feedback. Buckingham and Coffman (1999) found that people wanted to know how they were doing at least once every six months. Alvero, Bucklin, and Austin (2001) found that studies that provided feedback daily, monthly, and a combination of daily and weekly were the most effective. The emphasis here is on feedback as a constant process in the learning organization.

*Believing That People (Staff) Can Learn, Grow, and Change,
and Their Desire for an Opportunity to Grow*

Workers value learning and growth (Buckingham and Coffman, 1999). When performance is not what is expected it is easy to forget this important point. One mistake often made by a supervisor is not giving feedback immediately, instead waiting until the behavior continues to a point where the supervisor is angry. When a supervisor waits until experiencing anger to give feedback, he or she typically stops believing that the person can and is motivated to learn, grow, and change. At this point, feedback is viewed as something to just get done and documented rather than as a learning tool for the purpose of helping the staff improve performance. Believing that the worker can learn, grow, and change gives the supervisor the promise that the feedback can result in change.

Belief in the Strengths of Staff

Workers want the opportunity to do what they do best every day and receive praise for doing good work (Buckingham & Coffman, 1999). Supervisors must also be able to identify the strengths of the staff and the areas where they perform efficiently, as well as the areas that require improvement in performance. This helps the supervisor place the problematic situation or behaviors in perspective and can decrease anger and frustration, which can increase the desire to help. At the time of giving feedback, the supervisor is able to verbally identify to the staff person those things he or she is able to do well in addition to those that need improvement.

Viewing Feedback As Helpful Rather Than As Punitive

Our view of feedback is important to our ability to give it in an effective way. If a supervisor and/or supervisee views feedback as punitive, it will be seen as a negative activity. If supervisors focus on the goal of helping their staff be as effective and good as they can be, feedback will be easier to give as well as more satisfying.

Be Specific When Giving Feedback

Comparing performance to expectations requires specificity. The supervisor's ability to clearly articulate observed behavior that needs to be changed, and then clearly describe the replacement behavior is paramount. This is easier to do when the supervisor is able to observe firsthand the behavior or skill in question. However, oftentimes a supervisor gets information secondhand from another staff or consumers. In these cases, getting specific information from the informant and then finding opportunities to observe similar behavior in the field is desired.

Mental Exercise: Specific versus Nonspecific Feedback

Compare the following examples. In which case would the worker better understand what was expected?

Nonspecific: *You need to improve your ability to engage with clients. You are having a lot of no shows by clients because you do not spend enough time getting to know them as a person.*

Specific: *When you meet with John, you focused on the assessment form without looking at him, you rushed through the questions, writing down the answers without spending time on what he was actually saying and gaining details. To better engage with consumers during your first contact, I need you to (1) keep eye contact with the person through the majority of the session, and (2) not focus on the assessment; ask the question in your own words and then spend time understanding the response by asking at least two follow-up questions that give you more details, but are not on the form.*

Formal Feedback Mechanisms: Performance Appraisal

Most of the emphasis in this section has been on the interaction between a supervisor and a worker. Every organization also has formal feedback systems. Chapter 6 was devoted to these information system reports. Performance appraisal is another mechanism for providing feedback to workers on their performance albeit one that has a history of management-and-worker discontent. Consequently, it is good to be reminded of some of the following characteristics of these systems that are essential for them to be effective.

- Performance feedback provided through graphs with written or verbal messages is the most effective (Alvero, Bucklin, & Austin, 2001). Remember the old adage that "a picture is worth 1,000 words."
- Feedback was effective when it was provided to a group (Alvero, Bucklin, & Austin, 2001).
- Performance feedback is most effective when it is provided both privately and publicly (Alvero, Bucklin, & Austin, 2001). In other words, when the supervisor meets with the team, gives them the graph

showing their performance, discusses this with them, and then makes this more public, such as posting the chart on the bulletin board, the feedback tends to be more effective.

- Feedback is most effective when performance was compared to a standard, such as indicated by a goal or objective, or to previous performance (Alvero, Bucklin, & Austin, 2001).

Providing performance feedback under conditions that will help people learn and grow is an essential part of a social administrator's responsibility. As the review of the research on the use of feedback within organizations demonstrates, this is not something to be taken casually. There are clearly skills to be mastered to provide performance feedback effectively, whether it is within a rewards-based environment, weekly staff meetings, or periodic performance appraisal.

Conditions for the Most Effective Use of Feedback

Feedback is most effective when

1. *combined with an antecedent such as training, task analysis, supervisory prompts;*
2. *provided through graphs combined with written or verbal feedback;*
3. *given frequently, such as daily and weekly;*
4. *provided to the work team rather than to each individual;*
5. *provided both privately and publicly;*
6. *it compares performance to a standard or to past performance. (Alvero, Bucklin and Austin, 2001)*

The Process of Giving Feedback

1. *Identify the strengths of the person you are giving feedback to.*
2. *State the difficulty or situation that has come to your attention in a matter-of-fact manner. This should be the behavior described very specifically that needs to be changed.*
3. *Set a tone of "this is a discovery process that is tended to be helpful, not punitive" by finding out the staff person's perspective, exploring what the barriers are to changing the behavior or skills, identifying a mutual understanding of specifically what behaviors or skills need to be changed without debating expectations and offering assistance, problem solving, resource support, and/or information to support staff to change the behavior.*
4. *Brainstorm alternatives and strategies for reaching the mutually identified understanding of what needs to be different.*

Formal Performance-Appraisal Systems

The reader may think that the previous section adequately covers the topic of performance appraisal and we wish that were true. However, most organizations also have a formal performance-appraisal system. When these systems are well designed, they complement the features of effective feedback systems discussed in the previous section. However, all too often they are not based upon a model of a learning organization. In either case, every administrator must be able to navigate both systems.

Klingner and Nalbandian (2003) state, "Theoretically, the appraisal of performance provides employees with feedback on their work, leading to greater clarity regarding organizational expectations and to a more effective channeling of employee ability and effort" (p. 261). The choice to start the sentence with the work "theoretically" signals a general discontent with performance-appraisal systems. Price (2004) makes several relevant comments:

> Appraisals are generally disliked by employees and employer alike (Armstrong & Baron, 1998). . . . Despite the fact that most assessors are completely unqualified to make judgments on anyone's personality, even in the most general terms, the traditional appraisal form asks for a numerical rating on a scale of 1-4 or 1-7. Additionally, more detail is asked for as supplementary verbal comments, which could range from one word such as "good" to a paragraph or more of detailed criticism and/or praise. Moreover there is usually an overall rating that may be tied to promotability and a section to indicate areas for development or training. Finally, there are normally sections for comments by the person being appraised, possibly in the form of notes of a counseling interview and comments by the appraising manager's own supervisor.
>
> The document is usually signed by all the contributors and forms part of the company's personnel records. It can be used for promotion boards, training and management development programmes. What happens if an employee disagrees with the assessment? Despite its critical consequences for promotion prospects and, perhaps, remuneration, only a half of all organizations allow any form of appeal. (p. 518)

This extended quote identifies some of the displeasure with performance-appraisal systems. Yet the remainder of the Klingner and Nalbandian (2003) quote identifies the positive features such as providing workers with feedback, increased clarity of expectations, and directing their abilities and efforts. This is consistent with workers' desires as expressed in the Buckingham and Coffman (1999) "measuring stick" that identifies core elements to attract and keep the most talented employees. Through the "measuring stick," workers are clear on the elements of an effective performance-appraisal system. Workers want a system that includes

- clear expectations;
- recognition or praise for doing good work; and
- someone to talk with them about their progress.

Reconciling the problems and promises of performance appraisal is a daunting task. Workers, the authors, and many management scholars agree on the importance of systems of rewards and feedback as well as performance-appraisal systems. Performance appraisal is likely to succeed in a rewards-based environment and fail where this does not exist.

In large organizations, it is likely that the performance-appraisal system is directed by policy and procedures. In this context, managers need to develop expertise in the specified system. They also need to apply it in a manner that meets workers and organizational needs. Managers also need to take opportunities to advocate for improved performance-appraisal systems.

In small organizations, there is less likely to be a routine system. This is an opportunity to design a system that meets individual and organization needs. It is also an opportunity to ignore this need or to design a system with serious flaws. If you find yourself with the opportunity to design a performance-appraisal system for an organization, it is important to consult with an expert in personnel management to avoid costly mistakes. Given the problems identified by Price (2004), it is not surprising that this is a subject of legal action. Sims (2002) identifies the elements of legally defensible performance-appraisal systems based upon case law in the area as follows:

- Performance-appraisal criteria based on job analysis
- Absence of disparate impact and evidence of validity
- Formal evaluation criteria that limit managerial variability
- Formal rating instrument
- Personal knowledge of and contact with appraised individual
- Training of supervisors in conducting appraisals
- Review process that prevents one manager acting alone from controlling an employee's career
- Counseling to help poor performers improve (p. 212)

A comprehensive evaluation of all possible performance-appraisal methods is beyond the scope of this book. However, a list of some of the most common methods is presented in Exhibit 8.3. If you find yourself in an organization that has an established system, it is a good idea to learn all you can about its strengths and weaknesses so that you can use it as effectively as possible. If you are having a personnel consultant assist you in designing a system for your organization, it is useful to have some familiarity with the various systems. The references identified Exhibit 8.3 are two good sources for additional information.

EXHIBIT 8.3. Example Performance-Appraisal Methods

- *Graphic rating scale:* This is a list of traits, job criteria, or behaviors accompanied by a rating scale for each item. The evaluator rates the worker by identifying the relevant point on each scale.
- *Critical incidents:* The rater writes a list of examples of the person's good (successful) or bad (unsuccessful) performance in relation to each work objective.
- *Ranking:* A rater rank-orders each worker in the unit on each of a list of job traits. This is sometimes done without a list of job traits. In this case, the rater constructs a rank-order list of workers in the unit from highest performing to lowest.
- *Forced choice:* An expert determines which traits or behaviors contribute to high job performance. These are then presented as a multiple choice list from which the rater selects the one that best describes the worker.
- *Written essay:* The rater writes a statement of the employee's strengths, weaknesses, performance, and suggestions for improvement.
- *Behaviorally anchored rating scales (BARS):* A list of behaviors is developed for each job task that represents a range of performance from positive to negative. The rater selects the behavior that best represents the performance of the worker.
- *Management by objectives:* The worker and rater write a list of quantified goals for a coming time period. During the time period, the list is periodically reviewed. At the end of the time period, the appraisal is the degree of goal attainment.

Source: Examples drawn from Klingner, D.E. & Nalbandian (2003). *Public personnel management: Contexts and strategies.* (5th ed.) Upper Saddle River, NJ: Prentice Hall. Sims, R. R. (2002). *Organizational success through effective human resource management.* Westport, CN: Quorum Books.

Conducting the Performance Appraisal

The performance-appraisal event may be the most anxiety-provoking interaction within the organization for both supervisor and worker. Due to this anxiety, the event often does not go well. Consequently, it is important for both parties to be well prepared, and it is the supervisor's job to make certain that this happens. In an organization where expectations are clear and feedback and rewards are frequent, the performance-appraisal session should be a confirmation of what both parties have already shared. In fact, a supervisor who experiences less than satisfying performance-appraisal events may benefit from considering what may be lacking in the unit regarding clear expectations, rewards, and feedback.

Mental Exercise

Think about experiences you have had being evaluated in a job. Specifically identify one positive and one negative experience. If you have not had a performance appraisal, ask a friend to share their experiences.

1. Make a list of the features that contributed to the positive experience.
2. Make a list of the features that contributed to the negative experience.

The performance-appraisal session is an important time for the supervisor to use their best communication and interviewing skills, such as carefully formed questions and careful listening, as well as demonstrating direct knowledge of the worker's job performance. The session begins by putting the worker at ease. This is followed by giving the worker an opportunity to tell the supervisor what he or she believes he or she does best, as well as list skills the worker would like to acquire and define where he or she sees this career path leading. In the best session, this leads naturally into the supervisor confirming those strengths and additional skills that were agree upon. Talking about additional strengths that the worker has not identified as well as skills seen as increasing the worker's performance and career advancement are natural extensions of this conversation.

Asking the worker what work goals he or she would like to achieve during the next time period and using this to talk about what you think are important should lead to writing new and mutually agreed-upon performance goals. When a performance rating is required, it is important to explain the basis of the rating and what is needed to obtain a higher rating in the future. Finally, the session ends with restatement of the worker's major strengths, next steps, and possible timetable. These steps include writing a record of the session that is given to the worker with an opportunity for him or her to comment on its accuracy.

Performance Appraisal Session Reminder

1. *Prepare both parties for the session.*
2. *Take time to put the worker at ease.*
3. *Ask the worker regarding what he thinks he does well and skills that he would like to acquire.*
4. *Tell the worker what you agree with and what you would add in terms of strengths and skill acquisition.*
5. *Ask the worker for his job goals leading up to the next appraisal.*
6. *Talk about any additional goals that you would like to see become a part of the plan.*
7. *When rating the worker, tell him the basis for the rating and how he may achieve a higher rating in the future.*
8. *End the session with a restatement of the worker's strengths, goals, and timelines.*
9. *Write a record of the session and give it to the worker with an opportunity to comment on the accuracy of the record.*

This discussion of the performance-appraisal session has been framed as positively as possible. However, there are times when these sessions feel far less positive because they are a required part of a formal process of sanctioning the worker for poor performance and eventual termination. This is a careful process of documenting performance and steps required to demonstrate adequate improvement. Naturally, this is not a process to be taken lightly and it is recommended that you consult with a personnel or legal expert long before you think that this may be necessary.

TASK 5: ASSISTING WORKERS IN DEVELOPING SKILLS AND ENHANCING THEIR CAREERS THROUGH SUPERVISION: TRAINING

Helping workers acquire new skills is a theme throughout this chapter. This is also a clear manifestation of the consumer-centered value of learning for a living. Supervisors use a variety of strategies to accomplish this task. Field mentoring, group supervision, and training are all powerful strategies for assisting workers to develop skills. Due to the integrative nature of field mentoring and group supervision, these two powerful techniques are presented in detail in Chapter 10. These techniques are designed to assist managers to pull together virtually all of the ideas in this text in an efficient manner and are, therefore, presented last. In this section, we consider training as a supervisory technique for enhancing worker skills.

Unfortunately, training is sometimes an inappropriate reaction to an organizational problem. For example, workers may feel overwhelmed with meeting deadlines, so management might decide that time management training is the answer, when in fact a closer examination of expectations and caseload size may yield a better outcome. When expectations are clear and the requisite organizational supports are are already in place to allow workers to accomplish their jobs, then training is indicated. A variety of different types of training are required in the social service organization, from new worker orientation to policies and procedures. Although much of what we present in this section applies to all training in the organization, we focus on training that helps workers acquire the skills needed to produce consumer outcomes.

What to Train

In this section, we focus on training related to evidence-based practices. We think it is important to focus as much of agency training as possible on evidence-based practices. Recall from Chapter 4 that evidence-based practices are those helping technologies which have the highest level of evidence demonstrating effectiveness in achieving consumer outcomes. Levels of evidence refer to different types of research that more or less strongly demonstrate the relationship between the helping technology and consumer outcomes. The strongest level of evidence consists of findings of positive results from more than one randomized clinical trial (RCT). These are controlled experiments where consumers are randomly assigned to one of two groups, with one receiving the new helping technology and the other usually receiving the normal service.

Training content is dictated by the intervention that has been the subject of the most rigorous evaluation. When the intervention has been the subject of randomized clinical trials, there is almost always a manual that describes the intervention in great detail. This is the manual that is to be used to train people to replicate the intervention.

When to Train

Following are essentially the three situations in the social service organization that determine a training need.

1. When workers are new to the organization and have not previously done the work
2. When a new evidence-based practice is being implemented
3. When the information system (e.g., fidelity instruments) shows that consumer outcomes previously achieved are falling below expectations

Research has shown that the transfer of training to the job does not occur easily. For example, certain workers' beliefs and attitudes are prerequisites to conducting training. Fortunately, there is an increasing body of research, albeit not randomized clinical trials, that focuses on characteristics of trainees, the training, and the organization that are associated with training being used on the job.

Two characteristics of workers that have been associated with using the new skills on the job are self-efficacy and the perceived utility of the training (Wehrmann, Shin, & Poertner, 2002). In other words, workers are more likely to attend training with a positive attitude and use new skills in their work, if they think that they have the ability to do it and if they think that the training will be useful. In the organization with an environment where rewards for performance are common and where supervisors are using a variety of skills to help people achieve, workers are likely to feel that they have the ability to do the work. In the consumer outcome focused unit where there is constant searching for better evidence-based ways to help consumers achieve desired outcomes, evidence-based training is likely to be perceived as useful. If these conditions do not exist within the work unit, managers need to assess workers' perceptions of both their own abilities and the usefulness of the training before it is undertaken.

How to Train: Instructional Design

The way that training is designed and delivered has been shown to contribute to training transfer (Wehrmann, Shinn, & Poertner, 2002). Reviews of research on changing practice conclude that passive educational approaches such as dissemination of clinical practice guidelines and didactic presentations are ineffective (Bero et al., 1998; Grimshaw et al., 2001). Managers need to assess the instructional design of the training to ensure that it will have the best chance of fulfilling workers' expectations. Specifically, an effective training curriculum has clear objectives and presents the content in a variety of ways. Learning processes that involve interaction with participants, goal setting, role-playing, behavior modeling, and performance feedback are important. Finally, trainers who are perceived as being trustworthy, skilled, and credible are associated with training transfer.

What to Do After the Training Event

Returning to the job after a training event is a critical time for managers to facilitate the transfer of training to the work. The research conducted by Wehrmann, Shinn, and Poertner (2002) found the following post-training factors to be important in transferring new skills to the job:

- Opportunity to perform or practice new skills
- Supervisor support including incentives to use new skills
- Supervisor feedback on the use of new skills
- Peer support
- Work environment

This list shows that supervisors have an important role to play in the transfer of training after the training event, yet research suggests that this role goes largely unfulfilled (Gregoire, Propp, & Poertner, 1998). Structuring the time to have workers practice new skills with consumers in the presence of the supervisor is one step in encouraging use of new skills on the job. Following this with discussion of the worker's perception of the usefulness of the new skill and what she or he might want to improve is another. Continual reinforcement of the consumer-centered value of learning for a living within the work unit provides a work environment that includes peer support to encourage the use of new skills.

Supervisor's Training Checklist

1. *Is the training based upon an evidence-based practice with the highest level of available evidence?*
2. *Do my workers think that they can apply it with consumers?*
3. *Do my workers think that this training will be useful for working with consumers?*
4. *Are the training objectives clear?*
5. *Is the material presented in a variety of ways including modeling and role playing?*

6. *Will participants be expected to practice the new skill and be provided feed-back as part of the training?*
7. *Does the trainer have the background and experiences so that he or she is likely to be seen as credible by my workers?*
8. *What obstacles exist for workers using the new skills with consumers and how will I remove them?*
9. *What incentives will I provide for my workers to use the new skills?*
10. *How will I provide opportunities for workers to use the new skills?*
11. *When will I schedule time to observe the workers use the new skills and provide them feedback?*

TASK 6: USING STANDARD PROCEDURES, SPECIFIC TO A FIELD OF PRACTICE, TO MAINTAIN POLICIES, PROCEDURES, AND TRAINING THAT FOCUS ON WORKER AND CONSUMER SAFETY

Social workers are frequently in situations where there is potential for violence. Child welfare workers visit angry or distraught parents in their homes. Mental health case managers are in the community working with consumers who may have a violent episode. Shootings in schools that have appeared far too frequently in the news put school social workers at risk.

Exercise

Talk with three social workers you know about their experiences with clients and violence. Here are some possible questions:

What violent acts initiated by clients have you experienced?
What was the context (practice, physical)?
What did you do?
How did your agency prepare you for this occurrence?

Violence is not just a theoretical concern. The findings of a recent survey of social workers' experience with violence by Jayaratne, Croxton, and Mattison (2004) found that 23.8 percent of agency workers reported being physically threatened by a consumer. Not surprisingly, child protective services workers and those in institutional mental health settings experienced these threats most frequently. Physical assault was reported by 3.3 percent of all respondents. In a survey of social workers in California and Pennsylvania, 58 percent of the respondents reported they had directly experienced one or more incidents of consumer violence at some point in their careers (Newhill, 2003). Twenty one percent of these respondents reported verbal threats only, 5 percent reported property damage only, and 12 percent reported property damage, threats, and attempted or actually carried out physical attacks.

The social administrator has an important role in assuring that her or his organization has the training, policies, and procedures in place to equip workers to be as safe as possible. Child protective service agencies' training, policies, and procedures will be very different from the mental health inpatient unit, which will be different from the community mental health outreach unit. The safety training and policies for your agency need to be specifically tailored to your field of practice and agency.

There are a couple of sources for useful general guidance on developing agency training and policy regarding violence and consumers. The NASW Massachusetts Chapter (1996) developed safety guidelines that provide general guidance for what to consider in an agency safety training and policy. Their recommendations include the following:

1. Safety plan of action including
   a. how to recognize signs of agitation and what to do about them
   b. code words to signal for help
   c. format for ongoing assessment and intervention
2. Exterior and physical layout
3. a. maintaining and furnishing the facility
   b. ensuring adequate lighting
   c. being aware of traffic patterns
   d. establishing a risk room
   e. safety equipment such as buzzers
   f. attention to individual office layout and furnishings
4. Rules, regulations, and procedures
   a. establish a format for taking a required history of violence
   b. establish a format for communicating when danger exists
   c. communicating safety policies to consumers, policies on guns, consumers under the influence of alcohol and other drugs
   d. ongoing supervision, consultation, and training.
   e. policies on home visits.
   f. relationships with police.
   g. log all work-related incidents of violence

Newhill's (2003) work *Client Violence in Social Work Practice* is helpful for administrators who need to review current agency training and policy or to develop new materials. This book includes material on the short-term prediction of violent behavior, assessing the client environment, engaging and talking with the violent client, intervention modalities, and prevention strategies. She includes a concrete summary list of dos and don'ts for home visits.

Chapter 9

Fiscal Management

Consumer-centered social administration comprises working with consumers of social work service to achieve mutually desired results or outcomes. These results are largely achieved when a social worker engages with a consumer to work on tasks linked to results. This interaction requires many types of resources. It is one of the social administrator's responsibilities to assure that workers and consumers have the resources they need to succeed.

This text is mainly about resources needed to assist consumers. This chapter concerns fiscal resources. This text starts with the principles of client-centered management that guide managers in their everyday decision making. Skills in managing change are a resource used daily with a variety of people to help assure that everyone plays their role in assisting consumers. The program model is a resource for everyone in the enterprise to make the necessary arrangements for consumer success. This success would not be possible without hiring, equipping, and directing the best people to do the job. Knowing that everyone is doing their job and that this is resulting in consumer benefits requires managers to have the resource of information and the skills to use it to keep the program functioning at a high level.

Many social administrators work within an organization where someone else has the responsibility of acquiring funds and monitoring expenditures. The large state social service bureaucracy maintains a specialized unit to track expenditures and only the agency director can advocate for funds from the director of the budget, the governor, or the legislature. The hospital or school social worker works in a different context, where the social work unit depends on the larger organization for resources. In either of these contexts, the social administrator becomes an advocate for resources. In these cases, the change skills identified in Chapter 2, together with a solid understanding of budgeting and resource management, are the foundation for fiscal advocacy.

Textbook of Social Administration: The Consumer-Centered Approach
© 2007 by The Haworth Press, Inc. All rights reserved.
doi:10.1300/5802_10

This chapter covers fiscal management basics. The acquisition and management of funds is easy to discuss. However, the manager confronted with a budget shortfall finds it very difficult to locate funds to continue to pay salaries. The manager confronted with responding to a request for proposal for services under a performance contract with fiscal penalties for not succeeding finds it difficult to determine the appropriate unit costs. Just as managers may need consultants to examine personnel policies, information systems, and evidence-based practices, fiscal management requires specialized expertise that is beyond the scope of this chapter.

Fiscal Management Objectives

- *Identify ways in which fiscal management implements consumer-centered management principles.*
- *Identify program costs and link them to consumer outcomes through budgeting (line item, performance, program budgeting).*
- *Identify sources of funds and how they may be acquired.*
- *Identify the major forms of social service contracting.*
- *Analyze a contract to identify the fiscal incentives, the associated risks, and the potential impact upon program operations.*

THE PRINCIPLES OF CONSUMER-CENTERED MANAGEMENT AND RESOURCE MANAGEMENT

Venerating the people we call clients or consumers translates to obtaining and allocating funds that will improve outcomes. With the difficulties associated with raising funds, it is easy to get distracted by available opportunities that may not be related to achieving results with consumers. There is always a danger of chasing dollars rather then outcomes. *Creating and maintaining the focus* becomes operational by this unwavering commitment to dollars for outcomes.

A healthy disrespect for the impossible is evidenced by the manager who, in a difficult fiscal environment, finds funding mechanisms that can be used for benefit of the client. For example, the child welfare manager who finds that many of the children in care are there due to behavior problems rather than abuse or neglect links with mental health services may use Medicaid to provide evidence-based services for this population. The mental health program manager who struggles with helping consumers find jobs partners with a variety of employment services to garner resources for job placement and support.

Every year, there are new forms of performance-based contracting that not only require disrespect for the impossible but *learning for a living.* There are risks and rewards with these new arrangements that are often not anticipated and require an inquisitive mind and constant monitoring to assure that they are working as intended. When they fail, the learning is used to advocate for necessary changes before disaster strikes.

Managers achieve results through their interactions with key people over time. This tenet of social administration is critical to the acquisition and management of fiscal resources. Most social programs are maintained by a few funding sources. Continued acquisition of funds requires frequent contact with these sources, whether they are government officials, legislators, or private individuals. Through constant contact the manager can provide these sources with information about consumers. Mutual identification of additional sources to broaden the range of services in order to achieve consumer goals can result from this contact. In this age of experimentation, with various performance-based contracting systems, frequent contact helps everyone involved in contract management know what features are working and which ones need revision either immediately or through the next contract cycle.

IDENTIFYING PROGRAM COSTS AND LINKING THEM TO CONSUMER OUTCOMES: BUDGETING

The program framework (Chapter 3 to 5) is a necessary precursor to the acquisition and allocation of funds. It is through this framework that the manager knows the resource requirements for achieving desired consumer outcomes. The funds required to obtain these resources then make up the budget. There are a variety of different schemes for identifying these resource requirements. We will use Lawrence Martin's (2001) categories to present three types of budgets. A budget includes both income and expenses. We first discuss the expense side and then the sources of funds.

The Line-Item Budget

The line-item budget has been a staple of social agency budgeting for many years. It is easy to prepare and easy to read (Table 9.1). Development of the line-item budget involves identification of each type of resource

TABLE 9.1. Line-Item Expense Budget

Item	Cost
Elder Care In-home Service Component	
Personnel	
Caseworkers 7 @ $36,000 per year	$252,000
Clerical Assistance 1 @ $24,000 per year	24,000
Administrative Support 20% time @ $50,000	10,000
Fringe benefits @ 36% of salaries	94,320
Other staff costs	
Professional membership fees	4,500
Professional liability insurance	3,000
Staff Training	5,000
Travel	15,000
Supplies	
Office	3,000
Program	8,000
Equipment	
Computers	3,000
Networking maintenance	3,000
Copier	5,000
Space	
Rental	20,000
Cleaning and maintenance	1,800
Utilities	
Phone	4,000
Electric etc.	4,200
Postage	2,000
Printing	20,000
Total Program Costs	$481,820

needed (the line) and determining the number of dollars required for that resource. It also includes delineation of revenue sources along with the amounts expected from each source. The budget can be for one program or for an entire agency including several separate programs.

Exercise

Develop the expense portion of a line-item budget for a program you specified in Chapters 3 and 4.

The major advantage of the line-item budget is its simplicity. It is a straightforward way to determine the cost of a program. It facilitates communication with its format of a list of resource categories with their dollar amounts. It is also easy to read a list of revenue sources and make a general judgment about their adequacy.

The line-item budget can also play an important role in fiscal control and transparency. With a line-item budget established at the beginning of a fiscal year, a monthly check of expenditures and revenues is possible. If revenues are arriving and expenditures are proceeding as expected, the program should be on a sound fiscal footing.

However, a judgment that a program or an agency is on sound fiscal footing gives the manager no information regarding outcomes for consumers. This is one of the biggest disadvantages of line-item budgets. Neither can the efficiency of a program be assessed. Since this budget includes no information about amounts of service provided, it cannot be used to realign resources to produce more or better results at less cost. Similarly, the balance between administrative and service costs cannot be judged. As Martin (2001) observes, discussions of line-item budgets tend to focus on increasing or decreasing the amounts dedicated to particular line items in the absence of other critical information, such as how much service is needed to achieve a given outcome.

The Performance Budget

Management of social services is often criticized because there is little or no incentive to reduce costs and become more efficient. In an enterprise where profit is determined by the difference between income from sales and production costs, there is a natural incentive to cut as many costs as possible while maintaining sales income. The client/consumer-centered manager also has an interest in producing more at less cost. Their incentive is to serve more consumers. The performance budget is the major social administration tool for determining unit costs to focus on efficiency. As Martin (2001) comments, one of the major advantages of the performance budget is that it raises the level of discussion from line items to program services, program costs, and program efficiency.

A performance budget contains three parts. These are total program costs, outputs or service units produced, and costs per output (Table 9.2). Total program costs are easily determined by developing a line-item expense budget. The service units produced through the program are identified in the program analytic framework. If a program has existed for a period of time, count the number of service units that were produced during

TABLE 9.2. Performance Budget

Elder Care Agency In-Home Service Program Component	
Total Program Costs	$481,820
Unit of Service	One Visit
Total Units of Service	3,500
Cost per Unit	$138
Case Management Program Component	
Total Program Costs	$520,000
Unit of Service	One hour
Total Units of Service	7,000
Cost per Unit	$74

the preceding year or other convenient time period. If the program is being newly developed, in response to an RFP, for example, then the expected number of service units can be calculated through some formula such as considering how many staff will be delivering service units, how much of their time is expected to be devoted to producing service units, and the length of time for each service unit (e.g., hour). The final element of the cost of the units of service is the result of dividing total program costs by the number of service units.

Exercise

1. *Develop a performance budget for the program you specified in Chapters 3 and 4. Hint: Use your line-item budget from the previous exercise for total program costs.*
2. *Identify three ways that you could potentially increase the efficiency of your program (more units with no increase in costs or decreased costs with no decrease in units of service). Identify the advantages and disadvantages of each alternative and discuss these with a colleague.*

The Program Budget

While line-item budgeting delineates costs for items needed to operate the program and performance budgets identifies the costs of units of service, the program budgeting identifies the costs of program outcomes (Table 9.3). With consumer outcomes being the "bottom line" for the social administrator, this may be the most important budget. In addition, with

TABLE 9.3. Program Budget

Elder Care Home Living Program	
Total Program Costs	$1,001,820
Consumer Outcome	One consumer remains in home for one year
Total Outcomes	70
Cost Per Outcome	$14,312

some social service contracting systems now paying for results of outcomes, this type of budgeting can help align income and results.

Martin (2001) identifies one of the major advantages of program budgeting as raising the level of debate to discussion of producing results for consumers and the attendant costs. Program budgeting can also help focus several different program components on ultimate program results. For example, a child welfare agency may have a foster care program, an adoption program, and a family support program, all focused on assuring children a safe and permanent home. Program budgeting for this agency yields the total cost of a child achieving permanency, be that by returning home or through adoption. Consequently, all three program components, which may otherwise operate as distinct programs, are unified through one common outcome.

Another advantage is that this type of budgeting assists the social administrators to increased efficiency. Just as knowing the cost of a unit of service through performance budgeting can assist the social administrator to focus on ways to increase units of service with constant or fewer dollars, the focus on costs per consumer outcome can do the same. Over time, a manager who knows these costs and the relative contribution of each program component can experiment with different resource mixes to reduce the cost of an outcome.

Martin (2001) also points out that this type of budgeting can also assist benchmarking. That is, by knowing the cost of producing an outcome of a relatively efficient program, another program can set that cost as a goal. Similarly, a state agency that is funding a program by several different service providers can establish a benchmark cost per consumer outcome as a program standard. For example, let us say that I am managing Program A and I have a friend who is managing a similar Program B. In a statewide report comparing programs, I see that the cost per outcome in Program B is less than mine. I set as a target the same costs per outcome as that achieved in Program B so that I can use extra resources to serve more consumers.

Martin (2001) suggests that a major disadvantage of program budgeting is that there are many client service areas where there is no clear consensus on desired program outcomes. For example, within child welfare, there is much debate on older youth in care who are likely to exit care due to age rather then achieve a permanent home. Although some advocate for outcomes in the areas of education and employment, others say that participation in independent living skills programs is a sufficient goal. Comparing these costs would be like comparing a performance budget with the program budget. A clear consensus on consumer/client outcomes is a prerequisite for program budgeting to be useful.

Reminder: Types of Budgets and Major Uses

Line-item budgets identify that program costs are easy to read and assist fiscal control. They do not provide information-linking costs to consumer outcomes.

Performance budgets use the results of the line-item budget to identify costs of service units. They are useful for discussing service costs and increasing efficiency; they do not provide information-linking costs to outcomes.

Program budgets use the line-item budget to identify costs of consumer outcomes. This requires agreement on desired outcomes. Newer contracting systems may require the manager to have this information to keep expenditures in line with contract provisions. This information also helps increase efficiency and stretch funds to additional consumers.

Some people are also likely to be cautious about making the costs of achieving consumer outcomes public. Some might argue that if the public understood the cost of achieving a given outcome, then public support for such programs would decrease. This suggests the need to invest time and energy in educating agency staff and the wider public in understanding program budgeting and its uses.

Computing the program budget is straightforward. Total program costs are simply divided by the number of outcomes achieved. The line-item budget is the best way to identify total program costs, and the program specifications (Chapters 3-5) or experience are probably the best ways to identify the total number of consumer outcomes

---

Exercise

1. Develop a program budget for the program you specified in Chapters 3-5. Hint: Use your line-item budget for total program costs.

2. *Identify three ways that you could potentially increase the efficiency of your program (more units with no increase in costs or decreased costs with no decrease in units of service). Identify the advantages and disadvantages of each alternative.*
3. *Present the alternatives to your classmates and lead a discussion of the advantages and disadvantages.*

SOURCES OF FUNDS AND THEIR ACQUISITION

Without money, staff cannot be paid to work with consumers, travel to consumers' homes cannot be reimbursed, or rent cannot be paid to maintain office space. This is frequently the social administrator's most time-consuming task. In many cases, more of a manager's time is taken by acquiring funds and maintaining income than any other activity.

It is useful to distinguish between the source of funds and the method used to make them available to operate a social program. Taxes, voluntary donations, and client fees are the primary sources of funds. Contracts and grants are the primary mechanisms for passing these funds on to a social agency. This produces two distinct points of leverage or advocacy for the social administrator. Advocating for more funds usually means trying to obtain more dollars derived from taxes and increasing donations or fees. Advocating for a different allocation of funds to produce improved consumer outcomes means influencing the terms under which these funds are expended such as that of the contract.

The specific focus for these two resource acquisition tasks depend, in part, on the primary way that a program is funded. However, across programs and funding sources the interpersonal influence skills of the administrator are critical (Chapter 2). A manager of a program that is primarily funded through government contracts uses her or his skills to influence elected officials to dedicate more funds to a program category and improve the funding mechanisms to yield the fiscal incentives that will enhance outcomes for consumers. The program primarily funded through the local United Way devotes their influence skills to influencing local key actors to produce the same results.

In this section we provide the basics for understanding the primary sources of funds. The form in which they come to an agency will be covered in the next section.

Public Funds

The primary funding mechanism for social work services is some form of contract from an organization expending tax dollars. These funds may be from a city, county, state, or federal government. Most often the source is some combination of these. The agency that issues the contract is probably blending income streams to fund social services and is subject to requirements that they pass on to the contractor. At this time in our history, contracts from state government agencies is the primary source of public funds.

Understanding the sources of funds and the accompanying regulations supporting a contract is important to social administrators for their role in uniting with funding sources to increase the pool of available resources to benefit consumers. For example, while the Federal funding scene continues to change, many state-contracted social services are reimbursed, in part, by programs such as the Medicaid or child welfare funds under sections of the Social Security Act such as Titles IV-A and E. These are usually financial matching mechanisms that provide federal funds based upon the expenditure of state or local funds. Although these program provisions are very complex and require expert assistance to fully understand, a social administrator who is familiar with the basics can assist relevant state agencies in maximizing the capture of available federal funds and potentially increasing funding of their programs.

Reminder

Most social services are now funded through contracts with a state agency. The sources of these funds are usually a combination of local, state, and federal funds. Social administrators should know the following:

- *The sources of funds that support a contract*
- *The rules governing expenditures of these funds including state planning requirements, allowable services, and how these services are defined*
- *The experiences of other states in maximizing funds through changing state plans, services to be provided, or state definitions of services.*

For example, The Children's Bureau describes one such program funded under Title IV-B, subpart 2. The Promoting Safe and Stable Families program provides funds to states to provide family support, family preservation, time-limited family reunification services, and services to promote and support adoptions. These services are primarily aimed at preventing the risk of abuse and promoting nurturing families, assisting families at risk of having a child removed from their home, promoting the timely return of a child to his or her home, and placement of a child in a permanent setting, with familysupport services, when returning home is not an option. As part of this program, the Court Improvement Program provides grants to help state courts improve their handling of proceedings relating to foster care and adoption. After an initial assessment of court practices and policies, states use these funds for improvements and reform activities. Typical activities include development of mediation programs, joint agency-court training, automated docketing and case tracking, linked agency-court data systems, one judge/one family models, time-specific docketing, formalized relationships with the child welfare agency, and legislative change (downloaded 6/2/2005 from http://www.acf.hhs.gov/programs/cb/programs/state .htm).

The rules that states must comply with to receive such funds are included in the Code of Federal Regulations (45CFR1357). One section of these regulations is included in Figure 9.1. The reader can quickly see that these rules are very technical. One can also see some of the basics of this program including the matching or cost share provision of 75 percent of allowable expenditures. This raises questions about what can be used as matching funds. The regulations state that these funds can be cash, donated funds, and nonpublic third-party in-kind contributions. One of the categories of allowable expenditures is program costs. These costs are those expenditures in connection with developing and implementing the CFSP. The CFSP is defined in another section as the Child and Family Services Plan prepared by the state.

Exercise

1. Identify a program in an agency that you are familiar with that operates under a contract from a state agency.

2. Identify the state and federal funding sources.

3. Locate the legislation and regulations that govern one such source.

4. Identify what can be reimbursed.

5. Identify the terms of the reimbursement.

This example is presented as simply an introduction to a few of the features of federal funding sources to the states. This example points out some of the potential points of leverage including what to use as the states match, carefully examining what an allowable expense is and influencing agreements between states and the federal government through documents like state plans. There are a large number of these types of sources with some

---

TITLE 45--PUBLIC WELFARE
CHAPTER XIII--OFFICE OF HUMAN DEVELOPMENT SERVICES, DEPARTMENT OF HEALTH
AND HUMAN SERVICES

Sec. 1357.32 State fiscal requirements (title IV-B, subpart 2, family
preservation and family support services).
    (a) Scope. The requirements of this section apply to all funds
allocated to States under title IV-B, subpart 2, of the Act.
    (b) Allotments. The annual allotment to each State shall be made in
accordance with section 433 of the Act.
    (c) Payments. Payments to each State will be made in accordance with
section 434 of the Act.
    (d) Matching or cost sharing. Funds used to provide services in FY
1994 and in subsequent years will be federally reimbursed at 75 percent of
allowable expenditures. (This is the same Federal financial participation
rate as title IV-B, subpart 1.) Federal funds, however, will not exceed
the amount of the State's allotment.
    (1) The State's contribution may be in cash, donated funds, and non-
public third party in-kind contributions.
    (2) Except as provided by Federal statute, other Federal funds may not
be used to meet the matching requirement.
    (e) Prohibition against purchase or construction of facilities. Funds
awarded under title IV-B may not be used for the purchase or construction
of facilities.
    (f) Maintenance of effort. States may not use the Federal funds under
title IV-B, subpart 2, to supplant Federal or non-Federal funds for
existing family preservation and family support services. For the purpose
of implementing this requirement, ``non-Federal funds'' means State funds.
ACF will collect information annually from each State on expenditures for
family support and family preservation using the State
fiscal year 1992 as the base year.
    (g) Time limits on expenditures. Funds must be expended by September
30 of the fiscal year following the fiscal year in which the funds were
awarded.
    (h) Administrative costs. (1) States claiming Federal financial
participation for services provided in FY 1994 and subsequent years may
not claim more than 10 percent of expenditures under subpart 2 for
administrative costs. There is no limit on the percentage of
administrative costs which may be reported as State match.
    (2) For the purposes of title IV-B, subpart 2, ``administrative
costs'' are costs of auxiliary functions as identified through as agency's
accounting system which are:
    (i) Allocable (in accordance with the agency's approved cost
allocation plan) to the title IV-B, subpart 2 program cost centers;
    (ii) necessary to sustain the direct effort involved in administering
the State plan for title IV-B, subpart 2, or an activity providing service
to the program: and
    (iii) centralized in the grantee department or in some other agency,
and may include but are not limited to the following: Procurement;
payroll; personnel functions; management, maintenance and operation of
space and property; data processing and computer services; accounting;
budgeting; auditing.
    (3) Program costs are costs, other than administrative costs, incurred
in connection with developing and implementing the CFSP (e.g., delivery of
services, planning, consultation, coordination, training, quality
assurance measures, data collection, evaluations, supervision).
[61 FR 58661, Nov. 18, 1996]

FIGURE 9.1. A Section of the Code of Federal Regulations.

being far more flexible and amenable to states' efforts to increase funding than others. We believe that it is useful to have a basic understanding of funding mechanisms and that expert advice is frequently needed to understand the technical details and funding possibilities. For any particular federal funding mechanism, finding out which states are doing the best job of capturing funds and contacting fiscal people in that state can lead to deeper understanding of funding mechanisms and ideas for increasing a state's share of available resources.

Charitable Contributions

Although state and federal funds are a major income source for social programs, charitable contributions are the lifeblood of many community organizations. Working with the local United Way or organizing a fundraising event takes a major time commitment from the organization. It also requires a great deal of interpersonal and organizational skill. It is not unusual for a fund-raising approach to fail simply because it took more resources to carry out than it generated. Knowledge of the community and its many resources is the starting point for raising funds through charitable contributions.

United Way of America

For many local social service agencies, funds from the local United Way provide a significant portion of the program budget. As the United Way of America Web site indicates (Figure 9.2), this is a significant funding source with more than $3.5 billion generated in 2003/2004. The emphasis of this national organization is on the local affiliate and community, with the national office setting standards and providing technical assistance.

Essentially the local United Way is an annual community fund-raising campaign with the proceeds used to support programs of member agencies. The United Way seeks to involve all potential donors in the community with strong connections to employers and the use of individual pledges that may be fulfilled in a variety of ways including payroll deductions. A strong local United Way affiliate generally has a board of directors of business leaders and other influential members of the community. In addition to fund-raising, staff of the local affiliate are frequently involved in bringing interested groups together to work together on community problems and solutions.

United Way Mission and Vision

Mission

The mission of United Way is to improve people's lives by mobilizing the caring power of communities.

A Community-Based National Movement

United Ways across the country activate community resources to make the greatest possible human impact. The United Way system includes approximately 1,400 community-based United Way organizations. Each is independent, separately incorporated and governed by local volunteers.

As community leaders, United Ways address the most critical local issues and mobilize resources beyond the dollars that are pledged through their fund-raising efforts. Community partners often include schools, government policy makers, businesses, organized labor, financial institutions, voluntary and neighborhood associations, community development corporations and the faith community.

Mobilizing the Caring Power of Communities

United Ways bring communities together to focus on the most important human needs-building partnerships, forging consensus and leveraging resources to make a measurable difference. Focus areas are identified at the local level and vary from community to community.

Common focus areas include: helping children and youth succeed, strengthening and supporting families, promoting self-sufficiency, building vital and safe neighborhoods and supporting vulnerable and aging populations.

In 2003/2004, United Ways generated $3.59 billion in revenue, from the annual campaign and gifts beyond the campaign. United Ways leveraged a total of $4.05 billion in resources to build stronger communities. A vast network of volunteers keeps administrative expenses low, averaging 13 percent of all funds raised at the largest United Ways. This figure compares favorably with Better Business Bureau guidelines of up to 35 percent. [Downloaded 6/3/05 from http://national.unitedway.org/aboutuw/mission.cfm]

FIGURE 9.2. United Way Information

To receive United Way funds, a local organization must become a member agency. Each affiliate has a set of criteria for member agencies with United Way of America setting some basic requirements including the following:

1. Each organization in which they invest is a non-profit, tax-exempt charity governed by volunteers
2. Submits to an annual, independent financial audit

3. Provides services at a reasonable cost, and
4. Maintains a policy of non-discrimination. (Downloaded 6/3/05 from http://national.unitedway.org/aboutuw/)

For the social administrator in an established agency that is a member of the local United Way, membership provides potential access to influence as well as funds. Participation in local affiliate meetings and events brings influential community members together. These meetings become venues for developing relationships that can be a source of support or influence in other activities such as advocating or education local or state elected officials.

For the social administrator implementing a program in a new community agency that is not yet a member of the United Way, it will take time and effort to become a member. Although this is frequently frustrating knowing that funds may become available in a year or two after becoming a member, it is usually worth the wait. The road to membership requires a good program (Chapters 3 and 4) and the use of the same relationship and influence skills that are a theme of this text (Chapter 2). Developing relationships with local United Way affiliate staff and board members are keys to acceptance as are the formal requirements of member agencies.

Foundations

There is an immense number of foundations in this country that give away a great deal of money. The Chronicle of Philanthropy (June 23, 2005) reports that foundations gave $29.8 billions in 2004. A Google search using the words charitable foundations resulted in more than 1.5 million references. With all of these resources and all of this money the prospects of obtaining money from foundations looks promising. However, it is never that easy.

Most foundations target their money toward specific interests. For example, the Ewing Marion Kauffman Foundation of Kansas City Missouri specializes in entrepreneurship and education. With more than $1.7 billion in assets, they have substantial ability to make a difference in their area of focus (www.kauffman.org).

Some foundations specialize in a geographic area either solely or in addition to a special interest. For example, in addition to several specialized topic areas such as conservation and science; population; and children, families, and communities, the David and Lucile Packard Foundation has an interest in the northern California counties of San Mateo, Santa Clara, Santa Cruz, and Monterey (www.packard.org). This foundation reports

$5.2 billion in assets with approximately $200 million available for grants in 2005. If your agency is in one of the aforementioned counties, you have a distinct advantage.

Some foundations only fund large programs; others fund only small programs. Some large foundations that grant hundreds of millions of dollars per year may favor larger projects because they may see more of an impact. They may also see funding large projects as more cost efficient. Fewer larger grants generally require fewer foundation staff to manage the projects. On the other hand, a small foundation that only grants several thousand dollars a year may wish to spread its resources around to smaller projects. The foundation's annual report is a key document for determining the usual sizes of funded projects.

The tremendous variation in foundation types and giving means that the social administrator wanting to explore this funding source must do her or his homework. The Chronicle of Philanthropy is a good source for news related to foundations, including helpful books and workshops on important topics such as proposal writing. Many local libraries have reference material that can assist people in identifying relevant foundations. The first task is to identify foundations that support your type of program, at the size you want to request, and in your geographic area. Foundation annual reports are a good source for this information and much of this is available on their Web sites.

Examination of the programs funded by the foundation in the last year can tell you a great deal about how they actually apply these guidelines. A foundation may state that it funds programs in the area of education. This is a very broad category. A list of actual programs funded last year under the heading of education provides concrete examples of what the current group of decision makers includes in this category.

Once you have identified foundations that meet these requirements, note that each one has its own procedures for seeking funding. However, in general an introductory letter that introduces your agency, program, and funding request is a next step. This is an opportunity to "sell" your idea in a page or two. The extensive and careful process of working through the program framework of Chapters 4 and 5 provides the material for the letter and any subsequent proposal. The challenge is to capture the essence of your idea in an introductory letter of a couple of pages.

The old adage to think globally and act locally applies to foundations. Start by learning about foundations and their key decision makers in your area. Your colleagues will know what foundations are active on the local scene. If your city is home to one of the large foundations, you may have an opportunity to tap into their local interests.

Personal relationships are also important in the foundation world. Finding out who is on the staff and board of the foundation provides an opportunity to develop personal relationships which might provide you with information for better targeting your funding request, as well as potentially giving you an advocate on the inside. There are also a large number of small foundations that may not have offices or staff but which are administered through the trust department of a local bank. Finding out all you can about these foundations, who manages them, and where their interests lie may result in a small but reliable source of funds for your program. Frequently you and your great program ideas are then sold on an individual basis. Once you know who is making the funding decisions you can begin the process of developing personal relationships and selling the success of your program.

The community foundation is another local opportunity. The Council on Foundations identifies community foundations as

> a tax-exempt, nonprofit, autonomous, publicly supported, philanthropic institution composed primarily of permanent funds established by many separate donors of the long-term diverse, charitable benefit of the residents of a defined geographic area. Typically, a community foundation serves an area no larger than a state. Community foundations provide an array of services to donors who wish to establish endowed funds without incurring the administrative and legal costs of starting independent foundations. There are more than 500 community foundations across the United States today. The Cleveland Foundation is the oldest; the New York Community Trust is the largest. (http://www.cof.org/Content/General/Display.cfm?con tentID=120#c [downloaded 6/28/2005])

Naturally the size and complexity of these foundations varies with the size of the community. The Chicago Community Trust is a large enterprise that funds a wide variety of programs and granted $62 million in 2004 (www.ctt.org). In contrast the Douglas County Community Foundation is only five years old and recently awarded $186,000 to local agencies (www .dccfoundation.org). Since community foundations are concerned with the local area they are a good source of funding, frequently short term, for social services. Getting acquainted with your local foundation guidelines and decision makers is once again the first step.

Exercise

1. *Identify two foundations that fund programs in your community.*
2. *Locate their funding guidelines and identify one of these that funds programs similar to yours.*
3. *Draft a one- to two-page introductory letter that describes your program in general and states a request for a specific amount.*
4. *Share the letter with a colleague and obtain feedback on its impact.*

Campaigns

You do not have to have lived in a community very long to begin to hear about the variety of ways that organizations raise funds through special campaigns and events. Letters arrive informing residents about the good work of agency X and asking for financial support. Auctions, telethons, walkathons, dinners, and raffles are just a few fund-raising activities.

A critical part of any campaign is having something important to sell. Your program, the changes in peoples' lives that your staff facilitate, the social problems that your program addresses, and yourself are what you have to sell. Effectively communicating this to people in the community takes skill. Having materials that effectively tell the story of your program is essential to any fund-raising activity.

Some organizations enlist public relations firms to help them develop fund-raising materials. These agencies may be hired or you may be able to have this service donated. Identifying someone in your community from a public relations firm who has an interest in your agency and its programs may yield a board member who will donate the resources of his or her firm to help you sell your program. The Chronicle of Philanthropy (May 26, 2005) reported that $1.7 billion of exposure was donated in 2004 for public service announcements alone. In one community a public relations firm donates their services to every tenth client. When they obtain nine new paying clients they offer free services to a local nonprofit organization.

It is easy to come up with ideas for fund-raising activities. It is another matter to have the income from such an event greater than the costs. An organization that one of the authors was involved with had an annual auction and one year decided to compare costs and income. The income over expenses turned out to be only a few hundred dollars and this did not include the value of the time that many volunteers spent organizing the event. Once the organization faced this reality, planning took on a very different focus and within three years the event was both the place to be in this community and raised $15,000 over expenses.

Martin (2001) includes the fund-raising/expense ratio in his financial analysis for human service administrators. This ratio goes beyond the single fund-raising event to consider the cost of all fund-raising events for the organization. This is the ratio of total fund-raising expenses to total expenses. This ratio is easily turned into the percentage of all expenses that it took to yield current funds. For example, if an agency experienced a ratio of .15 last year this means that 15 percent of all expenses were needed to raise last year's funds.

This ratio is important to calculate for the agency to judge its efforts. It is also important to have this figure available for those donating to the agency. Most people who give money to an agency want as much of that as possible to have an impact on consumers. Martin (2001) cautions that a ratio of .15 or higher should cause an agency to examine its fund-raising activities and try to identify more efficient methods to acquire needed funds.

There is no single best fund-raising method. Many agencies find their fund-raising niche in the community through experience. In some communities a particular event becomes associated with a particular agency and is very successful. The following are a few notes regarding some of the more popular fund-raising activities.

Individual Gifts

People in the community who will open their checkbook and write a check to your agency are a wonderful resource. Finding these people is another matter. Membership, direct mail campaigns, and telethons are all mechanisms that attempt to find community donors.

All roads to individual gifts start with a list of people to solicit. Most of these lists are constructed by identifying people in the community who have an interest in your agency and the social problems that it addresses. These may be board members, both past and current, consumers, friends and family of consumers, or simply people in the community who are concerned citizens.

There are considerable costs associated with reaching donors regardless of how it is done. Therefore, it is important to have as good a list as possible and keep it updated. A direct mail campaign to a "good" list may generate a response from 10 percent of the people. An outdated list may yield a 1 percent response. Agency staff need to keep track of people on the list who have moved from the community, died, or not donated for several years.

Although this is costly in terms of someone's time, it is essential for updating the list and maximizing efficiency.

Once someone has donated to your program, there is a special relationship developing and it is in your interest to nurture it. The person who donates $20 may give that amount only once, every year, or may substantially increase the donation over time. Periodic communication with all donors regardless of level of giving is important in maintaining and developing this relationship.

Some organizations use membership and levels of membership to maintain the relationship and increase donor levels over time. A person who "joins" at $25 this year may become a "sustaining member" at $1,000 in the future. Some agencies keep close track of the giving of donors and use the size of the last donation to suggest a level for their next donation. For example, someone who gave $100 last year may be encouraged to increase their donation to $200 this year.

Some administrators identify "large" donors and maintain that relationship differently. What is considered large depends on the agency director's experience in raising funds through donations. For example, an agency director may target people who give $1,000 or more a year to visit individually. They may invite them to lunch or breakfast periodically recognizing the importance of their contribution and keeping them informed of the work of the agency. These larger donors may receive special individualized fundraising appeals and be excluded from the annual mass mailing or telethon, so that the special relationship can be recognized and even larger donations may be encouraged.

Special Events

The auction, pancake breakfast, or golf tournament are just three possible fund-raising events. These events take a great amount of time, energy, and money. There is also substantial competition in most communities. However, if an organization can find an event niche it can be a major venue for annually informing the community about program successes; it may be the "event of the year" in terms of community participation, leading to identifying important individual donors, and it may produce substantial dollars.

Finding the event niche in a community requires creativity as well as time and effort. Allowing sufficient time to adequately plan the event is one consideration. Trying to have a community breakfast next month may fail simply due to insufficient time to accomplish all of the necessary tasks rather than for any other reason.

Preparation time requires people. People are needed to accomplish all of the tasks. These people can be paid staff or volunteers.

Events also require materials. Auctions require items that people want to buy. Golf tournaments require a golf course. A breakfast requires food. Fundraising efficiency is greatly increased when good quality materials are donated. It takes time and energy to find these donors. In some cases it may be possible to find a single donor to pay all of the costs associated with the event.

Exercise

1. *Pick a fund-raising event that you would like to attempt.*
2. *Identify all of the resources that you will need to have a successful event.*
3. *Identify a time line for planning the event.*
4. *Share the resource list and time line with someone who has conducted fundraising events and ask for feedback.*

Client Fees

Charging fees for services rendered is a time-honored tradition in social services. However, unlike accountants or lawyers who charge fees to cover all costs and include a profit for the firm, most social service agencies are reluctant to charge fees; at most they only want to cover costs and they prefer to charge reduced fees for low-income consumers. As a result, client fees make up only a part of the agencies' total revenue.

The process of setting a fee schedule involves determining costs, how much consumers with different income levels will be charged, and what proportion of the budget these fees might generate. Determining costs can become very complex and the agency may want to hire an accountant to do a special study. However, the program and performance budgets from the early part of this chapter are very informative in determining costs and can be useful in the fee-setting process.

Recall that the performance budget determines the cost per output. Program outputs are those service transactions that produce the benefit to the consumer. If the event that produces the consumer benefit is a case management home visit, then this is the output. The cost of this unit of service is the total cost of the program for a time period, such as a year divided by the total number of case management home visits during the same time period. A program could use this as the starting point for fee setting, recognizing that if every consumer paid this amount the program would generate 100 percent of the needed income.

Program budgets on the other hand determine the cost per outcome. The desired outcome of the case management home visits might be maintenance of older citizens needing assistance with certain activities of daily living in their own home with a specified quality of life. The cost of this outcome is the total program cost for a specified period of time divided by the number of consumers served during the year who achieved this outcome. This could then be used to begin the fee-setting process. As was apparent in the budgeting section, costs per output and costs per outcome are very different figures.

Although the aforementioned example is described in a straightforward manner, costs per outcome can become very complex. For example, in some cases outcomes are achieved over longer time periods. If a public child welfare agency were to determine the cost of a child achieving permanency through adoption, these costs would accumulate over several years. Another difficulty is determining the point in the child's experience at which costs are to be considered part of the adoption. One might start counting costs when the child is placed with an adoptive family, when the goal for the child is changed to adoption, or when the child is first placed into foster care. One might even make the argument that costs should be considered from the time of the initial contact with the public child welfare agency. There is no correct answer to the question. This is simply presented to demonstrate some of the complexities of determining program costs.

It is worth mentioning a couple of categories of costs that are sometimes overlooked. Indirect costs and depreciation do not always receive the consideration that they deserve. Martin (2001) defines indirect costs as "any item of cost in an agency's line item budget that benefits two or more programs." Note that if an agency has only one program and the budget includes all necessary costs then the line-item budget necessarily includes both direct and indirect costs. It is when an agency has several programs which share costs that these become indirect. For example, the office space that houses three different programs is likely to pay a single rent. This is an indirect cost that might be allocated across programs by the number of square feet used by each program. Various types of insurance, computer networks, and copying machines are other examples.

Depreciation is the cost of an asset divided by its useful life. For example, a copying machine that cost $5,000 might be expected to last five years. Consequently, it is considered to depreciate $1,000 per year. This concept also applies to items such as phone systems, computer networks, and buildings. To determine the total cost of a program these costs must be included. Lack of consideration of depreciation can lead to a fiscal shock when confronted with a $5,000 expense for a copy machine that has broken down.

For an organization that owns a building, lack of consideration of depreciation can produce even larger shocks. The unbudgeted $50,000 for a new roof is just one example.

Once the performance budget (costs per output) and the program budget (costs per outcome) are determined the fees can be set. Theoretically, either of these could be used to charge consumers for either the specified output (case management visit) or the outcome (maintenance at home with a specified quality of life). If properly computed, and if every consumer paid, the program would be self-sustaining. There are a couple of considerations in taking the next step of determining a fee schedule.

The first consideration is the limit on consumer fees that might be placed on the organization. These may come from agency policy or from other funding sources. Some funding sources place limits on client fees or forbid their use entirely.

If fees are allowed, most social service agencies do not expect consumers to pay full costs and most consumers could not afford to pay them. Consequently, most agencies that charge fees have a sliding scale related to the consumer's income. One consideration in determining such a fee schedule is determining what consumer fees in a given community are likely to generate in income. The administrator considering charging consumer fees should examine existing fee schedules in the community and the results of these schedules in terms of income generation. It is likely that many of these fee schedules will be similar. Likewise, the amount of these fees that are actually collected will probably be similar across agencies in a given community. This analysis results in an estimate of the amount of program income that might result from using a fee schedule. This is an important piece of information in deciding whether the amount of income generated is worth the effort.

Reminder

Regardless of the source of funds social administrators need

- *knowledge regarding the funding source (rules, customs, key actors),*
- *skills to influence key actors (Chapter 2).*

SOCIAL-SERVICE CONTRACTING

When a wealthy individual writes a check to your agency for $10,000, he is supporting your "good work" and trusting you to use the funds wisely.

This is a grant and the individual is a patron. This person is willing to give your agency the money because he or she believes that your work is important based upon some information received. This form of fund acquisition, although still important, is increasingly being replaced with a variety of types of contracts. There are also forms of fund acquisition in addition to grants and contracts, such as cooperative agreements. However, given the current importance of contacts in the funding of social services we will limit our focus to them.

Every form of fund acquisition creates financial incentives that influence the behavior of everyone in the agency. The patron assumes that the $10,000 will encourage staff to continue to do "good work." Some types of contracts make the link between funds and desired behavior more explicit. It is important for social administrators to understand the fiscal incentives inherent in any form of fund acquisition so that they can make a considered decision as to the desirability of accepting funds under the prescribed conditions. Although fiscal incentives go beyond contracts, we discuss incentives and contracts in the same section for purposes of simplicity.

There is tremendous variation in provisions of contract and there is no standard nomenclature for types of contracts. Different authors have different names for similar types of contracts. For the purposes of this chapter we discuss three major types of contracts:

- Purchase of service
- Performance
- Capitated—managed care

Purchase of Service Contracts

A contract places the entity initiating it as a purchaser and the other party as a supplier. When a state contracts with Family Services of OZ to provide foster care services, the state is buying the services supplied by the agency. This is the essence of purchase of service contracts. This is similar to contracting for the delivery of computers or staples. The only difference is that the commodity in this example is foster care.

Just like any other contract to purchase a commodity, purchase of service contracts specify a number of conditions for the transaction. Ezell (2002) compared several types of family preservation contracts used by the state of Kansas. The original contract system that he compared to a grant in aid contract is also a type of purchase of service arrangement, in that it specified an annual contract amount along with a number of children to be served.

All purchase of service contracts also specify other conditions, conditions under which a contractor may refuse to serve someone, termination of service, reporting of abuse or neglect, and so on. Some contracting conditions have to do with case flow such as referral sources and procedures, and others are thought to be related to the quality of the service provided. Some require the providing agency to meet some minimum conditions to be an eligible contractor, such as being accredited by a professional association or having staff with certain qualifications.

Another type of purchase of services contract specifies a flat rate to be paid for the service. In Ezell's family preservation example, a second type of purchase of service contract specified that the contractor would receive $5,054 per family, up to a specified number of families to be served. The usual purchase of service case flow and "quality" provisions were also included in the contract.

Still other purchase of service contracts specify that the actual and allowable expenses incurred during delivery of services will be reimbursed. Although this sounds like an open-ended font of funds, a total contract dollar amount for the fiscal year is normally specified, along with definitions of allowable expenses. There is also an end-of-year process to audit expenses and determine whether all claims fall within the definition of allowable expenses.

These examples of different types of purchase of service contracts do not exhaust the universe but they are illustrative. What they all share from the point of view of the contractor is (1) the delivery of a service, (2) in a specified amount (number of units of service or consumers), (3) that is provided under conditions specified in the contract (case flow and quality), (4) up to a specified amount of money. They also influence behavior through fiscal and other incentives discussed in a later section of this chapter.

Performance Contracts

Martin (2001) defines a performance contract as one focusing on the outputs and outcomes of service provision. Consequences such as payments or contract renewal are linked to these outputs or outcomes. If the contract only specifies the output as a unit of service, then this is a purchase of service contract. What makes a performance contract different is the link to a consumer outcome.

Recognition of the lack of fiscal connection to consumer outcomes has generated a great deal of interest in performance contracts, with considerable experimentation in attempting to make this connection. Martin (2005) provides a good review of several examples of performance-based contracting systems in the human services arena. He reports that at least ten state government human service agencies were experimenting with performance-based contracts. These cover a range of service areas, including substance abuse, job placement, child welfare, and rehabilitation.

The essence of performance contracts is pay for performance. The work of Martin (2005) and others documents that these contracts influence the behavior of service providers. Yet there is no single definition or set of specifications for performance contracts. For example, in Maine, contractor compensation is based upon reimbursement of costs, but contract renewal or extensions is based upon achieving performance standards (Martin, 2005). On the other hand, the Oklahoma Department of Rehabilitation Services uses a "milestone" achievement mechanism to reimburse providers for employment services. Under their system, a contract amount per client is established and the contractor earns part of that fee each time a consumer achieves one of the milestones, such as vocational preparation, job placement, job retention, and case closure (Martin, 2005). In still another example, the Illinois Department of Children and Family Services (DCFS) used a performance-based contracting system to increase the number of children achieving permanency. In this system, agencies were reimbursed for caseloads of twenty-five children per worker, with the expectation that five children would achieve permanency each quarter. When contracts performed as expected, caseloads remained at twenty-five. When they underachieved (fewer permanencies), caseloads increased until DCFS stopped making referrals. If an agency overachieved (more permanencies achieved), caseloads decreased, with referrals and funding continuing based upon the twenty-five. In this system, the fiscal incentives were for agencies to achieve permanency for more children and reward workers with smaller caseloads (Martin, 2005). There were many other provisions in all of these contracts but these descriptions identify the essence of these systems.

Just as these brief descriptions of different performance-based contracts probably generated questions from readers, the social administrator examining a performance-based contracting scheme needs to carefully examine all of the provisions of these contracts. This is not a trivial task. The last request for proposal (RFP) issued for reintegration and foster care services in Kansas ran eighty-eight pages, not counting related documents, and reading and absorbing all of the conditions took a considerable variety expertise. It is essential to consumer and agency success to understand all contract provisions as fully as possible and to align agencies' operations with them.

Capitated or Managed Care Contracts

Capitated contracts can be a type of performance contract and get their name from the provision that a contractor is provided a specified amount of money per person served, for a specified period of time or to achieve a specific outcome. The payment is per person or head; consequently the name "capitated." These are also called managed care contracts because they have been thought to help control the use of services and costs.

The agency operating a managed care contract receives a set amount of money each year for everyone eligible to receive services. For example, a mental health agency operating an employee assistance plan (EAP) under a capitated contract receives a set amount of money for each person employed in the organization. When someone in this organization has mental health problems, the contracted agency provides the service.

When this hypothetical contract was designed, the amount of money per employee was determined, in part, by estimating the types of mental health services that might be needed and the number of people in the organization who are likely to need the service in the next year. If these assumptions underestimate the types or extent of problems, then the providing agency loses money. Consequently, it is in the contracting agencies' interest to be as accurate as possible in estimating these costs and controlling expenditures during the life of the contract. These agencies manage costs by managing care.

Many managed behavioral health care organizations rely on evidence-based practices to manage care in what they see as an ethical manner. These organizations require that specific conditions be addressed by their service providers through the use of therapies for specific durations based upon evidence that they achieve the desired outcomes.

Capitated and managed care contracts in social services is controversial, and there are many important and technical issues to be addressed for these contracts to work effectively. A full discussion of these issues is beyond the scope of this text.

RISK MANAGEMENT AND FISCAL INCENTIVES

The reader gets some sense of risks and financial incentives from the brief discussion of capitated contracts. However, risk management in organizations is traditionally discussed in terms of having adequate insurance to cover events such as accidents and lawsuits. Any good insurance agent can identify the major types of insurance needed by an agency and the usual amounts needed to cover a variety of unfortunate events. Risk in this sense is the possibility of suffering harm or loss. In addition to the electrical and plumbing risks of buildings or worker error, contract provisions also present the possibility of harm or loss as well as the possibility of generating positive results for consumers. In this section we discuss some of the risks inherent in major types of contracts. Social administrators are responsible for understanding and managing these risks. We briefly discuss program risks associated with the following:

- Referrals
- Allowable expenditures
- Consumer outcomes
- Fiscal incentives

Referrals

It is an obvious point that a program operating under either a purchase of service or performance contract will fail without consumers. All contracts for social services must specify how the contractor is to obtain consumers. The risks here are fiscal as well as fail to produce benefits to consumers. When considering a new contract it is important to be clear on referral methods and criteria. With an executed contract it is important to monitor referrals and case flow.

Under a purchase of service contract a lack of referrals shuts off income. Similarly, providing service to more consumers that the contract amount allows depletes agency resources. Monitoring referrals and flow of consumers to ensure that these meet contract expectations is part of the agency information system (Chapter 6). When numbers fall below expectations, the social administrator will need to engage referral sources and problem solving to identify ways to increase referrals. On the other hand, an excess of referrals involves engaging with referral sources and the funding source regarding either expanding services or establishing criteria as to which consumers will receive services first.

Allowable Expenditures

All contracting entities have categories of allowable and non-allowed expenditures. The risk here is that someone in the agency will purchase something that is not an allowed cost and the agency will not be reimbursed. For example, using state social service funds for lobbying, gifts to state employees, or construction of buildings may be prohibited. In other cases there may be a ceiling on some types of expenditures. The Kansas family preservation contracts included a provision that up to a maximum of $300 per family can be spent on concrete services (Ezell, 2002). Expenditures beyond this amount would not be reimbursed by the state.

Monitoring allowable costs should not be difficult and agency fiscal controls over purchases are normally adequate. However, occasionally a worker determines that a consumer needs something that is not an allowable cost per the contract but that other programs in the community cannot provide. In Ezell's example of Kansas family preservation services, the $300 per family limit on concrete services can easily be overspent. Suppose that a worker determines that a family needs a refrigerator and an electrical bill paid, amounting to more than $300. Some agencies maintain a special fund generated from fund-raising activities to cover such situations. However, these funds are usually limited, and meeting a consumer's unanswered need when the fund is depleted presents a difficult situation.

Consumer Outcomes

Another type of risk for social administrators relates to outcomes for consumers. The risk here is the possibility of not achieving desired results. Some of this risk may be related to contract provisions. For example, there may be no contract link of service to consumer outcomes; the contract may specify the wrong service or an evidence-based service may not be operating as intended.

Consumer outcome risks are inherent in the purchase of service contracts because there is no fiscal link to results for consumers. This increased attention to providing services so that income is generated makes it difficult for the social administrator to maintain the agency's focus on results for consumers. Under these conditions, the administrator must devote increased attention to other mechanisms, such as the organizational culture and values, to maintain the focus on consumer benefits.

Another type of consumer outcome risk is that the specified service may not be effective; it may be the wrong service. For example, a public child welfare agency may contract for the provision of parent education services and require a particular model for which there is no evidence of producing the desired result. In other words, it is not known whether the required service can achieve the intended results. The contracting agency undertakes the contract and subsequently the information system (Chapter 5) fails to demonstrate that consumers are achieving intended results. This situation calls for the social administrator's advocacy efforts using the change skills of Chapter 2. The goal is to influence the contracting agency to submit the model of parent education to rigorous testing or to adopt a model that has shown to be effective. The time and effort required to influence the contracting agency can be frustrating but is worth the effort.

It is also possible that the service is an evidence-based practice but does not produce desired results for consumers. This situation is probably internal to the agency. The use of fidelity instruments to determine whether the service is being delivered as intended was discussed in Chapters 3 and 4. Fidelity instruments may indicate a need for retraining in elements of the service using the original manuals. The use of fidelity instruments may also indicate that the service is being delivered as intended and therefore the administrator must look elsewhere to address the problem. For example, it may be that the consumers referred for service do not possess the characteristics of those who can benefit from the service. The parent education program may not have been designed for parents struggling with a drug addiction. These parents may need to be in recovery for several weeks before they can begin to benefit from the service. Here again is an opportunity for the social administrator to engage in advocacy with the contracting agency and referral sources to address the specific needs of consumers, so that those who are referred can benefit from the service.

Fiscal Incentives

Since a contract is an agreement to deliver something (e.g., a service) in return for money, most of the risks have to do with income. However, the fiscal incentives that are inherent in every contract are worthy of separate discussion. The more clearly that everyone understands the fiscal incentives included in a contract, the better chance there is that resources can be aligned with agency resources and consumer outcomes.

The fiscal incentive under purchase of service contracts is to provide as much of the service as possible. Although there may be contract provisions that cover other elements of service delivery, by their very nature these contracts are not concerned with issues such as quality or results. For example, an old-fashioned foster care purchase of service contract pays the contractor for each child in care each month. As long as the contractor has children in care there is income. If all of these children return home or are adopted, then income dries up.

There is so much experimentation with performance contracts that the specific provisions of each contract need to be examined to determine the fiscal incentives. For example, in Martin's (2005) description of the Maine Department of Human Services performance contracts, he describes them as cost reimbursement contracts with extensions or renewals dependent upon the contractor achieving specified performance standards regarding service outputs, quality, and outcomes. The fiscal incentive is to stay in business by achieving these standards. However, since the "payoff" comes later, there may be less urgency in achieving these results.

Exercise

Use a contract in an agency that you are familiar with

- *Identify the incentives (explicit or implicit)*
- *Identify the various types of risks*
- *Suggest methods for managers to respond to these incentives and risks*

In Martin's (2005) description of the Oklahoma Department of Rehabilitation Services, the contractor receives a part of the total payment per client at specified milestones. The first 10 percent is paid upon determination of need, another 10 percent on job placement, and so on, through case closure, which generates 25 percent of the fee. The fiscal incentives here are to move consumers along from opening the case through job placement, retention, stabilization, and case closing. Some of the results of this contract system included a 53 percent decrease in time consumers waited to be served and a 100 percent increase in case closures.

The DCFS foster care performance contracts attempted to reward permanency for children. Contractors were reimbursed for a caseload of twenty-five children and expected to find permanent homes for five each quarter. At the beginning of the next quarter the agency received five new children per caseload. Where the contractor exceeded expectations, the reward was having the same amount of funds available to work with fewer children. Where the contractor fell behind in achieving permanency, caseloads increased until DCFS stopped referring children. The fiscal incentive in this system is for workers to have a smaller number of children to work with. However, this performance contract also includes the risk of increasing caseloads, ultimately resulting in being excluded from receiving referrals and having the contract canceled.

The fiscal incentive under capitated contracts is to control costs so that the agency does not exceed the allocated amount per person. There are many ways to control costs. One way is to use services that are less expensive. Another is to attempt to exclude from service the people with the most severe needs. Rapp (2002) comments that capitated contracts in mental health have led to some providers using more naturally occurring community resources which in some cases are more effective than more traditional and expensive services. However, the results of fiscal incentives may be negative as well as positive. He concludes that the fiscal incentives in capitated community mental health contracts have resulted in

1. controlling costs;
2. reducing the use of hospitals and other forms of segregated institutional care;
3. increasing dramatically the amount of money diverted from services to administrative costs and profits;
4. not serving the people with the most serious disabilities;
5. under-serving some (perhaps, many) clients;
6. shifting costs to other entities (e.g., nursing facilities, jails, police);
7. reducing individualized care (p. 41).

This discussion on fiscal incentives does not intend to be all inclusive. It is possible to design an immense number of contracting systems with different fiscal incentives. Since fiscal incentives influence the behavior of service providers, it is important for the social administrator to understand the incentives that exist in various types of contracts. Beyond understanding fiscal incentives, social administrators need to work to align these incentives with desired outcomes for consumers. In some cases this occurs naturally because of contract provisions. In addition, the administrator may have to try to overcome the fiscal incentives inherent in a contract so the desired outcomes for consumers are achieved. Finally, social administrators need to be involved in the design of fiscal incentives. The advocacy role using skills described in Chapter 2 is required to influence decision makers to align fiscal incentives with consumer outcomes.

Configuring Incentives

Engaging in efforts to change policies that contain misdirected incentives is a responsibility of client-centered managers. Another set of strategies is focused on reconfiguring incentives within the agency or team. In a fee for service system, the incentives to the agency encourage more hours of service or more clients. Agency policy would require some standard that programs and workers had to meet. In addition, the agency could establish "bonuses" tied to outcome. For example, in an employment program, a worker or team could receive a bonus of $100 per job placement (that lasted at least ninety days) above a certain baseline. Instead of a bonus system, perhaps annual raises would be largely determined by placements (as long as hours of service targets were met).

In some situations, the social policy has configured incentives in a way that encourages the agency to strive for consumer outcomes through performance contracting. The Oklahoma Milestone System for vocational rehabilitation services described earlier is one example. In this situation, an agency could develop a bonus system for workers that parallel the system that reimburses the agency. Perhaps a worker would receive 5 percent of the agency payment for achieving each milestone. In this way, those who actually do the work are incentivized to achieve the same outcomes as the agency.

Financial incentives are powerful influences of the behavior of individuals, agencies, and entire systems. The significant trend toward performance contracting with agencies has not met with parallel efforts to use financial incentive within agencies. It is a fertile ground for experimentation.

Chapter 10

The Inverted Hierarchy

In this chapter, we integrate the concepts and skills from previous chapters, *conceptually* using the framework of the inverted hierarchy and *in practice* through three methods: group supervision, field mentoring, and performance-enhancement teams. The inverted hierarchy posits that a manager's job is to help personnel do their jobs more effectively and efficiently. The manager does this by providing the direction and the tools to do the job, creating a reward-based environment, and by removing obstacles and constraints to performance. Social administrators apply these skills in naturally occurring events through opportunity finding, which is the basis for action.

Learning Objectives: The Inverted Hierarchy

1. *Recognize opportunities to use the skills and knowledge of consumer-centered social administration to improve outcomes for consumers.*
2. *Provide direction to a social program through vision, program specifications, organizational culture, personnel management, information management, and modeling.*
3. *Provide workers the tools they need to be effective with consumers through the use of information, structural supports, reward-based environment, and other tangible resources.*
4. *Remove obstacles to performance by simplifying organizational structures and recognizing and eliminating psychological barriers.*
5. *Implement the components of inverted hierarchy through the use of field mentoring.*
6. *Implement the components of the inverted hierarchy through the use of group supervision.*
7. *Implement the components of the inverted hierarchy through the use of performance-enhancement teams.*

Textbook of Social Administration: The Consumer-Centered Approach
© 2007 by The Haworth Press, Inc. All rights reserved.
doi:10.1300/5802_11

The most resilient symbol of management is the organizational chart. Originally devised for the military and borrowed by manufacturing companies during the Industrial Revolution, the hierarchical and pyramidal organization chart (sometimes referred to as a table of organization) is ubiquitous in human service organizations. The basic configuration is portrayed in Figure 10.1. The chart typically includes three types of personnel. The first is line staff, the people who actually make the product or deliver the service. The second type is supervisory and management personnel who are responsible for controlling and coordinating the work to be done. The third is support personnel who perform specialized roles for the organization, such as budgeting and accounting, legal services, information technology, housekeeping, and so on. In the pure sense, these support personnel have no direct authority over the line and managerial personnel, although they do have control over knowledge and information.

This traditional organizational configuration was designed to enhance the manufacture and distribution of products. Efficiency was the ultimate criterion, and control was the principal function of management. The organizational chart portrays existing positions, how these are grouped into units, and how formal authority and communication flow among them. This vertical hierarchy depicts the division of labor and establishes the fact that control is centered at the top.

The criticisms of this organizational configuration are legion. For the consumer-centered performance manager, an important problem is the separation of managers from frontline workers and consumers. Furthermore, the larger the organization, the greater the distance between day-to-day consumer contact and the policy decisions affecting them. Although this

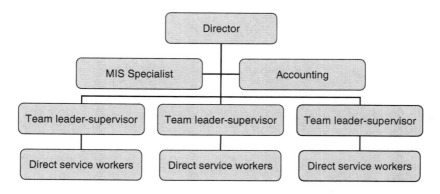

FIGURE 10.1. The Hierarchal Organization.

seems to occur in business with profound consequences, human services with its plethora of constituencies makes it that much easier to "forget" about the consumer. The typical organizational structure reinforces the tendency to maximize nonresponsiveness to consumers and their welfare.

A second consequence of this configuration is that control remains the major managerial function with its assumption that "employees in the trenches" will do badly or inadequately unless their behavior conforms to policies and procedures and is closely monitored. Unfortunately, many organizational rules (i.e., policies and procedures) were not developed based on the needs of consumers but on the needs of the organization. For example, most "paperwork" was not designed to help frontline workers provide better service but to control who is to receive what form of help for how long in order to please other constituencies. Another problem with policies in human service organizations is that they assume all consumers are the same or at least similar enough that a rule can be implemented uniformly with rather uniform results. The worker trying to help a particular consumer knows that this is a questionable assumption. The agendas are discrepant. Managers seek to control and maintain adherence to the policy manual, while workers seek to help individuals who are unique. It is no wonder that management in so many human service organizations is seen as irrelevant or as an obstacle to quality service.

A third consequence of the typical organizational configuration is symbolic. Consumers are not even included in the chart. The power is at the top and all others are subordinate. Subordinate has the following meaning: "Belonging to a lower or inferior class or rank; secondary; subject to the authority or control of another" (Dictionary.com, 2005). These concepts are abhorrent to the consumer-centered performance manager. The need is for a new symbol, a new metaphor for the social administrator.

A NEW METAPHOR

How does a social administrator "venerate consumers" if they are not an explicit part of the organization? Human service organizations that are producing superior rates of outcomes for consumers turn the typical organizational configuration upside-down in everyday practice. It is from this observation that the inverted hierarchy was created as depicted in Figure 10.2. This organizational configuration is a more accurate portrayal of a consumer-centered organization and has more fidelity with concepts underlying the consumer-centered performance model of management. First, the pinnacle of the chart is the consumer and all organizational personnel are

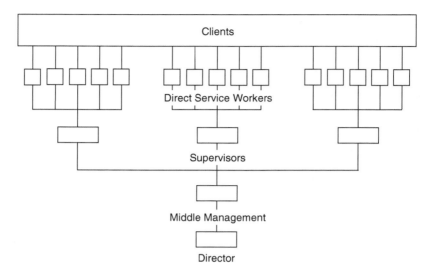

FIGURE 10.2. Inverted Hierarchy

subservient. In fact, supervisors are subservient to frontline workers and the "boss" is subservient to supervisors and frontline workers.

The assumption central to the inverted hierarchy is that the principal function of management at any level is not to control but to help the next higher rung do their jobs more effectively. "Subservient" then relates to service. The service is to help others who want to do the best job possible for consumers do their job better. However, how do social administrators help? The concepts and skills in this text are organized into the following four major categories of organizational helping:

1. Specifying the job to be done and the expectations of how it should be done
2. Providing the tools to get the job done
3. Creating reward-based environment and organizational culture
4. Removing obstacles and constraints to the desired performance

With the host of competing, nonconsumer demands placed on the manager, how can the social administrator use the skills and strategies identified in the text? The inverted hierarchy requires highly developed skills in finding opportunities to be consumer and worker centered. Opportunity finding is the foundation for successful implementation of the inverted hierarchy.

FINDING OPPORTUNITY:
THE FOUNDATION OF THE INVERTED HIERARCHY

Social administrators achieve results for consumers through interactions with others. For the consumer-centered administrator, there is no "throw away" behavior. All behavior affects others in the work environment and it is through structured interactions over time that people and organizations learn and grow. As Lawler (1996) observes; "Managers do things right; leaders do the right thing. Managers influence through bureaucratic system; leaders influence through vision and challenge. Managers motivate through rewards and punishment; leaders motivate through values and shared goals" (p. 40). A key to leading is finding opportunities to implement the principles and tools of consumer-centered social administration.

Opportunity is defined as "a favorable or suitable occasion or time. A chance for progress or advancement" (Dictionary.com, 2005). For the social administrator, it is a suitable occasion for advancement of results for consumers and for shaping a consumer-centered organizational culture. This then implies at least the following three-step process:

1. Environmental sensing
2. Comparing the sensing to purpose
3. Exploiting those events or circumstances that are favorable to the purpose.

Environmental Sensing

Opportunities are present in virtually all situations, from writing a memo or getting a cup of coffee to responding to a grant announcement or testifying before a legislative committee. The consumer-centered performance manager is highly skilled in exploiting everyday events, tasks, and situations to move the organization and its personnel to higher levels of consumer-centeredness. This demands a high level of perceptiveness. The performance manager is constantly surveying the environment for cues. Although the range of environmental cues is infinite and rather amorphous, there are five identifiable categories.

Problems

The first set of problems comprises those events that have already been defined as such by some player. Often these take the form of complaints or dissatisfactions. At times, they emerge as messes: a configuration of events and opinions in which the "problem" has not yet clearly emerged. The Chinese character for opportunity is the same as the one for problem (see Figure 10.3). This connotes that embedded in every problem is an opportunity.

In terms of sensing, problems are the most straightforward since they are usually communicated orally or occasionally in writing. The difficulty comes when the manager must analyze the contours and textures of the problem so that an opportunity can emerge. An element of "learning for a living" and creating a learning organization is disentangling problems by listening to the perspectives of all of those who define the problem. The social administrator has the difficult but necessary task of keeping the consumer at the center of attention while identifying different perspectives on the problem. As Friedman, Lipshitz, and Overmeer (2001) observe, this is a part of organizational learning where seemingly contradictory strategies combine advocacy and inquiry. Listening and speaking for consumers is one step in disentangling problems.

Strengths

A second category of environmental cues are strengths of people in the organizations. This includes identifying high-performing people and units, locating the factors that have contributed to this performance, influential relationships between people (e.g., staff, key players, etc.), special talents of people, strong consumer-centered beliefs, and so on. The sensing and storage of strengths is important to the social administrator for several reasons.

1. It provides the basis for rewards. Behavior that is rewarded tends to increase in frequency, thereby replacing behavior that is ignored.
2. The performance manager is constantly trying to disseminate "what works" to other organizational units and people who are not using the effective methods.
3. People tend to grow and prosper based on exploiting their strengths. Once aware of these strengths the manager can facilitate this growth.
4. Identified strengths can be used by the manager to help turn problems and other environmental cues into opportunities.

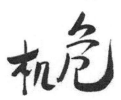

FIGURE 10.3. Chinese Character for Opportunity/Problem

Inconsistencies and Discontinuities

A third category of environmental cues is inconsistencies and discontinuities between events, behavior, and beliefs. Argyris (1999) observes that one of the necessary conditions for organizational learning is a mismatch between intentions and results. The search for discrepancies requires a higher level of conceptual skill than does the search for problems and strengths, because the manager needs to find two or more items to compare and often these are not obvious. In addition, this requires an organizational climate that fosters inquiry, openness, and trust (Friedman, Lipshitz, & Overmeer, 2001). This does not always exist in an organization where a social administrator may be directing a program. However, the emphasis on "learning for a living" drives the manager to find these discontinuities. The inconsistencies are endless, but here are a few, prevalent, general types:

- A person's statements and his or her behavior
- An organization's statements and its behavior
- A person's behavior or statements and the organization's purpose
- Social work values and a person's behavior

Other Effective Programs and People

A fourth category of environmental cues concerns what others are doing. "Learning for a living" includes learning about effective program strategies, evidence-based interventions, management techniques, and so forth. A sense of privacy, envy, and competition is replaced by a spirit of inquiry and learning from others. This also includes learning from seemingly unrelated events and enterprises. The manager, for example, can learn much about public speaking by watching politicians and skilled orators. Similarly, although most management fads should be avoided, many business management techniques are worth investigating for their usefulness to social administration.

Social Trends

The fifth category of environmental cues concerns societal trends, stable societal beliefs and values, and some wisdom about the future. This cluster is by far the most challenging, demanding a high level of intelligence and acuity. The manager is called on to see the larger environment and how the organization and its purpose are consistent with this context. For example, our larger society places a value on individual responsibility. Another value is the safety of members of the community. Most people also value community assistance for those members who are vulnerable due to age, some form of disability, or illness. The social administrator who is "venerating consumers" finds opportunities to educate the community about consumers in ways that are consistent with influential values.

A few examples include the following:

- Expressed concern with the most vulnerable and disadvantaged consumers
- The over 100-year trend toward normalization and integration of consumers, and how this is consistent with personal responsibility
- The fact that the costs of solving social problems will continue to be a consideration

---

Opportunity Finding

1. Environmental sensing
   a. Problems
   b. Strengths
   c. Inconsistencies and discontinuities
   d. Other effective programs and people
   e. Social trends
2. Comparing the sensing to purpose
3. Action

Comparing the Sensing to Purpose

The performance manager is constantly comparing circumstances and environmental cues with organizational purpose. It is from this cognitive process that managers identify opportunities. Organizational purpose is linked to the five performance areas: consumer outcomes, service events, resource acquisition, efficiency, and staff morale. Performance in these areas is directed by the mission to make the organization as consumer-centered as possible. Some of this comparison is captured by the following questions:

- What about the identified problem related to the performance areas (consumer outcome, service events, resources, staff morale, efficiency)?
- Whose behavior or performance (strengths) has contributed to performance or consumer-centeredness?
- To what performance area does the discontinuity that I am sensing contribute?

- Which organization, program, or person is doing the best in producing results that I can learn from?
- How can I respond to what the community is valuing to enhance consumer-centeredness or performance?

These are examples of sensing and then comparing to purpose. Other times, you start with purpose then sense. For example, you will be representing your agency at a ribbon cutting ceremony for a new homeless shelter. Your agency's goal is to get permanent housing for homeless individuals through outreach case management. One obstacle has been that many landlords will not rent to people who use Department of Housing and Urban Development (Section 8) housing vouchers. You know that the head of the landlord association will be there. You decide to engage her in a conversation and request an opportunity to attend the next members' meeting. You have sensed that this ceremony presents an opportunity to engage a key actor in a series of conversations, potentially increasing housing opportunities for your consumers.

Exploiting Those Events or Circumstances That Are Favorable to the Purpose

Once the opportunity is identified, leadership requires action. Chapter 2 was devoted to a variety of ways to exercise influence to increase performance. The landlord association meeting of the previous example is a perfect place to use a variety of influence skills. These influence skills are linked to the perceptions, attitudes, and behaviors of people required to increase performance, and often require blending the agendas of a variety of internal and external constituents. Social administrators use these influence strategies in persistent interactions with constituents to implement strategies that turn opportunities into performance. The remainder of this chapter contains strategies that can be employed once opportunities have been identified.

STRATEGIES FOR TURNING OPPORTUNITIES INTO PERFORMANCE

Social administrators operate in a context that is producing an existing level of performance. In fact, one can say that every system is perfectly designed to achieve the results it is achieving. The administrator has a host of analytic skills at her or his command to implement the inverted hierarchy and increase performance, including use of program specifications, information, personnel, and resource management. Opportunities are found to make this happen through the managers' abilities to influence people, organizational culture, and learning. The strategies to pull together this nearly overwhelming array of tools include the following:

1. Providing direction
2. Providing the tools
3. Creating a reward-based environment and organizational culture
4. Removing obstacles

Providing Direction

Much of this text is about clearly laying out the job to be done and the expectations of how it should be done. Detailed program specifications are about defining the work to be done. Information management is about obtaining and productively using feedback on expectations and performance; most of personnel management is about clearly defining the job and providing rewards and feedback to those doing the work. Clearly defining expectations is also the first concept that Buckingham and Coffman (1999) discovered "the world's greatest managers do differently." This includes clearly describing how a particular employee's job fits into the larger program, agency, or societal context. Managerial strategies for providing direction include the following:

1. Vision
2. Organizational culture—bringing meaning to everyday events
3. Program specifications
4. Managing people
5. Managing information
6. Modeling

Vision

Vision is the key to leadership. Unless you have a vision of where you are going, you are not going to get there.

> Where there is no vision, the people perish. (Proverbs 29:18)

> A vision without a task is a dream. A task without a vision is drudgery. But a vision with a task can change the world. (Black Elk, Oglala Sioux)

> To accomplish great things, we must not only act but also dream, not only plan but also believe. (Anatole France)

The inverted organization is guided by a vision of consumer achievements. It is the social administrator who venerates consumers and focuses everyone's attention on results by articulating a vision. Visions that influence tend to have the following characteristics:

1. The vision captures the central reason for the organization's existence and describes its fundamental business. It defines the consumer as the reason for the organization but does so by speaking directly to the interests of not only consumers but also staff and a larger society as well.
2. It is future oriented and has a timeless quality to it. It invokes feelings of optimism and hope. It has a certain universality of appeal. It is both inspiring and realistic.
3. It uses a language that eschews jargon and professional terminology, and often employs analogy, metaphor, and personification. The use of symbols is prevalent.
4. It is personal. It is something the manager owns, and it derives its passion from that ownership.

At its core, a vision establishes and communicates the organization's values. As Lawler (1996) says: "Managers influence through bureaucratic system; leaders influence through vision and challenge" (p. 40). Shared values are the principal control mechanism, not hierarchy, and policy and procedures manuals seem to be the mechanism of choice in human service organizations.

A vision serves several important functions for the manager and the organization. First, it acts as a guide to managerial and staff behavior. It provides a benchmark for selecting priorities, identifying opportunities, and making decisions. Second, a vision acts as a tool for unifying potentially disparate agendas of multiple constituencies. The vision is something the manager seeks to share with others. Third, a vision should answer two important questions. For consumers, "Why would I want service from the organization?" For employees, "Why would a person want to work for this program?" It seeks to create a shared meaning. Fourth, a vision is a symbol for the organization and a basis for developing other symbols. In fact, the vision is quickly turned into symbols by the best managers. The vision is communicated in myriad ways—it becomes ubiquitous. It is a way of stating what the organization stands for.

Program Specifications

The program specifications as developed in Chapters 3 through 5 identify the many behaviors and conditions required to achieve results with consumers. Program specifications are a blueprint for action and a living document that is revisited often as everyone in the program continues to learn for a living. A well-specified program sets direction. The program theory defines the goal, what consumers and workers need to achieve to reach the goal, and identifies the behavioral expectations of consumers and workers. The program specifications identify the most likely emotional reactions of consumers and workers and the most useful responses; the minimum behaviors required of key players for the program to meet its goals; and the environment that is most likely to produce consumer outcomes. As illustrated at the end of each of the program specification chapters, the consumer-centered performance manager uses these specifications as a ready source for directing behavior.

Managing People

Two critical vehicles for setting direction, task analysis and job descriptions, were described in Chapter 8. If done with precision and tied to outcomes for consumers, job descriptions are the most direct source of direction for the individual employee. The focus in Chapter 8 was direct service worker positions, but it is important to write supervisory and managerial job descriptions that are equally precise.

One strategy for developing supervisor job descriptions is to use the inverted hierarchy concepts in the following order:

1. Establish the perspective that a manager's job is to make the work of others more effective and efficient and that there are clusters of ways this can be accomplished.
2. Take each cluster sequentially and have three to ten people brainstorm a list of ways that cluster could be put into operation.
3. Edit the lists by grouping similar items together and removing ones not seen as relevant.
4. Convert the remaining lists into job description format.

Managing Information

The information management concepts described in Chapters 6 and 7 are tools for keeping organizational personnel directed. If "what gets measured gets done," then the data collected and reported by personnel send a powerful message concerning what is important to the organization. The selection and reporting of consumer outcomes venerates consumers and defines the priority domains of the work. The selection and reporting of those worker behaviors most influential in producing these outcomes focuses attention on these behaviors. Data helps guide and direct behavior. Feedback, when used prospectively, reinforces desired behavior and is a tool for directing behavior that improves performance.

Modeling: Management Behavior As a Resource

A powerful technique for directing behavior is modeling by supervisors and managers. Chapter 2 identified modeling as a powerful strategy for exercising influence. In that context modeling was identified as a way to increase perceived behavioral control by showing that the behavior can be performed. For social administrators, modeling is not only a conscious decision to demonstrate a desired behavior; it is also a day-to-day management activity. Managers model through their behavior, whether they are aware of it or not. Management behavior demonstrates the values of the organization. Modeling helps guide others in how to make decisions and how to behave. There is no element more destructive in an organization's culture than supervisors and managers pronouncing one set of values or prescriptions while they themselves behave in incompatible, inconsistent, or opposite ways. Social administrators might ask themselves: How does my behavior model consumer-centeredness?

The modeling of consumer-centeredness is particularly important. The following are but ten examples that are often within the control of managers:

1. Interact with consumers in the hallway and waiting rooms; find opportunities to do so—have an open-door policy.
2. Institutionalize a variety of consumer feedback mechanisms (e.g., client satisfaction surveys, focus groups, suggestion boxes) and respond to them.
3. Insure consumer representation on the board of directors or advisory board.
4. Provide membership dues to staff and consumers so they can join consumer organizations and advocacy groups.
5. Arrange for advocacy group representatives to regularly address staff meetings.
6. Donate honorariums to consumer organizations.
7. Talk about consumers in every interaction; make them heroes.
8. Insure that the manager's personal staff acts as an extension of that manager in treating consumers with the highest degree of courtesy, respect, and dignity.

9. Hire former consumers.
10. Involve consumers in the design and implementation of program evaluations and share results with them.

Providing the Tools

With expectations clarified and reinforced, the tools required to meet the expectations need to be provided. It is often the discrepancy between expectations and available tools that causes job dissatisfaction and ineffectiveness. For example, setting ambitious goals for consumers and workers, and then requiring service to a caseload of fifty is a recipe for failure.

The consumer-centered performance manager should constantly be asking employees, "How can I help you with your job?" The question is meaningless unless acted upon. The responses need to be written down and become an agenda for action. An eminently worthwhile question the manager could ask every day while driving home is: "What did I do today that made the jobs of my workers more effective or easier?" There are three categories of tools:

1. Information
2. Structural supports
3. Tangible resources

Information

Information provides direction and is also a tool for accomplishing the work of the program. The management information system designed in Chapters 6 and 7 is a tool. Workers also need information regarding their practice with consumers. This includes training, technical assistance, and the latest evidence-based practices.

Performance reports. Data reports are provided by the organization's information system. They are designed according to the criteria of Chapter 6 and are relevant and self-correcting. If designed according to the criteria, reports are tools for frontline workers to receive information on the results of their prodigious efforts.

Feedback. Feedback is part of the formal information system as well as the normal day-to-day activities. Interpersonal feedback provides information concerning behavior on the part of those in the organization. Behavior is, in part, determined by the reactions of others. We grow and learn from what others tell us about ourselves. Field mentoring and supervision discussed later in this chapter are a particularly powerful mechanism for feedback. The reward-based environment is rich with feedback.

The learning organization includes cultural elements that encourage and facilitate ongoing exchanges. Mechanisms for feedback need to be established to make this happen. Focus groups and exit interviews with consumers, group and individual supervision, written notes and evaluations, and even coffeepot conversations are opportunities for feedback.

Training. Training is frequently an inappropriate organizational response to a problem more effectively solved by better policy or more resources. Yet it is an indispensable tool for assuring that workers are not asked to do something they do not know how to do. This includes such activities as orientation and preservice training, in-service training, and continuing education. Given the inherent difficulty of human service work and the fact that the lowest credentialed, most inexperienced personnel are often placed in direct helping roles, the training imperative is clear.

The key to determining when training is indicated is employing this strategy when workers truly need to learn new skills, not when workers know how to do the work but need other tools, such as increased resources and lower caseloads. Training has been discussed in Chapter 2 as a way to increase perceived behavioral control and again in Chapter 8 as one of the personnel management tasks. Once training has been determined to be useful, it is critical to do it properly or it is a waste of resources. The training checklist included in Chapter 8 is a tool that social administrators should use to assure the maximum impact from training.

Technical assistance and consultation. This refers to the provision of help in the technical application of helping strategies to consumers. It is one thing to know how to do a specific method of assessment or intervention and another to skillfully apply that methodology to the myriad case situations that a frontline worker confronts. Ready and continuous access to such a resource can help insure that training is applied in practice. The most continuous source of such help is the immediate supervisor or peers, but access to outside experts is often valuable. Group supervision and field mentoring (both discussed later in the chapter) are arenas particularly suited to technical assistance and consultation. One aspect of learning for a living is learning from others. Social administrators seek out high performers wherever they find them. These people are an important source of consultation and technical assistance.

Evidence-based practices. The learning organization continually scans the environment for the latest most effective interventions. However, neither workers nor managers have the time needed to locate effective interventions and transfer them to the organization. Gray (2001) confronts this difficulty by suggesting that every organization establish an evidence center. An evidence center is staff with the skills and resources to continually scan the research literature, classify it according to its level of evidence, and disseminate this knowledge within the organization. Although this may sound like a large organizational unit, it can be a part of the job of an existing person or carried out through an agreement with a local university.

Information As a Tool

- *Performance reports*
- *Feedback*
- *Training*
- *Technical assistance and consultation*
- *Evidence-based practices*

Structural Supports

It is unlikely that consumers will be successful unless workers have the time to devote to them. Time is a finite organizational resource of infinite importance to consumers. There are many demands on a worker's time, including paperwork, consultation with other community professionals, and meetings. Social administrators seek to maximize the time that workers have with consumers. One way to do this is by paying attention to caseload size. Others include creating intragency synergy, interagency agreements, forms as tools, and supportive policies and procedures.

Caseload size. Given the established expectations, a frontline worker's caseload must allow for these to be met. Protective service caseloads of fifty are common, as are caseloads of forty for community mental health case managers. The protection of children and improving the community integration of people with severe mental illness is both too important and too demanding to be prohibited by unworkable caseload size. The simple truth is that the outcomes that we seek with consumers simply cannot be achieved under such a yoke.

Evidence-based interventions are one source of caseload size expectations. The specifications of the testing of the intervention include the size of the caseload while the project was evaluated. Adopting an evidence-based intervention but increasing the caseload of workers expected to deliver the intervention will render it useless. Consumers will just not achieve under those conditions.

In areas where interventions do not yet have high levels of evidence, professional organizations frequently recommend caseload sizes that they feel are most likely to be effective. For example, the Child Welfare League of America has suggestions for caseloads for different types of child welfare practice. These are a type of practice wisdom where many professionals contribute their experience to the question. Social administrators can use these guidelines to advance arguments for increased resources that focus on effectiveness by increasing worker time with consumers.

In some situations, managers need to be creativite and courageous to provide some consumers more time with workers. For example, a team of five frontline workers is expected to provide case management services to 200 frail elderly. Instead of having each worker responsible for fifty clients, whereby four workers are overwhelmed and only day-to-day crises can be responded to, assign twenty consumers to one or two workers and assign the other consumers to the remaining workers. This configuration provides at least one worker and twenty consumers a chance to receive the benefits promised by the service. The other workers would continue to be overwhelmed and only be able to provide crisis intervention services. However, this clarification of expectations and the entire unit celebrating the success achieved by all consumers may mitigate the effects of the overwhelming caseload.

Reducing caseloads may mean not serving everyone who is eligible or who could benefit from the service. Rather than being seen as irresponsible, this choice is often the most responsible decision and consistent with the NASW Code of Ethics. This requires "straight talk" to elected officials, those providing the funds, and other constituencies. An analytic process for defining who will be served was described in the chapter on program design and would be helpful in establishing reasonable caseloads.

Intra-agency synergy. Many human organizations provide multiple services to a particular target population. An agency serving the elderly may provide case management, home-delivered meals, socialization opportunities through a senior center, home-based assistance with activities of daily living, and so on. Community mental health centers often serve people with psychiatric disabilities through crisis services, day treatment, case management, medication services, supported employment and housing services, personal care attendants, individual and group therapy, and so on. To achieve the desired consumer outcomes, these separate services must be working in a compatible manner. For example, achieving high levels of consumer employment is the primary responsibility of the supported employment team within the mental health center but if psychiatrists, nurses, therapists, and case managers perceive of work as "too stressful" for clients or in some other way see the client as "not ready," clients will doubt their ability to work and referrals to the employment team will be slow in coming.

The manager's job is to align the beliefs and behaviors of involved units, teams, or departments so that everyone is fulfilling their necessary roles. Among the tools that can be used include the influence strategies presented in Chapter 2 are the following: specifying necessary behavior of these parties as described in Chapter 8 concerning key actors, providing research results concerning the benefits of working, organizing training, arranging a visit to a program where everyone works toward employment, monitoring referral behavior and regularly providing feedback results to them, presenting successful examples of consumers who were employed. A structural strategy is to create multidisciplinary or multiprogram teams in which the psychiatrist, therapist, and supported employment worker are assigned to a case management team and take part in weekly group supervision.

Interagency agreements. The increasing specialization of our service programs combined with the complexity of human life and problems means that consumers can rarely have their needs met through one agency. Many consumer problems are not "client problems" but problems at the transaction between consumers and societal institutions (e.g., schools, courts, employers). This means that help is provided by multiple agencies and the targets of change are often institutions rather than consumers. The close working relationships between agencies is indispensable for effective and efficient helping.

Workers who have to negotiate the interactions between these institutions for each case lose valuable time with consumers. Interagency agreements can be a time-saving tool for workers. We are not referring to agreements with their vague references to cooperation and collaboration, nor are we referring to twenty-six-page "continuity of care" agreements. Rather, one- or two-page working documents that detail the reciprocal responsibilities in behavioral language is the recommendation. The document should answer the question: "Who will do what when?" This is a document that can literally, if needed, be placed on the table between workers of two agencies to guide their work with a consumer. The program specification section on key actors in the Chapter 5 can guide the content of such agreements.

Forms as tools. Paperwork is a major time user for workers. The importance of the paperwork burden is demonstrated by its repeated treatment in this text. Chapter 2 addressed paperwork as an obstacle removal strategy to increase perceived behavioral control. Here, we address paperwork as forms for helping and return to the topic later in this chapter.

When workers retreat to their offices to complete paperwork, they are not available to consumers. One way to protect worker time is to make certain that whenever possible forms are tools to do the job. Forms as tools require that the form is directly related to the specific job a person is being asked to do and provide some notion about how it is to be done. Furthermore, the form needs to help the worker help the consumer by identifying the work focus, making specific decisions about consumers, and/or serving as a means of feedback.

The two "forms" that are ubiquitous in every agency are assessment and case (treatment) plan. These forms should, more than any others, be supportive of good helping. For example, a case plan should be designed to include the consumer goals, the tasks needed to accomplish the goals, time frames for accomplishment, who is responsible, and a place for worker and consumer signatures.

To act as a tool, a case planning form must be able to be used with consumers. It should act as an agenda between worker and consumer, laying out the areas to be discussed and the agreements to be reached. It should be a document that both worker and consumer can work from and each should have a copy.

The form should not be isolated from the helping task. In other words, a case plan should be completed with the consumer, not before or after a consumer encounter in the worker's office. If workers are not using the case plan with consumers regularly, then the form is wrong (it is not a tool), or the work is not being done properly. The case planning form should not include superfluous information except when adding an item allows another form used for documentation to be eliminated. If it is to guide the work, it cannot pose distractions to that performance.

Similarly, assessment recordings should help structure the information collection. It should help workers and consumers identify the information needed to develop a case plan and organize it in a way that conclusions and directions become clear. It should not include information that will not be used. For example, some agencies still require rather long social histories as part of the assessment process, but little of this information is ever used to form a case plan. Assessment should be relevant to the form of help the agency is offering.

Both case plans and assessments should be designed to be as dynamic as actual helping. Assessment is ongoing—it is not a one-shot event. Workers learn something about consumers with each encounter. Case plans change as situations change and often tasks are added or time lines altered weekly. Forms and policies that do not allow or facilitate changes detract from their helpfulness. For example, agency policies requiring a treatment plan update every three or six months is simply not reflective of actual helping.

Helpers for the helpers. Many workers have too much to do for too many people. Some of the work involves little skill but is constant, if not predictable (e.g., consumers needing emergency transportation, a reassuring phone call, or help balancing a checkbook). Managers who arrange for volunteers, casework extenders, emergency transportation services, or student help, and adequately structure their work, may free workers for tasks requiring their skills and assist in managing the workload.

The case manager at an inner-city mental health center found that workers there, despite reasonable sized caseloads, were devoting all their time to resolving crises concerning housing, medications, substance abuse, and law enforcement. Despite their desire to do so, workers had difficulty finding time to focus on individual skill building, locating community opportunities for recreation or social supports, and otherwise helping consumers build a decent life. Consumers were often placed in their day treatment program where they attended various groups. The staff felt that these groups were not being helpful, but instead further segregated people from the community, and therefore reinforced low expectations rather than a pursuit of recovery. The managers downsized the day treatment program and converted the staff to community integration specialists responsible for ensuring that goal-directed work continued with consumers. They worked individually with consumers to help them access normal community resources and opportunities. The use of task analysis described in the Chapter 8 will help guide the meaningful structuring of such roles.

Supportive policies and procedures. Policies and procedures are important for the control of hierarchical organization. Policies and procedures are also obstacles to the consumer-centered organization. Organizations often develop policies and procedures in response to a case with an unfortunate outcome, a perceived problem that no longer exists, or something that is contradictory to expectations of workers. For example, a crisis that leads to a negative outcome may result in an agency developing an expectation that workers will be available for these situations after hours. However, other policies place limits on the use of compensatory time. If the expectation is for an outreach mode of service delivery, yet billable service hours do not include transportation time, major disincentives are created.

The best source for identifying these organizational anomalies is the workers themselves. Listening to workers often results in identifying the areas of change. Asking workers about policies what make the work more difficult is a useful prompt for this information. Another source is the program specifications that identify the conditions required for consumer success. Existing policies should be examined to determine how they support program requirements.

Structural Supports As Tools

- *Caseload size*
- *Interagency agreements*
- *Forms*
- *Helpers for helpers*
- *Supportive policies and procedures*

Tangible Resources

Information, caseloads, forms, and rewards are all tangible resources. Here we are simply reinforcing the idea that the social administrator seeks to place as many resources as possible in the trenches where the help occurs. In many agencies, especially public bureaucracies, there are simply too many employees for whom providing service is not their primary responsibility. Overhead costs should be kept to the minimum. This usually means reducing levels of managerial and staff positions. The social administrator's attention to efficiency is driven by the desire to put as many resources as possible where they will have the largest effect on consumer outcomes, and that is generally with frontline staff.

For the worker. Tangible resources for workers vary widely depending on the agency and the job. A classic situation concerns the outreach worker who is expected to do his or her work outside of the agency. Resource supports include cars, adequate travel reimbursement, liability insurance, a beverage holder and trash bag for the car, lap top computers, and cellular phones or beepers. For many workers, easy-to-use resource guides, rolodexes, adequate office supplies, and so on would help them do their jobs more effectively or efficiently.

For the consumer. These too can vary widely, but in many agencies access to a fund for emergencies would be critical. These are monies not bureaucratically encumbered (e.g., requiring forms, permissions, meetings, and several layers of review) and almost immediately available for such things as rent deposits, food, clothing, and registration fees for community activities. It could mean a "lending closet," where consumers could borrow some items such as vacuum cleaners, kitchen supplies, furniture, or even fishing poles.

Organizational Culture: Meaning and Rewards

The third category of managerial behavior within the inverted hierarchy is developing and maintaining an organizational culture that reinforces the principles of the consumer-centered organization. Organizational culture includes the values and norms of the unit that are communicated in many ways including heroes, stories, and symbols. It communicates and reinforces the work to be done and the outcomes to be achieved, as well as fostering a learning atmosphere and creating a satisfying work environment.

Bringing Meaning to Everyday Events

Workers encounter challenges to achieving outcomes with consumers on a daily basis. These challenges can lead workers to become fatigued and cynical, or once again mount extraordinary efforts on behalf of consumers. Social administrators employ the elements of organizational culture in the myriad interactions that fill each day to link these events to the vision of the unit and energize workers to continue their efforts. The most obvious opportunities of this type are those in which workers seek advice and suggestions. Others are more subtle.

A worker frustrated by a consumer who has not followed through on a series of agreements will have a tendency to be angry. Although acknowledging the frustration, the manager can reframe the consumer's behavior as resulting from fear or lack of confidence. The manager can emphasize the heroic mission the program has established to work with consumers confronting the most difficult situations. The manager can use stories of similar consumers who, after repeated attempts, have succeeded. These stories demonstrate that a healthy disrespect for the impossible is an organizational norm.

Another example is that a worker frustrated by helping a consumer complete onerous financial assistance forms can be placed in a perspective that emphasizes their need for money and the importance of the worker arranging it. Once the assistance is arranged, the worker and consumer can begin work on other tasks such as job training or parent education. These examples demonstrate how common day-to-day interactions are used to reinforce values and norms.

Another method of bringing meaning to everyday events is to create a book of agency stories. Stories are an important way to transmit organizational norms. These are short descriptions of consumers, events, and worker actions that reflect the specifics of how work is conducted in this organization.

Stories can be solicited from workers, colleagues, supervisors, or consumers, or can be generated by the manager. New additions can be included in newsletters or posted for some period before being formally entered into a storybook. The stories themselves can be used in speeches and training sessions, and made a formal part of employee orientation. The storybook could also be used as a recruitment device for new staff; it becomes one source of the heroes and symbols of the organization.

The Reward-Based Environment

The concept of the reward-based environment has been discussed in several places in this text and is an integral part of the consumer-centered learning organization. Rewards are a tool that managers use to recognize and reinforce the work that leads to outcomes for consumers. This includes creating winners, principles of reinforcement, menus of available awards, and getting other organizational members involved. However, beyond these ideas is a simple notion that work should be fun!

Ideally the fun should come directly from the work or be symbolic of the work. This does not preclude birthday parties, agency softball teams, or Friday afternoon "Happy Hours;" these can help build camaraderie and make people feel special as well. However, fun that comes from the actual work offers the added benefits of increasing performance and making the work itself enjoyable.

Awards not only provide public recognition of meaningful achievement but are a source of much laughter. The power is seen in the response of one mental health center executive director whose agency had not received an award, "What do you think we need to do in order to receive an award next year?"

Every organization should celebrate failure with something like a "Perfect Failure Award." One agency calls it the "Boner Award," which is a large bone with a yellow ribbon around it. The nature of human service work means that despite Herculean efforts by workers, consumers will still not achieve all their goals and will endure other "failures." Given the complex nature of social problems and the lack of social work knowledge linking worker behavior to consumer benefits, managers must encourage worker creativity. For workers to succeed with consumers, they must experiment and risk failure. This is not risk taking that endangers consumers or workers but has the promise of achieving results for consumers. Workers who do everything correctly and go beyond normal efforts deserve as much recognition as those who achieve "success." Celebrating this kind of failure encourages the kinds of creativity required of the worker.

Two other highly recommended awards are the "Extra Mile Award" and the "Mission Impossible Award." The former would recognize effort well beyond the call of duty. The latter award would recognize the solution of some chronic or seemingly incorrigible problem (e.g., a consumer who has made significant gains but who everyone had given up on; getting an uncooperative judge to follow agency recommendations). Such awards would help encourage risk taking and extra effort by organizational members.

Fun and celebrations should also include consumers. Award ceremonies, pictures on walls, and alumni involvement in current programs are all examples. Why not enshrine the heroes in an agency Hall of Fame? Our social programs should have an element of joy to them.

The prerequisite of recognizing and celebrating achievement is observation and listening. Managers must simply place themselves in a position where they can see or hear incidents of good or superior work and achievement. One cannot hide in an office and still identify performance worth rewarding. The use of consumer satisfaction surveys, focus groups, information system reports, and contact with key factors are traditional sensing devices.

Removing Obstacles and Constraints

The fourth category of managerial behaviors in the inverted hierarchy is the constant and conscientious removal of barriers to performance. Obstacle removal was presented as linked to organizational change and perceptions of behavioral control in Chapter 2. People who perceive that there are obstacles to doing something are less willing to try. There are a variety of reasons that people in organizations do not do some of the things necessary to produce the best outcomes for consumers. In this section, the focus is on managers anticipating those barriers to performance common to social service bureaucracies.

Social administrators operating from a consumer-centered and inverted hierarchy perspective anticipate obstacles and work to remove them. In a sense, the lack of any of the previously mentioned behaviors and strategies is an obstacle. For example, job descriptions that do not detail work expectations are an obstacle. Lack of rewards is an obstacle. This section will not repeat these but rather will focus on a few of the most ubiquitous obstacles in human service organizations. A major theme in this section is "less is more": less paperwork, fewer meetings, fewer priorities, fewer permissions, fewer organizational levels, fewer excuses, less noise. The obstacles are addressed under two categories:

1. Organizational structures
2. Psychological obstacles

Organizational Structures

These obstacles are created by the organization. The primary function of bureaucracies is control. There are levels within traditional hierarchal organizations to control the behavior of those at the next lower level. Since it is thought that one person can only "control" seven to nine other people, each level is built upon the idea of having one position supervising seven to nine people in the previous level. This continues until there is one person on top who is the executive director. Paperwork is a control mechanism. Supervisory control is tenuous, so documentation is needed to assure that behavior is within specified boundaries. When there is a perceived anomaly in the organization or something does not seem to be as it should, a meeting is required to solve "the problem." In the inverted hierarchy, this type of control is a barrier to performance and social administrators seek to reduce or eliminate its effects.

Hierarchy. The performance manager must remove needless organizational levels. The goal is to push responsibility, authority, resources, and problem solving to the lowest possible level of the organization. This can only be done by removing managerial levels whose major purpose is unnecessary control. The test needs to be as follows: How does this position directly enhance performance? How does it help the people "above?"

What responsibilities are redundant with other levels? Where is authority shared when it could be vested in one person at the next level? In many human service organizations, managers are not helping but in fact get in the way. Jobs should be redesigned to be helpful, and the remainder phased out. This removes an obstacle to performance and allows the organization to commit the resources to frontline positions where the help to consumers occurs. The result is a more efficient and effective organization.

Paperwork. Paperwork is the most onerous task for frontline practitioners; the burden can consume over 35 percent of an agency's time and resources, and the benefits accrued to the organization are slight even when identifiable. More specifically, the link between performance and every form now being required of staff is unclear. Paperwork within human service organizations has reached crisis proportions, with studies and estimates suggesting that over 30 percent of a worker's time is consumed by such requirements. It is a major factor in reduced productivity, efficiency, job satisfaction, and even effectiveness. The reduction of paperwork, however, seems particularly incorrigible.

Forms can serve three legitimate purposes. First, forms provide the information needed for documentation, a record of what was done to whom, for instance. This information can help the agency meet professional standards set by accrediting bodies, protect itself against complaints and lawsuits, and satisfy requirements for funding. The majority of forms in agencies are devoted to this purpose.

Second, forms can act as tools for staff to help prompt and guide their work and as an aid in supervision. For example, a model of intervention that depends on an assessment of consumer strengths requires an assessment device that helps guide the practitioner and consumer through this process. Requiring social histories, listings and analysis of problems, deficits, and weaknesses, in addition, will not only consume a large amount of time but will distract the practitioner from the desired focus. Assessment and case planning forms are the most common manifestations of forms for this purpose.

Third, forms can act as the collector of performance information. Chapters 6 and 7 address this topic.

Paperwork reduction success stories. The process that a manager needs to follow to reduce paperwork varies by purpose, so forms for documentation and forms as tools will be treated separately. Our experience suggests that 90 percent of agencies are overdocumented and/or incorrectly documented. In other words, too much needless information is collected and some valuable information is still missing. Over time, some external group (e.g., state or federal government, insurance carriers, accrediting bodies) adds and occasionally deletes data requirements, while internal groups (managers, planners, information system specialists, supervisors) are doing the same. Managers have all too often assumed a passive position as these new intrusions occur by viewing the new demand as nonnegotiable or unchangeable.

One program manager took a different strategy. In trying to improve case management services to persons with psychiatric disabilities, she wanted to confront the need for intensive service with limited resources but did not want to be consumed with unnecessary paperwork. She collected all the forms being used and quickly observed that many were redundant in whole or in part, while others appeared useless. In answer to her question, "Why are we using this form?" her staff most frequently stated that it was required by the State Department of Mental Health, the County Mental Health Board, the Joint Commission on Accreditation of Hospitals, or all three. The manager called each organization and reviewed their requirements form by form. She found that some forms and information were not required at all; other information was required but could be collected much more simply or not as frequently; and other forms and information were negotiable. An example of the latter situation was a form required by the state to assess a consumer's functional status. When the supervisor demonstrated that this information in a different format was duplicated in their case assessment forms, the demand was withdrawn and one form was eliminated. When she was done, the required forms for case management were down to six pages. These six pages were designed to act as "tools" and still meet all documentation requirements.

Strategies for paperwork reduction. The following are strategies for reducing documentation requirements. First, the manager should establish a benchmark such as the following: no more than 10 or 15 percent of frontline staff's time can be consumed by paperwork. The burden then falls on the management to set documentation requirements that would accommodate such a goal.

Second, the manager can analyze the paperwork demands on frontline staff by creating two lists. The first list contains all of the "assumed" data and forms required by external agencies (e.g., accreditation, granting agencies, legislature). The goal of this list is to meet (or change) the requirements of the external agencies at the minimum acceptable level. This means the manager talks directly with people from these agencies, asking the following:

> What are the minimum requirements?
> How often must it be completed?
> What is the intent of the information?
> What is done with it and why is it important?

Many human service agencies are laboring under false assumptions about such requirements. Once this information is gathered, the manager orders people to only complete forms that meet the minimum requirements. Then the manager designs the simplest, least redundant way of collecting it.

The second list contains the forms and data requirements developed by the agency itself. With this list, the manager tests each data element and each form in terms of its presumed effects on the performance areas. The questions are as follows:

> How is this piece of information helpful to the work?
> What decisions or actions need to be informed by this data?

If the answers do not meet *explicit* tests of helpfulness, performance, action, and decision, they are automatically dropped. Another approach with this list is to do a zero-based paperwork review in which staff are to pretend that there are no requirements and develop needed forms as if the agency is new.

Third, exploit the power of the computer. Although the full potential of computers to reduce or eliminate paperwork is far from being achieved in social services, gains are being made. This is a long-term and perhaps costly strategy but one that is worth continually revisiting.

Memos and policies. Although forms seem to be the major culprit, the use of other kinds of paperwork can also needlessly consume resources. Some people rely on memos where a short e-mail or phone call would suffice or be more effective. Others believe that memos should include *all* the relevant information, which leads to several pages for each document. They are not only time consuming to write but the receivers also have to devote time to reading, thereby multiplying the time consumed.

Another paper producer is the predilection of many organizations to construct policies as a solution to organizational problems, which then means having them committed to paper, reproduced, distributed, read, and stored. The nature of bureaucracies, especially public ones with their concern with equity and rules, seems to encourage such practices. In such settings, thick policy and procedure manuals evolve quickly, and because of their size, density, and detail, are rarely used. In some human service organizations, separate units are established to design policies. Policies are seen as inflexible prescriptions for behavior and probably should be, but organizations and consumers are often not amenable to uniform prescriptions. The pattern is often that a policy is identified as not working as it does not handle all situations or handles them poorly, at which time a new one needs to be written to help cover these disparate situations. This pattern continues but the newer policies never seem to apply to all situations. In these cases, a policy is not needed but rather more staff training, better supervision, or a stronger organizational culture, in which people will make "correct" decisions and actions as they relate to particular situations.

Meetings. Many years ago, Drucker (1967) stated that every meeting is a waste of time.

> Meetings are by definition a concession to deficient organization. For one either meets or one works. One cannot do both at the same time. In an ideally designed structure there would be no meetings. Everyone would know what he needs to know to do his job. (p. 45)

This statement is as true today as it was in 1967. There is no perfectly designed organization and Drucker realized that. Meetings are a reality of organizational life and much of our precious time gets spent in them. Keeping Drucker's admonition in mind should be a first step in using meeting time more constructively. However, this is not enough. You need to know how to diagnose meeting time and what to do about it. The first step is to decide how much intra-organizational meeting time you are willing to tolerate, knowing that whatever time spent cannot be used to serve consumers. Ten percent of a worker's time seems like a reasonable amount to shoot for. The following are some useful guidelines for the use of meetings.

When Not to Have a Meeting

1. If the meeting is a substitute for action, do not have it. Can the next steps be taken without the meeting? Could the decision be made without the meeting? The key is knowing the goal of the meeting and determining whether the goals could be accomplished in another, more efficient manner.
2. If the meeting does not have an agenda, do not have it. This is an old and obvious point, but how many meetings have you attended that have not had agendas? Do not assume someone else has an agenda. If the agenda is not explicit, do not have the meeting.
3. If the meeting does not enhance performance, do not have it. This requires a clear link between the goals of the meeting and the goals of the organization. If the link is not obvious or seems forced, the meeting is not necessary.
4. If the purpose of the meeting is to convey information, do not have it. Announcements are more efficiently handled by memo.

What to Do to Prepare for the Meeting

1. Remember the chairperson does not do it alone. Frequently people "leave the running of the meeting to the person in charge." Do not do it! Help out. The behavior expected of someone who is designated as chairperson is also the responsibility of everyone else.
2. Prepare for the meeting. Look at the agenda. Think about the items. Do you need to take something with you? A few minutes of preparation can help save a lot of time at the meeting.
3. Set expectations. For a meeting to run efficiently, everyone needs to know and perform their role. You need to perform your role and also help establish expectations for everyone else. All of the points in this list are expectations for people's behavior. Follow this guide and expect it of others.

What to Do When the Meeting Starts

1. If the link between agenda items and performance is not explicit, question each item and delete those with no connection.
2. If someone only needs to be at part of the meeting, schedule them accordingly.
3. If the meeting does not begin on time, start it. You do not have to be the chair of the committee to get it going. Just suggest that the meeting begin and keep it up.
4. If someone wants you to come out of the meeting for a phone call or anything else, tell them later.
5. If someone is talking, listen. This is easier said than done. The mind loves to ramble. Test yourself as someone talks. Can you summarize what the person has said? Can you connect what they are saying to the central issue under discussion?
6. If the person talking begins to ramble, do not reinforce their behavior. Use nonverbal behavior consciously: Look away or attend to something else. When the person finishes, bring the group back to the question or agenda.
7. If closure on the point of discussion is evasive, push it. Help to reach closure by reflecting back on what has been said; summarize the points or positions presented, probe by asking follow-up questions.
8. If closure on an item is occurring, make certain that the action is explicit. What is the decision? Who is going to follow up? What is the next step?

What to Do After the Meeting

1. Make certain someone has summarized the meeting and distributed the summary to everyone who needs it.
2. Do your part. Take whatever next step you agree to and report back to the chairperson.

Organizational Structures As Obstacles

- *Hierarchy*
- *Paperwork*
- *Meetings*

Psychological Obstacles

This entire book is about new managerial methods and new perspectives. Given this, it is logical to identify obstacles that reside in the minds of managers and their staff. Chapter 2 is focused on organizational change and includes a model of behavioral intention that is equally applicable to managers. Social administrators are subject to the same barriers to action as other people. Many of these are created and sustained by structural features of the human service organization, but etiology is not the concern here. Rather, the concern is that there are personal and psychological stances that greatly impede organizational performance.

The absence of the managerial perspective reflected in the consumer-centered principles of Chapter 1 acts as a major barrier. For example, it is simply impossible to manage according to the inverted hierarchy if one does not have a healthy disrespect for the impossible. If you think that you cannot reduce paperwork, you will not. If you think that you cannot arrange training opportunities with such a limited budget, you will not.

Blaming and excusing. Many of the negative descriptors (e.g., complacent, defensive, rigid) of organizations, specific organizational units or people reflect a certain psychology characterized by feelings of impotence and insecurity at its roots. The most prevalent behavioral manifestations are in blaming or excusing. Common excuses for not performing are "not enough money," "not enough time," "not enough staff," or "not enough community resources." Blame is often focused on families, court personnel, other agencies, funders, administrators, and, most disturbingly, on the consumer. Some human services have even developed professional-sounding phrases for blame such as "the client is resistant to therapy." Blaming and excusing deflect responsibility from the agency and its personnel and reinforce feelings of impotence.

High-performing managers simply will not and do not tolerate blaming and excusing. The perspective is to identify obstacles that, for example, may be the behavior of court personnel. Obstacles, however, are meant to be attacked, removed, or attenuated. Where excuses and blame lead one to passivity, obstacles are susceptible to analysis, problem solving, and intervention. Every small increment of success can, therefore, produce an increment of confidence, control, and empowerment.

Detachment of personnel. Organizations unresponsive to employee needs, organizations that place a premium on control and permissions, organizations that ignore or punish extra effort or risk-taking on behalf of consumers, and organizations that place a premium on form rather than results come to be viewed as the enemy.

Employees, especially those in frontline positions who have the least power and responsibility, often become psychologically detached from these programs or organizations. It is a coping strategy—a protective device against feelings of low worth and hostility by the organization. The organization is not "me" but is personalized as upper management or the board of directors. The goal for the consumer-centered performance manager is to have each employee see themselves as the agency. They share responsibility for each success and each disappointment. In their contacts with consumers and key players, they realize that they not only represent the agency but they are the agency. Their names could just as easily be placed on the agency letterhead as the executive director. Part of their work identity is the organization, much like a part of a person's identity is the family or church.

Strategies for creating such feelings include the constant sharing of credit for agency successes, maintaining nurturing work environments, treating employees as adults by giving them responsibility and authority, permitting autonomy, encouraging risk taking, learning from failure, encouraging interdependence, creating winners, rewarding risk taking, and establishing an inspiring vision and concomitant values. The manager can also create other opportunities for linking personal and organizational identities: have frontline workers speak to community groups on behalf of the organization, arrange for workers to do presentations at statewide conferences on the agency's programs, encourage workers to attend board meetings or legislative hearings, involve workers on temporary task forces and work groups, have the organization be a regular source of prestige and rewards for the worker, place pictures of workers in annual reports, include stories of workers in newsletters, regularly ask everyone for their opinions and take them seriously, give frontline workers business cards, fill their offices with agency awards.

This section identified a large number of strategies for using the inverted hierarchy to improve outcomes for consumers. Managers begin the process of diagnosing a program when they become aware that there is a gap between expectations and performance. Exhibit 10.1 is a diagnostic tool that summarizes the ways that the inverted hierarchy can be used to improve results for consumers.

EXHIBIT 10.1. Diagnosing Inadequate Performance

The inverted hierarchy is a useful diagnostic tool when one perceives a gap between expectations and performance. Here is one way to organize the information into a diagnostic tool.

Expectations (direction):

Are they clear and unambiguous?
Are there conflicting expectations?
Is there consensus on the expectations?
Do people agree?
Who does not?
Are job descriptions, mission statements, program descriptions, evaluation procedures consistent with the expectations?

Tools:

Are the tools in place to help people meet the expectation?
Are people receiving meaningful and consistent feedback relevant to the expectation?
Do they have enough time to meet the expectation?
Are time-wasters (needless meetings and paperwork) minimized?
Are supportive policies and procedure in place?
Are resources adequate to meet the expectations?
Do people have the authority to meet the expectation?
Do the people have the skills in their repertoire to meet the expectations?
Do they have easy access to assistance for applying expectations to idiosyncratic case situations?

Rewards and Consequences:

What are the consequences for meeting the expectations?
Are adequate and meaningful rewards in place?
Is failure to meet minimum expectations treated in an unambiguous and direct manner?
Do people have the confidence to meet their expectations?
Do they believe that the expectations are "nice in theory" but really cannot be met? Are mechanisms in place to build people's sense of self-efficacy and make them feel like winners?

Obstacle Removal:

Are the mechanisms and responsibilities clear when obstacles to meeting expectations are confronted?

(continued)

(continued)

Do people have sanction to pursue obstacle removal?
Do supervisors help others translate complaints and excuses into
obstacles that can be addressed?
Are obstacle removal efforts publicized and celebrated?
Have people received training in diagnosing and addressing obstacles?
Are there means for reducing complexity?

POWERFUL INTEGRATING MECHANISMS: FIELD MENTORING, GROUP SUPERVISION, AND PERFORMANCE-ENHANCEMENT TEAMS

This chapter has organized and integrated the wide range of methods and tools into the *conceptual* framework of the inverted hierarchy. The *practice* of the consumer-centered manager benefits greatly when structures are created which allow and encourage the application of multiple methods of turning opportunities into action on a continuous basis. Three powerful structures for doing so are field mentoring, group supervision, and performance-enhancement teams. Each of these allows the supervisor to employ methods covered in this book: modeling, feedback, training, process monitoring, setting and reinforcing expectations, creating and sustaining a positive consumer-centered work culture and sense of esprit de corps, reward-based environment, and identifying and removing barriers. Furthermore, if done properly, group supervision, field mentoring, and performance-enhancement teams manifest and reinforce the following four principles of the consumer-centered model:

1. Venerating consumers
2. Focus on consumer outcomes
3. Learning for a living
4. A healthy disrespect for the impossible.

Field Mentoring and Supervision

Another indispensable component of helpful supervision is that which occurs while staff are actually doing their work in the field. The supervisor accompanies the case manager, for example, on visits with people or in meeting with particular community resources. The supervisor can observe the case manager and provide feedback on his or her skills in assessing strengths, formulating goals, and building relationships. The supervisor could model strengths-based methods in real-life situations or provide job coaching. Too often supervisors are unaware of exactly how case managers present themselves to others. This is a great opportunity for the supervisor to see the strengths of the case manager in action (use this information for rewarding and celebrating) as well as areas in which a person struggles.

This kind of field mentoring is very powerful. In the national Evidence-Based Practice Implementation Project (Drake et al., 2001), several sites had dramatic increases in fidelity after such efforts were made. There is nothing more difficult than taking skills taught in formal training and applying them in real practice. It is one of the reasons why the results of formal training on actual practice are so limited (Grinshaw et al., 2001). The supervisor acts as the helpful translator for such skills.

Many supervisors initially feel uncomfortable doing field mentoring because they think their staff will perceive it as overly intrusive. It is often threatening to have your skills be on display. If approached properly, we have found that most staff find field mentoring to be helpful and instructive.

Employment staff at a mental health center involved in the implementation of supported employment had been struggling with developing their skills in the area of job development. In fact, many of the staff had avoided going out to contact employers because of their fears and lack of skills. The staff involved in the project had been through training in job development and had some time to practice and role-play skills in training and team meetings. The employment staff's supervisor began to go out with her staff to observe how they were doing job development. The supervisor soon realized that her staff did not have the skills or the confidence to adequately engage and work with employers in order to help people obtain employment. The supervisor aggressively set a goal to spend 40 percent of her time for three months going out with her staff with the purpose to model skills, give feedback on skills, and build confidence. Six months later, one of the employment staff talked about the experience.

> After our training in job development, our supervisor set the expectation that we should be doing job development and set a certain number of contacts that we should be having with employers each month. I didn't really do it. I didn't like to do job development and did not feel comfortable doing it. I wasn't even sure about how to do it so I wasn't doing much. Later, my supervisor said she wanted to help us be more effective with our job development and would be going out regularly

with us to talk with employers. At first, I was really upset and did not want to do it. After a while, I realized that I was feeling more comfortable with talking with employers and that my supervisor was really helping me do it better. I really liked it when I started getting consumers jobs through my contact with employers. I realize now how helpful it was and how much better I am at job development.

Prior to a field-mentoring session, the supervisor and worker should define the purpose of the session. Is it for the supervisor to model certain skills? Is it to receive feedback on the worker's skills? For example, "I'm really having difficulty staying purposeful with Joe. Could you give me some feedback on what I could do differently" or "I would like for you to get a better picture of what is going on with Nancy so I can get more ideas during group supervision." The purpose could be what the supervisor would like to assess (i.e., "During our last training we talked about use of motivational interviewing techniques when discussing employment with people; I'd like to see how you are able to use some of these techniques in your practice.").

It is important that the goals of field mentoring are clear in order to keep it purposeful rather than being just a monitoring session. Being clear on the purpose of a particular field-mentoring session sets the stage for feedback following the session. The following is a suggested format for providing feedback on completion of field mentoring:

1. Restate the purpose of the particular field-mentoring session (i.e., to give you feedback on how you could be more purposeful with Joe).
2. Point out specific strengths of the case manager observed during field mentoring.
3. Point out specific words, behaviors, or actions that might have been obstacles to the case manager reaching his or her desired outcomes.
4. Make a plan for follow-up.

In order to give a staff good feedback following the session, it is important that the supervisor be an active observer during field mentoring and restrain from trying to do the work themselves (unless the purpose of the field-mentoring session was for the supervisor to demonstrate a particular skill). This does not mean that the supervisor does not interact in the session (i.e., distant observer), but rather is consciously allowing the staff to do their work so as to give them the feedback requested. Remember, the purpose of field mentoring is to help the worker improve their skills and not to demonstrate how great the supervisor is.

*Group Supervision**

The inverted hierarchy framework avers that the central purpose of supervision is to help case managers do their jobs on behalf of consumers in an effective, efficient, and satisfying way. Group supervision has been found to be a principal mechanism for achieving these supervisory purposes. In its most frequent form, group supervision involves a unit or team of direct service workers (usually four to six) and their supervisor. At times, specialists participate. Occasionally family members or key actors (e.g., friend, minister, employer) may be invited. The group meetings vary in length and frequency. The recommended and most frequent scheduling is once a week for two hours.

During this two-hour period, two to four difficult consumer situations are intensely discussed. The selection of situations is usually delegated to direct service workers with perhaps consultation by the supervisor. The selection is based on consumer situations on which the worker desires new ideas. Typically, these are consumers who have been unable to achieve their goals. Other situations particularly amenable to group supervision are:

1. Lack of progress in engaging with a person or developing a relationship.
2. Situations where workers are having difficulty identifying consumer strengths or developing a direction for helping as manifest in case plans.
3. Difficulties with particular key actors in gaining access or accommodation.
4. Consumer goals where identification of community resources has been lacking.

Crisis situations are rarely appropriate for group supervision; instead, the worker should consult directly with the supervisor or specialist at the time of the crisis.

Each discussion of a consumer situation begins with the distribution of the consumer's assessment and most recent case plan(s) and a presentation of the particular situation by the worker. This presentation should include the following:

1. A statement of the difficulty or problem
2. A statement of what the worker would like to see instead (desired state) and how the group can help
3. A complete list of strategies and efforts already tried to achieve the desired state.

---

*Much of this section is taken from Rapp, C. A., & Goscha, R. J. (2006). *The strengths model: Case management with people with psychiatric disabilities.* Reprinted with permission.

This presentation is then followed by questions from the group and brainstorming solutions or alternative. Statements of empathy and support are often exchanged. Minimum standards for brainstorming usually include that at least three potential alternatives be generated. Each discussion of a consumer situation closes with the worker repeating the alternatives and perhaps indicating the one believed to be most promising. The worker also tells the group what the next discrete step is (e.g., consult with consumer on Thursday; phone Ms. Harris at the Garden of Eden nursery; write on paper the information needed to employ a two-sided argument with the landlord). Each consumer situation discussion usually lasts between 25 and 40 minutes.

Group supervision also includes each worker sharing one or more achievements from the past week, some of which could be derived from past group supervision brainstorming. This kind of "celebration" is found to be uplifting and energizing for workers.

The Methods of Group Supervision

The session should start on time. Interruptions and distractions should be avoided, whether from other staff entering the room, telephone calls, or consumer demands. If interruptions cannot be totally eliminated, the *specific* situations warranting interruptions need to be written and all staff and perhaps consumers notified.

The setting for the group supervision should be large enough for the members to arrange themselves comfortably in a circle. Some teams benefit from having a chalk board or flip chart present. Although the location is most often a room within the case management agency, some group supervisions have occurred in a church or other community facility, or in the supervisor's home. One case management team held their weekly group supervision in a gazebo located in a cemetery across from the mental health center. The supervisor said that it was quiet, there were no interruptions, and it was convenient.

The selection of the situations to be presented and the order should be established before the group supervision or within the first few minutes of beginning. The worker should have copies of the consumer's assessment and recent case plan(s) sufficient for each person in the group. Group supervision is about consumers and the work with them. Discussion of policies, new procedures, or other agency topics should be rigorously avoided unless they directly pertain to the consumer situation under discussion. These topics need to be transmitted and often discussed but this should occur at some other opportunity.

Group supervision is to be an uplifting experience, enjoyable if not fun. Supervisors and workers should laugh. Efforts that workers make on behalf of consumers (whether they succeed or not), creative or particularly skillful methods that were employed (whether they succeeded or not), and specific achievements (including small ones) should be recognized if not celebrated. When group supervision is really working, the exchange of "pats on the back" come from all team members, not just the supervisor.

The ambiance of group supervision should be characterized as positive and optimistic. This does not mean that frustrations are not permitted or acknowledged. They surely must be. However, group supervision needs to help a particular worker get beyond that by reminding the person of how far the consumer has come, recognizing the efforts made to date, helping the worker "see the forest through the trees" and regaining a focus on consumer achievement, and generating alternative ideas and strategies.

There are certain conditions that facilitate creativity and idea generation, and obstacles. One facilitating condition is for everyone to be clear on the desired outcome. This is why the worker is required to tell the group what the desired state would be and how the group can be helpful. At times, this requires the worker to do some thinking ahead of time. It is often easier to say "Joe needs to stop swearing in the café" than to specify what Joe should be doing. Like work with consumers, setting goals as the presence of something rather than an absence is more conducive to achievement. At times, a case manager may have difficulty doing this. In these situations, the case manager should state this and instruct the group that this is what he or she wants help with.

Another facilitating condition is for members to have the necessary information. Over the last twenty-five years, we have found three pieces of information to be critical. First is a clear statement of the dilemma or problem and why it is a problem for the consumer and others. Second is information on the consumer's strengths, goals, efforts, and achievements reflected in the case plan. What the consumer wants in the particular situation is often forgotten, but is critical to generating ideas and selecting the ones to try. This is not always obvious. For example, the person who loudly swears in the café and therefore will not be permitted to return may want to continue eating lunch at the café or want to talk to someone while eating. Third is that all the strategies have already been tried by the worker with some level of detail. This last set of information is important to reduce or eliminate some of the "yeah—but I already tried that." "Yeah—buts" waste time and place a pall over brainstorming. Other information, specific to the situation being examined, can be gathered through questioning. Particularly productive sources of questions are the program design and other material (e.g., fidelity guides, methods covered in training) that specify the methods to be used. Often even the most skilled worker has not followed all the methods specified in the model.

Once the desired state has been precisely described and relevant information shared, only then does idea generation commence. The two stages of information gathering and idea generation should be kept separate when possible, otherwise time will be wasted—prematurely generating ideas just to have them discounted because all the information was not taken into account.

The brainstorming phase of consumer situation discussions should be characterized by the free flow of ideas. Evaluation of the ideas should be left to the next phase. If brainstorming is to flourish, evaluation and selection of ideas need to be kept separate from idea generation. The aim is to generate as many different ideas by as many people as possible and not to evaluate or select the best. Often the most "crazy" idea, if allowed to be shared, can provoke a similar but perhaps more feasible idea. Some teams even have an award as in the following example:

A case manager was having difficulty helping a person keep an apartment because the consumer always said the apartment was covered in roaches. Even after several moves to apartments that seemed to be "roach-free," the person would continue to complain of seeing roaches everywhere and would leave the apartment. The case manager brought this situation looking for ideas, since she had no idea of where to go next and was frustrated. After several minutes of brainstorming, one person on the team offered a very nontraditional idea. She stated that she heard that geckos kept roaches away. The case manager took this idea to the person she was working with, and the consumer wanted to try this in her next apartment. In fact, she wanted to get two geckos. We are still not sure whether there is any truth to geckos keeping roaches away, but in this woman's mind it was working and she never complained of roaches again. We started giving out "The Gecko Award" (a rubber gecko mounted on a piece of wood) to any team member who came up with a "wild and extremely nontraditional" idea that actually ended up working.

The worker is responsible for recording all the ideas generated. The use of a flip chart is often helpful because it allows everyone to keep track of ideas already generated. Brainstorming continues until the group has exhausted its ideas and the worker has at least three promising or "reasonable" ideas to try. The evaluation and selection of ideas are the workers' and consumers' responsibility. although the group surely can comment and suggest. Options that require the least change by the consumer and/or resource, *if they are attractive to the consumer,* should be given extra consideration. since they often have the most probability of success, both short term and long term. The discussion of a particular consumer situation concludes with the worker identifying the "best" ideas and specifying the first (next) discrete step he or she will take.

The group supervision format, with its difficult consumer situation focus and group involvement, enhances professional learning beyond that allowed by individual supervision. Learning is enhanced by the supervisor (or others), helping the group to generalize from the discussion of specific consumers. The supervisor points out similarities with other consumer situations or strategies used successfully by other workers. Learning also occurs in terms of community resources. Except in the smallest of communities, will any worker be fully apprised of all the resources available? Often a resource that is identified in group supervision is eventually rejected for that particular consumer situation but gets used for another consumer.

The Role of the Group Supervision Facilitator

The person who facilitates group supervision must be focused and able to stay on task. For many teams, the supervisor has the role of facilitating group supervision, but some teams decide to rotate responsibilities for facilitating group supervision discussions. It takes some discipline to facilitate quality group supervision, because for most people the group supervision process presented here is a departure from traditional formats. One supervisor stated that a facilitator has to be "a little obnoxious" in order to keep the various parts of the group supervision process separated and maximized to their fullest potential. It can take several months of weekly group supervision, with copies of the process (Exhibit 10.2) in front of each person, before it finally became part of their regular routine. Without a facilitator helping to maintain the discipline required, it will be easy for the team to revert to old ways of doing things.

The Power of Group Supervision

Group supervision is consumers, consumers, consumers. Nothing else should be allowed to intrude. Rather than "talk about" cases, the team works together generating specific alternatives to be implemented. The overall effect is one of empowerment, not continued frustration. The alternatives

EXHIBIT 10.2. Group Supervision: Structure and Process

Purpose:	1. Support and affirmation 2. Ideas/information 3. Learning
Who:	Supervisor and three to four case managers
When:	Once a week for 1.5 to 2 hours (starts on time, no interruptions
Agenda:	"Consumers, Consumers, Consumers" Two to four difficult consumer situations
	"Ticket to Group Supervision" Strengths Assessment/Personal Plans
Beginning:	1. Case manager distributes strengths assessment and personal plan 2. Describes the difficulty 3. Describes the desired situation and how the group can help 4. Lists what efforts and strategies have been used to reach the desired situation
The Middle:	1. Brainstorming 2. Case manager is responsible for recording all ideas
The Ending:	1. Case manager with group help selects three best ideas 2. Case manager identifies first step(s) 3. Notes of next tasks are recorded 4. Move to next case situations
Closing Group Supervision	1. Each case manager shares a consumer/ case manager achievements(s) during the last week

may not work, but the team will learn from it and other alternatives will be produced. The advantages of group supervision include the following:

1. Generate more ideas regarding creative alternatives in working with challenging circumstances
2. Ethnic and cultural diversity present in the group may help in understanding consumer behavior from a cultural perspective
3. Support and affirmation from colleagues who understand how challenging, frustrating, and disappointing the work can be

4. Having others with whom you can share successful helping efforts and consumer success stories
5. Can help with the "can't see the forest for the trees" phenomenon. One may get a different perspective from a colleague who is not as intimately involved with the consumer
6. When circumstances suggest difficult treatment decisions (e.g., petitioning for involuntary commitment or removing a child from their home), workers may feel a sense of sharing and consensus; in effect, the decision becomes a team decision rather than an individual one
7. May be more efficient in terms of time allotted to supervision and communicating information and ideas to each worker
8. The entire team becomes familiar with consumers, and on-call crisis coverage may be shared and individualized response delivered
9. Workers may gain support in the face of opposition from other providers regarding treatment decision
10. Team may enjoy sessions and have fun while helping each other
11. There may be generalized learning—ideas or resources discussed for one consumer may have relevance for others
12. Workers may feel a sense of respite—a time away from the telephone calls, consumer requests, other demands on their time.

At the end of this chapter are two tools developed to help guide and evaluate group supervision. The first one, "Case Manager's Group Supervision Feedback," was designed for case managers to evaluate the sessions and provide feedback to the supervisors and other case managers. The second one, "Supervisor's Group Supervision Monitor" allows the supervisor to evaluate the session and his or her performance. Teams are urged to use these as a basis for exchanging feedback and for fulfilling group supervision's promise of increased efficiency, satisfaction, and effectiveness.

This model of group supervision satisfies many of the conditions for adult learning and is an efficient means of conducting training. We suggest that learning through this type of supervision is often more effective than the normal workshop format. The following is a description of a group supervision session that has been greatly telescoped for purposes of presentation.

Performance-Enhancement Teams

The people who work directly with consumers are in the best position to know their successes and challenges. The group supervision model relies on this knowledge to have staff engage in learning, rewarding and empowering each other. Performance-enhancement teams have demonstrated a benefit to consumers, and are another model of supervision that we present here.

Yeaman, Craine, Gorsek, and Corrigan (2000) found that the use of a performance-improvement team model resulted in mental health consumers increasing their knowledge of medication skills, symptom management, leisure skills, and physical health by at least 25 percent. In addition, the number of aggressive incidents occurring in the facility decreased to 25 percent of the original rate. This research was conducted in an organization that was concerned with assisting consumers to return to the community and function with the appropriate help from the mental health system. The program achieved these results through teaching skills that help consumers cope with their illness and return to the community.

Performance-enhancement teams are a popular topic in the management literature. However, there are many different definitions for performance-enhancement teams. Wageman (2001) demonstrated that the design choices that managers make in creating these teams effects task performance. Consequently, to describe the performance-improvement team model employed by Yeaman et al. (2000), we will use Wageman's framework.

1. Defining the team as a group with clear membership that is stable over time. In the mental health example, the Psychiatric Rehabilitation Performance Improvement Team was a committee whose members were selected from the disciplines across the entire center.
2. Giving the team purpose that is stated clearly. If more than one purpose is stated, there should be few enough to be remembered by the team and the leader, focused on the ends to be achieved rather than on the details of the means to be used.

   The Performance Improvement Team was given the mission: "To assist patients to increase their success in coping with the environment so they can function in the community with the appropriate help from the mental health systems." This single purpose statement states clearly that the focus is on results.
3. An enabling team structure that includes
   a. Appropriate team size, meaning no larger than the minimum required to accomplish the work.

      This criterion is vague and the size of the Performance Improvement Team was not clearly indicated in the report. However it appeared to consist of 8 members representing the disciplines working in the Center.

b. Skill diversity with substantial heterogeneity of task-relevant skills but not so much that members have difficulty coordinating their efforts.

   The Performance Improvement Team consisted of a professionally heterogeneous staff from psychosocial rehabilitation, psychology, nursing, mental health technicians, social work, psychiatry, activity therapy, and vocational services.

c. Task interdependence.

   The professionally diverse staff of the Performance Improvement Team assured interdependence since no one discipline could achieve the mission by itself.

d. Challenging task goals.

   The Performance Improvement Team identified six task goals that included conducting a needs assessment by surveying staff and consumers; reviewing the results of the needs assessment with each unit; expanding skills training programs (an evidence-based practice) to day, evening, and weekends; recruiting a variety of disciplines to participate in skills training; regularly evaluating new skills training programs; and modifying programs according to regular assessment.

e. Articulated strategy norms that legitimize and support active strategizing and long-term planning by the team.

   The staff of the organization had a consumer orientation and knowledge of the principles and strategies of psychiatric rehabilitation as effective to improving the quality of life in persons with severe mental illness. These strategic norms along with the mission statement provided support for long-term planning by the team.

4. A supportive organizational structure that provides:
   a. A reward system that recognizes and rewards excellent team performance.
   b. An information system that provides information members require to plan their collective work.
   c. An education system that is available to provide training or technical assistance for the team.

Although the research report of the Performance Improvement Team does not specifically address each of these points, there is enough information to indicate that there was a supportive organizational structure. The director of the facility had an eighteen-month record of pursuing performance-improvement initiatives. A performance-improvement steering committee existed prior to initiation of the reported effort. Education of staff and consumers was an ongoing emphasis in the facility. Although rewards were not explicitly discussed, it is apparent that with the goal of consumer improvement and subsequent documentation of success, rewards to the team were produced. The information system did not apparently exist but became part of the team's efforts. It appears that a good deal of their efforts was expended on collecting, synthesizing, reporting, and reacting to information.

SUMMARY

The consumer-centered model of social administration is practiced within the structure of the inverted hierarchy as presented in this chapter. Consumer-centeredness is the degree to which consumers and their well-being intrude on or flavor all aspects of agency behavior. The model is built upon assumptions that consumers are the reason that social programs exist and therefore the focus of all organizational activities, that the criterion of organizational performance is producing consumer benefits, and that managerial performance is judged by organizational performance. This performance begins with outcomes for consumers and includes attention to service events, resource acquisition, staff morale, and efficiency. Emerging management research is beginning to support the idea that management behavior is linked to results for consumers.

To achieve the lofty goals of consumer-centered social administration, we posit that managers operate on a day-to-day basis with the principles of venerating consumers, establishing and maintaining organizational focus on consumer outcomes, having a healthy disrespect for the impossible, and learning for a living. The tools available to social administrators to operationalize these principles are their time and skills. These skills include influencing others to play their role in helping consumers achieve through carefully structured persistent interactions over time; creating and maintaining a consumer-centered, reward-based, and learning organization through carefully reinforced norms, values, and behaviors; creating program specifications that are most likely to produce consumer benefits; using information and feedback to pilot the program to success; acquiring and directing personnel to achieve personal and consumer success; and acquiring and managing funds to achieve the maximum benefit for consumers. These skills are integrated into practice through the mechanisms of field mentoring, group supervision, and performance-enhancement teams.

References

Achenenbach, T. (2001). *Child Behavior Checklist for Ages 6-18* [Online]. Available: www.aseba.org.

Adoption and Safe Families Act of 1997, Pub.L. No. 105-89, 42 USC 1305, 111 Stat 2115 (1997).

Agency for Healthcare Research and Quality (2004). *Closing the Quality Gap: Fact Sheet—A Critical Analysis of Quality Improvement Strategies* [Online]. Available: www.ahrq.gov/clinic/epc/qgapfact.htm.

Ahearn, K. K. (1999). *The impact of supervisory behavior on permanency rates for foster children in a child welfare context.* Unpublished doctoral dissertation, University of Illinois at Urbana-Champaign.

Alter, C. F. (2000). Interorganizational collaboration in the task environment. In R. Patti (Ed.), *The handbook of social welfare management* (pp. 283-302). Thousand Oaks, California: Sage Publications.

Alvero, A. M., Bucklin, B. R., & Austin, J. (2001). An objective review of the effectiveness and essential characteristics of performance feedback in organizational settings (1985-1998). *Journal of Organizational Behavior Management, 21*(1), 3-29.

Anderson, R. B. (1995). Cognitive appraisal of performance capability in the prevention of drunken driving: A test of self-efficacy theory. *Journal of Public Relations Research, 7,* 205-229.

Anderson, R. B. (2000). Vivacious and persuasive influences on efficacy expectations and intentions to perform breast self-examination. *Public Relations Review, 26,* 97-114.

Argyris, C. (1999). *On organizational learning* (Second edition). Malden, MA: Blackwell Business.

Argyris, C. (2004). *Reasons and rationalizations: The limits to organizational knowledge.* Oxford: Oxford University Press.

Argyris, C., & Schon, D. (1978). *Organizational learning: A theory of action perspective.* Reading, MA: Addison Wesley.

Argyris, C., & Schon, D. (1996). *Organizational learning II.* Reading, MA: Addison-Wesley.

Axelrod, S., & Wetzler, S. (1989). Factors associated with better compliance with psychiatric aftercare. *Hospital and Community Psychiatry, 40,* 397-401.

Textbook of Social Administration: The Consumer-Centered Approach
© 2007 by The Haworth Press, Inc. All rights reserved.
doi:10.1300/5802_12

Balcazar, F. E., Hopkins, B. L., & Suarez, Y. (1985). A critical objective review of performance feedback. *Journal of Organizational Behavior Management, 7,* 65-89.

Baldwin, T. T., & Ford, J. K. (1988). Transfer of training: A review and directions for future research. *Personnel Psychology, 41,* 63-101.

Barnoski, R., & Aos, S. (2004). *Outcome evaluation of Washington State's research-based programs for juvenile offenders* [On-line]. Available: www.wsipp .wa.gov.

Becker, D. R., & Drake, R. E. (2003). *A working life for people with severe mental illness.* New York: Oxford University Press.

Becker, D. R., Smith, J., Tanzman, B., Drake, R. E., & Tremblay, T. (2001). Fidelity of supported employment program outcomes. *Psychiatric Services, 52,* 834-836.

Becker, D. R., Xie, H., McHugo, G. J., Halliday, J., & Martinez, R. A. (2006). What predicts supported employment program outcomes? *Community Mental Health Journal, 42,* 303-315.

Bero, L. A., Grilli, R., Grinshaw, J. M., Harvey, E., Oxman, A.D., & Thomsom, M. A. (1998). Getting research findings into practice. Closing the gap between research and practice: An overview of systematic reviews of interventions to promote the implementation of research findings. *British Journal of Medicine, 317,* 465-468.

Bond, G. R., McGrew, J. H., & Fekete, D. M. (1995). Assertive outreach for frequent users of psychiatric hospitals: A meta-analysis. *Journal of Mental Health Administration, 22*(1), 4-16.

Bond, G. R., & Salyers, M. P. (2004). Prediction of outcome from the Dartmouth ACT Fidelity Scale. *CNS Spectrums, 9,* 937-942.

Bronfenbrenner, U. (1995a). Developmental ecology through space and time: A future perspective. In P. Moen, G.H. Elder Jr., & K. Luscher (Eds.), *Examining lives in context: perspectives on the ecology of human development* (pp. 619-648). Washington, DC: American Psychological Association.

Bronfenbrenner, U. (1995b). The bioecological model from a life course perspective: Reflections of a participant observer. In P. Moen, G.H. Elder Jr., & K. Luscher (Eds.), *Examining lives in context: perspectives on the ecology of human development* (pp. 599-618). Washington, DC: American Psychological Association.

Buckingham, M., & Coffman, C. (1999). *First, break all the rules: What the world's greatest managers do differently.* New York: Simon & Schuster.

Burger, J. M. (1999). The foot-in-the-door compliance procedure: A multiple-process analysis and review. *Personality and Social Psychology Review, 3,* 303-325.

Carli, L. L. (2004). Gender effects on social influence. In J. S. Sieter & R. H. Gass. (Eds.), *Perspectives on persuasion, social influence and compliance gaining* (pp. 207-222). Boston, MA: Pearson Education, Inc.

Cheney, D., & Osher, T. (1997). Collaborate with families. *Journal of Emotional and Behavioral Disorders, 5*(1), 36-44.

Chicago Community Trust (2005). *Reflection: 2004 annual report* [Online]. Available: www.cct.org/publications_research/2004_AR.pdf.

Cialdini, R. B., & Guadagno, R. E. (2004). Sequential request compliance tactics. In J. S. Sieter & R. H. Gass (Eds.), *Perspectives on persuasion, social influence and compliance gaining* (pp. 207-222). Boston, MA: Pearson Education, Inc.

Clegg, V. L., & Cashin, W. E. (1986). Improving multiple-choice tests. *Idea paper No. 16.* Manhattan, KS: Center for Faculty Evaluation and Development, Kansas State University.

Cohen, J. A., & Mannarion, A. P. (1997). A treatment study for sexually abused pre-school children: Outcome during a one-year follow-up. *Journal of the American Academy of Child and Adolescent Psychiatry, 36*(9), 1228-1235.

Cohen, J. A., & Mannarion, A. P., & Knudsen, K. (2005). Treating sexually abused children: One year follow-up of a randomized controlled trial. *Child Abuse and Neglect 29,* 135-145.

Cook, J. A., Toprac, M., & Shore, J. E. (2004). Combining evidence-based practice with stakeholder consumers to enhance psychosocial rehabilitation services in the Texas Benefit Design Initiative. *Psychiatric Rehabilitation Journal, 27*(4), 307-318.

Cooper, J., & Stone, J. (2000). Cognitive dissonance and the social group. In D. J. Terry & M. A. Hogg (Eds.), *Attitudes, behaviors, and social context: The role of norms and group membership* (pp. 227-244). Mahwah, New Jersey: Lawrence Erlbaum Associates, Publishers.

Corcoran, K., & Fisher, J. (2000a). *Measures for clinical practice: A sourcebook vol. 1: Couples, families and children* (Third edition). New York: The Free Press.

Corcoran, K., & Fisher, J. (2000b). *Measures for clinical practice: A sourcebook vol. 2: Adults* (Third edition). New York: The Free Press.

Corrigan, P. W., Giffort, D., Rashid, F., Leary, M., & Okeke, I. (1999). Recovery as a psychological construct. *Community Mental Health Journal, 35*(3), 231-239.

Corrigan, P. W., Lickey, S.E., Campion, J., & Rashid, F. (2000). Mental health team leadership and consumer satisfaction and quality of life. *Psychiatric Services, 51*(6), 781-785.

Council on Foundations (2005). *Community foundation* [Online]. Available: www .cof.org/Content/General/Display.cfm?contentID=120#c.

Curry, D. H., Caplan, P., & Knuppel, J. (1994). Transfer of training and adult learn-ing (TOTAL). *Journal of Continuing Social Work Education, 6*(1), 8-14.

David and Lucile Packard Foundation (2005). *Home page* [Online]. Available: www.packard.org/index.cgi?page=home.

Deal, T., & Kennedy, A. A. (1982). *Corporate cultures: The rites and rituals of cor-porate life.* Reading, MA: Addison-Wesley Pub. Co.

Deal, T., & Peterson, K. D. (1999). *Shaping school culture: The heart of leadership.* San Francisco: Jossey-Bass Publishers.

DiBerardinis, J., Ramage, K., & Levitt, S. (1984). Risky shift and gender of the advocate: Information theory versus normative theory. *Group & Organizational Studies, 9,* 189-200.

Douglas County Community Foundation (2005). *Foundation awards more than $186,000 in grants* [Online]. Available: www.dccfoundation.org.

Drake, R. E., Goldman, H. H., Leff, H. S., Lehman, A. F., Dixon, L., Mueser, K. T., & Torrey, W. C. (2001). Implementing evidence-based practices in routine mental health service settings. *Psychiatric Services, 52*(2), 179-182.

Drucker, P. F. (1967). *The effective executive.* London: Pan Books.

Eber, I., & Rolf, K. (1998). Education's Role in Systems of Care: Student/Family Outcomes. *10th annual research conference proceedings. A system of care for children's mental health: Expanding the research base* (pp. 175-180) [Online]. Available: http://www.fmhi.usf.edu/institute/pubs/pdf/cfs/rtc/10thproceedings/10thproctoc.html.

Ewing Marion Kauffman Foundation (2005). *About the foundation* [Online]. Available: www.kauffman.org/foundation.cfm.

Ezell, M. (2002). A case study of an agency's three family preservation contracts. *Family Preservation Journal, 6*(1), 31-50.

Fairweather, G.W. (1972). *Social change: The challenge to survival.* Morristown, NJ: General Learning Systems.

Fine, S. A., & Cronshaw, S. F. (1999). *Functional job analysis: A foundation for human resource management.* Mahway, NJ: Erlbaum Associates.

Frantz, J. P. (1994). Effect location and procedural explicitness on user processing of and compliance with product warnings. *Human Factors, 36,* 532-546.

Freagon, S. (2001). *Variables determining school and early childhood success* [Online]. Available: www.cedu.niu.edu.

Friedman, V. J., Lipshitz, R., & Overmeer, W. (2001). Creating conditions for organizational learning. In M. Dierkes, A. G. Antal, J. Child, & I. Nonaka (Eds.), *Handbook of organizational learning and knowledge* (pp. 757-774). Oxford: Oxford University Press.

Gambrill, E. (1999). Evidence-based practice: An alternative to authority-based practice. *Families in Society: The Journal of Contemporary Human Services, 80*(4), 341-350.

Gass, R. H., & Sieter, J. S. (2004). Theorizing about persuasion: Cornerstones of persuasion research. In J. S. Sieter & R. H. Gass (Eds.), *Perspectives on persuasion, social influence and compliance gaining* (pp. 45-64). Boston, MA: Pearson Education, Inc.

Gibbs, L., & Gambrill, E. (2002). Evidence-based practice: Counterarguments to objections. *Research on Social Work Practice, 12*(3), 452-476.

Glisson, C. (2000). Organizational climate and culture. In R. J. Patti (Ed.), *The handbook of social welfare management* (pp. 195-218). Thousand Oaks: CA Sage Publications, Inc.

Glisson, C., & Hemmelgarn, A. (1998). The effects of organizational climate and interorganizational coordination on the quality and outcomes of children's service systems. *Child Abuse & Neglect, 22*(5), 401-421.

Government Printing Office (1996). *Code of Federal Regulations Title 45–Public Welfare* [Online]. Available: www.gpoaccess.gov/cfr/index.html.

Grasso, A. J. (1994). Management style, job satisfaction, and service effectiveness. *Administration in Social Work, 18*(4), 89-105.

Gray, J. A. M. (2001). *Evidence-based healthcare* (Second edition). London: Churchill Livingston.

Gregoire, T. K., Propp, J., & Poertner, J. (1998). The supervisor's role in transfer of training. *Administration in Social Work, 22*(1), 1-18.

Grimshaw, J. M., Shirran, L., Thomas, R., Mowatt, G., Fraser, C., & Bero, L. (2001). Changing provider behavior: An overview of systematic reviews of interventions. *Medical Care, 39*(8), II-2-II-45.

Gummer, B. (2001). Innovate or die: The necessity for change in contemporary organizations. *Administration in Social Work, 25*(3), 65-84.

Hagan, J. (1990). Training income maintenance workers: A look at the empirical evidence. *Journal of Continuing Social Work Education, 5*(2), 3-8.

Hagen, K. M., Gutkin, T. B., Wilson, C. P., & Oats, R. G. (1998). Using vicarious experience and verbal persuasion to enhance self-efficacy in pre-service teachers: "Priming the pump" for consultation. *School Psychology Quarterly, 13,* 169-178.

Hale, J. L., Householder, B. J., & Greene, K. L. (2002). The theory of reasoned action. In J. P. Dillard & M. Pfau (Eds.), *The persuasion handbook: Developments in theory and practice* (pp. 259-288). Thousand Oaks, California: Sage Publications.

Harkness, D. (1995). The art of helping in supervised practice: Skills, relationships, and outcomes. *Clinical Supervisor, 13*(1), 63-76.

Harkness, D. (1997). Testing interactional social work theory: A panel analysis of supervised practice and outcomes. *Clinical Supervisor, 15*(1), 33-50.

Harkness, D., & Hensley, H. (1991). Changing the focus of social work supervision: Effects on client satisfaction and generalized contentment. *Social Work, 36*(6), 506-512.

Harms, T., & Clifford, R. M. (2000). *Family day care rating scale* [Online]. Available: www.fpg.unc.edu/~ecers.

Harris, G., Poertner, J., & Joe, S. (2000). The parents with children in foster care satisfaction scale. *Administration in Social Work, 24*(2), 15-27.

Hasenfeld, Y. (2000). Social welfare administration and organizational theory. In R. J. Patti (Ed.), *The handbook of social welfare management* (pp. 3-25). Thousand Oaks, CA: Sage Publications, Inc.

Henggeler, S. W., Schoenwald, S. K., Borduin, C. M., Rowland, M. D., & Cunningham, P. B. (1998). *Multisystemic treatment of antisocial behavior in children and adolescents.* New York: The Guilford Press.

Henggeler, S. W., Schoenwald, S. K., Rowland, M. D., & Cunningham, P. B. (2002). *Serious emotional disturbance in children and adolescents.* New York: The Guilford Press.

Hetts, J. J., Boninger, S. S., Armor, D. A., Gleicher, F., & Nathanson, A. (2000). The influence of anticipated counterfactual regret on behavior. *Psychology and Marketing, 17,* 345-368.

Hoagwood, K., & Erwin, H. D. (1997). Effectiveness of school based mental health services for children: A 10 year research review. *Journal of Child and Family Studies, 6*(4), 435-451.

Howard, M. O., & Jenson, J. M. (1999). Clinical practice guidelines: Should social work develop them? *Research in Social Work Practice, 9,* 283-301.

Jayaratne, S., Croxton,T. A., & Mattison, D. (2004). A national survey of violence in the practice of social work. *Families in Society: The Journal of Contemporary Social Services, 85*(4), 445-453.

Johnson, B., Morriss, L., & McElhiney, L. E. (1998). Impact of a Parent Liaison on a Special Day School Setting. *Tenth annual research conference proceedings. A system of care for children's mental health: Expanding the research base* (pp. 181-184) [Online]. Available: http://www.fmhi.usf.edu/institute/pubs/pdf/cfs/rtc/10thproceedings/10thproctoc.html.

Judge, T. A., Higgins, C. A., & Cable, D. M. (2000). The employment interview: A review of recent research and recommendations for future research. *Human Resource Management Review, 10*(4), 383-406.

Kansas Department of Administration (May 27, 2004). *Request for proposal–Reintegration, foster care services* [Online]. Available: http://da.state.ks.us/purch.

Kansas Department of Social and Rehabilitation Services (2005). *Portraits: A data album of families served through children and family services FY 2005.* Topeka, KS: Department of Social and Rehabilitation Services.

Kaplan, R. S., & Norton, D. P. (2001). *The strategy-focused organization: How balanced scorecard companies thrive in the new business environment.* Boston, MA: Harvard Business School Press.

Kaplan, R. S., & Norton, D. P. (1992). The balanced scorecard: Measures that drive performance. *Harvard Business Review, 70*(1), 71-79.

Kaplan, R. S., & Norton, D. P. (1993). Putting the balanced scorecard to work. *Harvard Business Review, 71*(5), 134-147.

Kaplan, R. S., & Norton, D. P. (1996). *The balanced scorecard: Translating strategy into action.* Boston, MA: Harvard Business School Press.

King, N. J., Tonge, B. J., Mullen, P., Myerson, N., Heyne, D., Rollings, S., Martin, R., & Ollendick, T. H. (2000). Treating sexually abused children with post-traumatic stress symptoms: A randomized clinical trial. *Journal of the American Academy of Child and Adolescent Psychiatry, 39*(11), 1347-1355.

Klingner, D. E., & Nalbandian, J. (2003). *Public personnel management: Contexts and strategies* (Fifth edition). Upper Saddle River, New Jersey: Prentice Hall.

Kotter, J. (1996). *Leading change.* Boston, MA: Harvard Business School Press.

Lawler III, E. E. (1996). *From the ground up: Six principles for building the new logic corporation.* San Francisco, CA: Jossey-Bass, Inc. Publishers.

Lewin Group (2000). *Assertive community treatment: A literature review* [Online]. Available: www.mentalhealth.samhsa.gov/cmhs/communitysupport/toolkits/community.

Lehman, A. F., Steinwachs, D. M., and the survey coinvestigators of the PORT Project (1998). Patterns of usual care for schizophrenia: Initial results from the Schizophrenia patient Outcomes Research Team (PORT) client survey. *Schizophrenia Bulletin, 24,* 11-20.

Littell, J. H., & Tajima, E. A. (2000). A multilevel model of client participation in intensive family preservation services. *Social Service Review, 74*(3), 405-435.

Locke, E. A., & Latham, G. P. (1990). *A theory of goal setting and task performance.* Upper Saddle River, NJ, U.S.: Prentice-Hall, Inc.

London, M. (1997). *Job Feedback: Giving, seeking and using feedback for performance improvement.* Mahway, NJ: Lawrence Erlbaum Associates, Inc.

Lopez, J. S., Ciarlelli, R., Coffman, L., Stone, M., & Wyatt, L. (2000). Diagnosing for strengths: On measuring hope building blocks. In C. R. Snyder (Ed.), *Handbook of hope: Theory, measures, and application* (pp. 57-84). San Diego, CA: Academic Press.

MacDonald, G. (1998). Promoting evidence-based practice in child protection. *Clinical Child Psychology and Psychiatry, 3,* 71-85.

Mackie, D. M., & Queller, S. (2000). The impact of group membership on persuasion: Revisiting "Who says what to whom with what effect?" In D. J. Terry & M.A. Hogg (Eds.), *Attitudes, behaviors, and social context: the role of norms and group membership* (pp. 135-156). Mahwah, NJ: Lawrence Erlbaum Associates, Publishers.

Maio, G. R., & Olson, J. M. (1995). Relations between values, attitudes, and behavioral intentions: The moderating role of attitude functions. *British Journal of Social Psychology, 33,* 301-312.

Mallon, G. (2005). What is family-centered practice? *Permanency Planning Today.* New York: Hunter College School of Social Work.

Martin, L. L. (2001). *Financial management for human services administrators.* Needham Heights, MA: Allyn and Bacon.

Martin, L. L. (2005). Performance-based contracting for human services: Does it work? *Administration in Social Work, 29*(1), 63-77.

Martin, M., Scott, J., Pierron, J., & Bauerle, B. (1984). The Kansas family and children's trust fund: Funding prevention programs in the eighties. *Child Abuse and Neglect, 8,* 303-309.

Martin, P. Y., & Segal, B. (1977). Bureaucracy, size and staff expectations for client independence in halfway houses. *Journal of Health and Social Behavior, 18,* 376-390.

McConnell, A. R., Niedermeier, K. E., Leibold, J. M., El-Alayli, A. G., Chin, P. P., & Kuiper, N. M. (2000). What if I find it cheaper somewhere else?: Role of prefactual thinking and anticipated regret in consumer behavior. *Psychology and Marketing, 17,* 281-298.

McDonald, T. P., Press A., Billings, P., & Moore, T. (2003). *Outcomes Research Report #4: Predictors of timely adoption-A cohort analysis.* Lawrence, KS: University of Kansas School of Social Welfare.

McGrew, J., & Griss, M. (2005). Concurrent and predictive validity of two scales to assess the fidelity of implementation of supported employment. *Psychiatric Rehabilitation Journal, 29,* 41-47.

McHugo, G. J., Drake, R. E., Teague, G. B., & Xie, H. (1999). Fidelity to assertive community treatment and client outcomes in the New Hampshire dual disorders study. *Psychiatric Services, 50,* 818-824.

Menefee, D. (2000). What managers do and why they do it. In R. J. Patti (Ed.), *The handbook of social welfare management* (pp. 3-25). Thousand Oaks, CA: Sage Publications, Inc.

Mishra, S. I., Chavez, L. R., Magana, J. R., Nava, P., Valdez, R. B., & Hubbell, F. A. (1998). Improving breast cancer control among Latinas: Evaluation of a theory-based educational program. *Health Education and Behavior, 25,*653-670.

Moen, P., Elder Jr., G. H., & Lüscher, K. (1995). *Examining lives in context: Perspectives on the ecology of human development.* Washington, DC: American Psychological Association.

Moore, T. (2003). *Results-oriented management in child welfare, Section II Managing for results.* University of Kansas School of Social Welfare ROM Web site [Online]. Available: http://www.rom.ku.edu.

NASW Massachusetts Chapter, National Association of Social Workers (1996). *Safety guidelines revised March 1996* [Online]. Available: www.socialworkers.org/profession/centennial/violence.

National Association of Social Workers (1999). *Code of ethics of the national association of social workers* [Online]. Available: www.socialworkers.org/pubs/code.

Newhill, C.E. (2003). *Client violence in social work practice: Prevention, intervention and research.* New York: The Guilford Press.

Ng, J. Y. Y., Tam, S. F., Yew, W. W., & Lam, W. K. (1999). Effects of video modeling on self-efficacy and exercise performance of COPD patients. *Social Behavior and Personality, 27,* 475-486.

Oestmann, J.(1996). Day Treatment for Children with Emotional and Behavioral Disorders: A Program Evaluation. *Eighth annual research conference proceedings. A system of care for children's mental health: Expanding the research base* (pp. 167-170) [Online]. Available: http://www.fmhi.usf.edu/institute/pubs/pdf/cfs/rtc/8thproceedings/8thproctoc.htm.

O'Keefe, D. J. (1999). How to handle opposing arguments in persuasive messages: A meta-analytic review of the effects of one-sided and two-sided messages. *Communication Yearbook, 22,* 209-249.

O'Keefe, D. J. (2002). *Persuasion: Theory & research* (Second edition). Thousand Oaks, CA: Sage Publications.

O'Keefe, D. J. (2004). Trends and prospects in persuasion theory and research. In J. S. Seiter & R. H. Gass. (Eds.), *Perspectives on persuasion, social influence and compliance gaining* (pp. 31-43). Boston, MA: Pearson Education, Inc.

Olds, D. L. (2002). Prenatal and infancy home visiting by nurses: From randomized trials to community replication. *Prevention Science, 3*(3), 153-172.

Ollendick, T. H., Alvarez, H. K., & Greene, R.W. (2004). Behavioral assessment: History of underlying concepts and methods. In S. N. Haynes, E. M. Heiby & M. Hersen (Eds.), *Comprehensive handbook of psychological assessment. volume 3: Behavioral assessment* (pp. 19-32). Hoboken, NJ: John Wiley & Sons, Inc.

Osborne, E., & Plastirk, P. (2000). *The reinventor's fieldbook: Tools for transforming your government.* San Francisco, CA: Jossey-Bass.

Patti, R. J. (1977). Patterns of management activity in social welfare agencies. *Administration in Social Work, 1*(1), 5-48.

Patti, R. J. (1985). In search of purpose for social welfare administration. *Administration in Social Work, 9*(3), 1-14.

Patti, R. J. (2000). The landscape of social welfare management. In R. J. Patti (Ed.), *The handbook of social welfare management* (pp. 3-25). Thousand Oaks, CA: Sage Publications, Inc.

Patti, R., & Resnick, H. (1985). Leadership and change in child welfare organizations. In J. Laird & A. Hartman (Eds.), *Handbook of child welfare* (pp. 269-288). Glencoe, IL: Free Press.

Perlmutter, F. D. (2000). Initiating and implementing change. In R. Patti (Ed.), *The handbook of social welfare administration* (pp. 445-458). Thousand Oaks, CA: Sage Publications.

Peters, T. J., & Waterman, R. H. (1982). *In search of excellence.* New York: Harper & Row.

Poertner, J. (2006). Social Administration and Outcomes for Consumers: What do we know? *Administration in Social Work, 9*(2), 11-24.

Poertner, J., Moore, T., McDonald, T. P. (in press). Managing for child welfare outcomes: The selection of outcomes measures. *Administration in Social Work.*

Posthuma, R. A., Morgeson, R. P., & Campion, M. A. (2002). Beyond employment interview validity: A comprehensive narrative review of recent research and trends over time. *Personnel Psychology, 55*(1), 1-81.

President's New Freedom Commission on Mental Health (2003). *Achieving the promise: Transforming mental health care in America.* Washington: DC: U.S. Department of Health and Human Services.

Price, A. (2004). *Human resource management in a business context* (Second edition). London: Thomson Learning.

Propp, K. M. (1995). An experimental examination of biological sex as a status cue in decision-making groups and its influence on information use. *Small Group Research, 26,* 451-474.

Rapp, C. A. (1998). *The strengths model: Case management with people suffering from severe and persistent mental illness.* New York: Oxford University Press.

Rapp, C. A. (2002). Incentive structures within mental health financing strategies: Toward an incentive based model. *The Social Policy Journal, 1*(2), 37-54.

Rapp, C. A., & Goscha, R. J. (2006). *The strengths model: Case management with people with psychiatric disabilities.* New York: Oxford University Press.

Rapp, C. A., Huff, S., & Hansen, K. (2003). The New Hampshire financing project. *Psychiatric Rehabilitation Journal, 26*(4), 385-391.

Rapp, C. A., & Poertner, J. (1992). *Social administration: A client-centered approach.* White Plains: New York, Longman Publishing Group.

Ridgway, P. (2001). Restoring psychiatric disability: Learning from first person narrative accounts of recovery. *Psychiatric Rehabilitation Journal, 24*(4), 335-343.

Rones, M., & Hoagwood, K. (2000). School-based mental health services: A Research review. *Clinical Child and Family Psychology Review, 3*(4), 223-235.

Sackett, D. L., Straus, S. E., & Richardson, W. S. (1997). *Evidence-based medicine: How to practice and teach EBM.* New York: Churchill Livingston.

Seiter, J. S., & Gass, R. H. (2004). *Perspectives on persuasion, social influence and compliance gaining.* Boston, MA: Pearson Education, Inc.

Schoech, D. (2000). Managing information for decision making. In R. J. Patti (Ed.), *The Handbook of social welfare management* (pp. 321-340). Thousand Oaks, CA: Sage Publications.

Sims, R. R. (2002). *Organizational success through effective human resources management.* Westport, Connecticut: Quorum Books.

Snyder, C. R. (1994). *The psychology of hope.* New York: Free Press.

Snyder, C. R. (2000). Hypotheses: There is hope. In C. R. Snyder (Ed.), *Handbook of hope: Theory, measures, and application* (pp. 3-18). San Diego, CA: Academic Press.

Sosin, M. R. (1986). Administrative issues in substitute care. *Social Service Review, 60*(3), 360-377.

State of Illinois Office of the Auditor General (2003). Report Digest: Illinois violence prevention authority. Downloaded 2/26/2003 [http://www.state.il.us/auditor/violence].

Stone, J., Wiegand, A. W., Cooper, J., & Aronson, E. (1997). When exemplification fails: Hypocrisy and the motive for self-integrity. *Journal of Personality and Social Psychology, 72,* 54-65.

Stroul, B. A., & Friedman, R. M. (1994). *A system of care for children and youth with severe emotional disturbances* [Online]. Available: http://rtckids.fmhi.usf.edu/publications.html.

Substance Abuse and Mental Health Services Administration, National Mental Health Information Center (SAMSHA) (2005). *Illness management and recovery fidelity scale* [Online]. Available: www.mentalhealth.samhsa.gov/cmhs/communitysupport/toolkits/illness/Fidelity/default.asp

Taber, M. (1987). A theory of accountability for the human services and the implications for social program design. *Administration in Social Work, 11* (3/4), 115-126.

Taber, M., & Finnegan, D. (1980). A theory of accountability for social work programs. Unpublished paper, University of Illinois School of Social Work. Urbana, Illinois. Reprinted with permission.

Terry, D. J., & Hogg, M. A. (Eds.) (2000). *Attitudes, behaviors, and social context: The role of norms and group membership.* Mahwah, NJ: Lawrence Erlbaum Associates, Publishers.

Terry, D. J., Hogg, M.A., & White, K. M. (2000). Attitude-behavior relations: Social identity and group membership. In D. J. Terry & M. A. Hogg (Eds.), *Attitudes, behaviors, and social context: The role of norms and group membership* (pp. 67-94). Mahwah, NJ: Lawrence Erlbaum Associates, Publishers.

The Chronicle of Philanthropy (June 23, 2005). *Giving Tick Up.*

Thomlison, B. (2003). Characteristics of evidence-based child maltreatment interventions. *Child Welfare, 82*(5), 541-569.

Thyer, B. A., (1995). Promoting an empiricist agenda within the human services: An ethical and humanistic imperative. *Journal of Behavioral Therapy and Experimental Psychiatry, 26,* 93-98.

Torrey, W. C., Finnerty, M., Evans, A., & Wyzik, P. E. (2003). Strategies for leading the implementation of evidence-based practices. *Psychiatric Clinics of North America, 26,* 883-897.

Trafimow, D. (2000). A theory of attitudes, subjective norms, and private versus collective self concepts. In D. J. Terry & M. A. Hogg (Eds.), *Attitudes, behaviors, and social context: The role of norms and group membership* (pp. 47-66). Mahwah, NJ: Lawrence Erlbaum Associates, Publishers.

U.S. Department of Education (2002). *No child left behind: standards and assessments* [Online] Available: www.ed.gov.admins/lead/account.

U.S. Department of Health and Human Services (2005). *Promoting safe and stable families* [Online]. Available: www.acf.hhs.gov/programs/cb/programs/state.htm.

U.S. General Accounting Office (2003). *Child welfare: most states are developing statewide information systems, but the reliability of child welfare data could be improved* (G.A.O.-03-809) [Online]. Available: http://www.gao.gov/new.items/d03809.pdf.

United Way of America (2005). *Basic facts about the United Way* [Online]. Available: http://national.unitedway.org/aboutuw/.

United Way of America (2005). United Way mission and vision [Online]. Available: http://national.unitedway.org/aboutuw/mission.cfm.

Wageman, R. (2001). How leaders foster self-managing team effectiveness: Design choices versus hands-on coaching. *Organization Science, 12*(5), 559-577.

Washington State Institute for Public Policy (2004). *Outcome evaluation of Washington state's research-based programs for juvenile offenders* [Online]. Available: www.wsipp.wa.gov.

Wehrmann, K. C., Shin, H., & Poertner, J. (2002). Transfer of training: An evaluation study. *Journal of Health and Social Policy, 15*(3/4), 23-37.

Weise, C. S., Turbiasz, A. A., & Whitney, D. J. (1995). Behavioral training and AIDS risk reduction: Overcoming barriers to condom use. *AIDS Education and Prevention, 7,* 50-59.

Yeaman, C., Craine, W. H., Gorsek, J., & Corrigan, P. W. (2000). Performance improvement teams for better psychiatric rehabilitation. *Administration and Policy in Mental Health, 27*(3), 113-127.

Yzer, M. C., Fischer, J. D., Bakker, A. B., Siero, F. W., & Misovich, S. J. (1998). The effects of information about AIDS risk and self-efficacy on women's intentions to engage in AIDS preventive behavior. *Journal of Applied Social Psychology, 28,* 1837-1852.

Index

Page numbers followed by the letter "f" indicate figures; those followed by "t" indicate tables.

Time parameters for objectives, 122-123
Time parameters for phases of helping, 144
Timeline for task completion, 217-218, 219, 221
Tools, providing, 9, 343, 346, 352, 356-363, 375
Total care services, 158
Traditional (site-based) services, 151
Training
  as administrator responsibility, 3, 263
  in appraisal conducting, 298
  behavior control, perceived, enhancing through, 60
  behavior eliciting through joint staff, 149
  content of, 302
  curriculum, components of effective, 57
  education and, 53, 54, 56-58, 72, 170, 275, 303, 387
  emotional response, dealing with, 161
  evidence-based, 302, 303, 304
  feedback combined with, 191, 292, 296
  follow-up of, 304-305
  impact of, 376
  instructional design of, 57, 303-304
  methods of effective, 303-305
  need for, determining, 303
  in performance-enhancement team, 387
  for performance improvement, 205, 213
  pros and cons of, 137, 357
  in safety, 263, 306
  services, impact on, 142
  support for, 57
  in technology, 248
  time available for, 136
  as tool, 357, 358
  transfer of, 56-57, 137, 280, 303, 304
  utility, perceived of, 303
  for volunteers, 157
Transitional employment programs (TEP), 142

Transportation, 151, 158, 159, 176
Treatment versus prevention programs, 99
Trial home placement of children, 144, 149
Truancy
  case studies of, 144-145
  of emotionally disordered, 164, 166
  sample problem analysis, 91-93, 92t
True/false questions, 236, 237, 239
Trust, fostering, 349
Typology for social problem analysis, 89-90

Under-serving of clients, 340
Understandable measures, 224-225, 229
Understanding, barriers to, removing, 61-62
Unions, 266
Unit of service, cost per, 249
United Way, 317, 321-323, 322f
Unmet expectations, consequences of, 124, 125t
Urgency, establishing sense of, 46

Validity of job interviews, 288
Validity of measures, 224, 225-226, 229, 236, 237, 243, 251
Values
  behavior compatibility with, 69, 138, 140, 149
  community, 76, 351
  cultural, 276
  framing problem through, 82
  job, 61, 251, 289-291
  motivation through, 347
  organizational, 215, 268-271, 286, 355, 364
  reinforcing, 388
  rites, rituals, and ceremonies depicting, 271
  social worker, 76
  societal, 349
  stories communicating, 272
  symbols depicting, 271-272
  vision role in establishing and communicating, 353